Community-Based Collaborative Action Research

A Nursing Approach

Carol Pillsbury Pavlish, PhD, RN, FAAN
Assistant Professor
School of Nursing
University of California
Los Angeles, California

Professor Emeritus
St. Catherine University
St. Paul, Minnesota

Margaret Dexheimer Pharris, PhD, RN, MPH, FAAN
Graduate Programs Director and Associate Professor
Department of Nursing
St. Catherine University
St. Paul, Minnesota

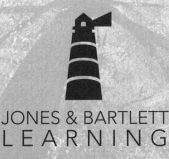

JONES & BARTLETT
LEARNING

World Headquarters

Jones & Bartlett Learning
40 Tall Pine Drive
Sudbury, MA 01776
978-443-5000
info@jblearning.com
www.jblearning.com

Jones & Bartlett Learning
Canada
6339 Ormindale Way
Mississauga, Ontario L5V 1J2
Canada

Jones & Bartlett Learning
International
Barb House, Barb Mews
London W6 7PA
United Kingdom

Jones & Bartlett Learning books and products are available through most bookstores and online booksellers. To contact Jones & Bartlett Learning directly, call 800-832-0034, fax 978-443-8000, or visit our website, www.jblearning.com.

Substantial discounts on bulk quantities of Jones & Bartlett Learning publications are available to corporations, professional associations, and other qualified organizations. For details and specific discount information, contact the special sales department at Jones & Bartlett Learning via the above contact information or send an email to specialsales@jblearning.com.

The authors, editor, and publisher have made every effort to provide accurate information. However, they are not responsible for errors, omissions, or for any outcomes related to the use of the contents of this book and take no responsibility for the use of the products and procedures described. Treatments and side effects described in this book may not be applicable to all people; likewise, some people may require a dose or experience a side effect that is not described herein. Drugs and medical devices are discussed that have limited availability controlled by the Food and Drug Administration (FDA) for use only in a research study or clinical trial. Research, clinical practice, and government regulations often change the accepted standard in this field. When consideration is being given to use of any drug in the clinical setting, the health care provider or reader is responsible for determining FDA status of the drug, reading the package insert, and reviewing prescribing information for the most up-to-date recommendations on dose, precautions, and contraindications, and determining the appropriate usage for the product. This is especially important in the case of drugs that are new or seldom used.

Production Credits

Publisher: Kevin Sullivan
Acquisitions Editor: Amy Sibley
Associate Editor: Patricia Donnelly
Editorial Assistant: Rachel Shuster
Production Editor: Amanda Clerkin
Associate Marketing Manager: Meagan Norlund
V.P., Manufacturing and Inventory Control:
   Therese Connell

Composition: DataStream Content Solutions, LLC
Cover Design: Kristin E. Parker
Cover Image: © Satori13/Dreamstime.com
Printing and Binding: Malloy, Inc.
Cover Printing: Malloy, Inc.

Library of Congress Cataloging-in-Publication Data
Pavlish, Carol P.
   Community-based collaborative action research : a nursing approach / Carol P. Pavlish, Margaret D. Pharris.
       p. ; cm.
   Includes bibliographical references and index.
   ISBN 978-0-7637-7112-6 (pbk.)
   1. Community health services—Research.   2. Community health nursing—Research.
I. Pharris, Margaret Dexheimer.   II. Title.
   [DNLM: 1. Community-Based Participatory Research.   2. Ethics, Research.   3. Financing,
Organized.   4. Minority Health.   5. Nursing Research—methods.   6. Research Design.
W 84.3 P338c 2011]
   RA440.85.P39 2011
   362.12072—dc22
                                                                                    2010025305
6048

Printed in the United States of America
15 14 13 12 11   10 9 8 7 6 5 4 3 2 1

Dedication

While writing this book, we each lost a parent. Their spirits are woven in these pages.

In memory of my mother, Caroline Marie Pharris, who whispered humble, earthy dreams in my ears and in memory of my father, Charles Nikolas Pharris, who taught me the beauty of simplicity and common people.

—MDP

In memory of my father, Wilbur Fiske Pillsbury II, whose integrity, generosity, humility, and scholarship inspire me and in memory of my mother, Katherine Wheeler Pillsbury, whose wisdom, joy, love, and laughter inspirit me.

—CLP

Contents

Acknowledgments

Many brilliant minds shaped our journeys with the community-based collaborative action research process. Research participants, nurse theorists, action research pioneers, representatives of community-based organizations—and particularly colleagues at St. Catherine University, the University of California, Los Angeles, and the University of Minnesota challenged our thinking, smoothed our road, and urged us forward.

The editors and staff of Jones & Bartlett Learning resuscitated the idea of this book and nurtured it along the way to publication. Their responsive professionalism throughout the publication process has been exceptional.

We specifically thank Dr. Margaret Newman for her profoundly transformative theory and relational presence. We are also grateful for the example of another nurse, Dr. Susan Smith, who went to Mexico 15 years ago for a visit and never left the people in the mountains of Guerrero with whom she has been engaging in multiple cycles of participatory action research to reclaim culture, health, and access to the basic necessities of life, particularly clean water. Dr. Paulette Sankofa was an early partner in the creation of CBCAR, along with wise women from North Minneapolis, particularly Mrs. Doloris Irwin, Mrs. Nothando Zulu, and Ms. Jewelean Jackson, and former nursing graduate students, Linda Amaikwu-Rushing, Deborah Fitzgerald, and Krista Ollom. We appreciate Connie Kamara who believes so strongly in participatory approaches and all our community partners in both local and global offices. Dr. Anita Ho, who authored Chapter 8, has deepened our intellectual thought, stretched and enlarged our concept of ethical action, and been a conscientious, faithful friend.

Our families provided much-needed and deeply-appreciated support and encouragement. In particular, we thank our husbands, Chuck and Bill, who believed in this book as much as we did. We are deeply grateful.

CPP and MDP

Introduction

*T*he intent of this book is to propose an easily understand-able framework of community-based collaborative action research (CBCAR) that can be used by nurse researchers, clinicians, leaders, and graduate students in partnership with communities experiencing health disparities or with organizations needing system improvements. This research framework identifies and analyzes entrenched barriers to health and well-being and provides opportunities to design systemic and structural improvements so all human beings can flourish. The CBCAR process aims to promote healthcare equity and quality. Sometimes that means listening to the experiences of marginalized people, hearing from other key stakeholders, and engaging entire communities in actions that improve people's health and well-being. Other times, in an effort to generate high-quality and evidence-based care management decisions, CBCAR means listening to the experiences of multiple actors in complex healthcare organizations, hearing not only about institutional resources and successes but also attending to data on health outcomes, service gaps, practical challenges, and contextual stresses.

We situate this research framework within a unique kaleidoscope that blends the unitary participatory paradigm, the socio-ecological perspective, and action-based science with the tenets of human rights and social justice. Because nurses work in numerous settings and with many populations, we define community broadly as "all who will be affected by the research" (Horowitz, Robinson, & Seifer, 2009, p. 2634). Communities, therefore, can refer to groups with a common identity or condition such as children at the end of life or Mexican Americans with diabetes or survivors of natural disasters. Communities can also be defined as geographic or organizational settings. Wherever nurses interact with people, communities exist.

With this research approach, we also emphasize the unique talents and collective responsibilities of nurse leaders, scholars, and clinicians in creating and advancing knowledge to address the contextual backdrop of health—with health defined as much more than simply the absence of disease. The socio-cultural, political, economic, and environmental influences on individual and community health and well-being flow from community and social structures and policies (Falk-Rafael, 2005; Commission on Social Determinants of Health, 2008). The proposed research framework creates an opportunity for community-academic partnerships to form and collectively analyze how systems and structures contribute to and/or detract from people's health and well-being (**Figure I-1**). Furthermore, these partnerships can also form to analyze how organizational systems and structures influence efficiency, effectiveness, and quality of healthcare services. Within this multi-use framework, CBCAR examines important issues, such as social injustices or system inadequacies that affect not only people's health but also the nation's health. Specific root causes and branching impacts are carefully and systematically considered. Chosen actions address both.

In contrast to many traditional research methods, CBCAR is a relationship-based research process that requires partnered planning, sustained commitment, equitable benefits, and a common desire to address structural health barriers. CBCAR assumes that wisdom surrounding solutions to health problems and system inadequacies reside in the groups of people most affected by the concern. Falling into a participatory and constructivist inquiry paradigm, CBCAR values multiple realities, transactional findings, dialectic processes, and textual hermeneutics (Lincoln & Guba, 2000). As such, CBCAR gathers individual and community narratives about particular health experiences or quality of care concerns. To verify or expand what is being learned, CBCAR might also employ positivist and critical research methods to understand health patterns and their meanings. Once the issues are well understood, research partners engage multiple, diverse groups to find solutions. As an action-based and relational process, CBCAR assumes that knowledge is related to power and that power is related to change. CBCAR exemplifies "pragmatic solidarity"—standing with those in need and together finding practical ways to improve their situations (Farmer, 2005, p. 26).

Figure I-1   Community-Based Collaborative Action Research Framework

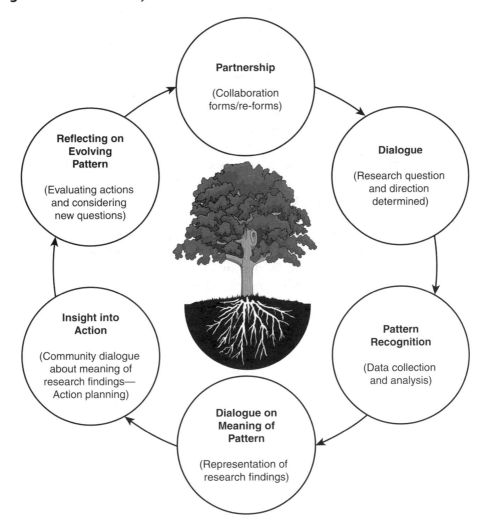

In this book, we provide essential theoretical perspectives and research techniques to enact CBCAR. With this research process, we urge nurses to join voices and share leadership responsibilities with others who are creating equitable health opportunities and crafting high quality health systems.

■ Why a Different Approach?

Current research frameworks and strategies have produced vital knowledge, important innovations, and significant health improvements. However, if nurses rely solely on traditional forms of research, several gaps result. First, most health research remains biomedically and individually focused whereas most health advancements emerge from improvements in the social determinants of health (Commission on Social Determinants of Health, 2008; De Negri Filho, 2008; Marmot, 2007; Sanders, Labonte, Baum, & Chopra, 2004; Semenza & Maty, 2007; Yamin, 2008). Research approaches, such as CBCAR, that engage multiple social sectors in exploring and intervening on social determinants and root causes are required for health equity, healthcare quality, and human flourishing.

Second, while we have learned more about health disparities, interventions to correct these disparities have lagged behind (Horowitz et al., 2009). Additionally, evidence-supported interventions, which are sometimes disseminated as standards of care, do not necessarily consider the historical and social roots of health disparities or fit into the complicated lives of people from underserved populations. As a result, health disparities stubbornly persist, people and communities suffer needlessly, and nurses and other healthcare providers experience a dissonant pull in their work which potentially contributes to moral distress.

Third, healthcare organizations have become increasingly complex and more interdependent with their external environment. These complexities often challenge the translation of research findings into clinical practice (Haines, Kuruvilla, & Borchert, 2004; Leykum, Pugh, Lanham, Harmon, & McDaniel, 2009). Furthermore, relatively little financial support is available for assisting organizations to apply research findings, such as those that could improve access, help clinicians make more informed decisions, strengthen relationships, and enhance system effectiveness (Woolf, 2008). Traditional research designs often disseminate findings without moving forward to action and easing translation. However, CBCAR projects incorporate action within the process, and therefore, make translation of findings into practice more possible (Horowitz et al., 2009).

Finally, many current research practices, while producing very important information, sometimes miscalculate relevance. Traditional research methods are usually planned and driven by "outside" experts—many of whom do not remain in touch with communities after data are collected. These "outsider" efforts are insufficient in addressing multiple factors that differentially impact populations (Seifer & Sisco, 2006). In community-partnered research, relevance is determined in partnership with communities that are most affected by the concern or issue being studied. Discussing the importance of community-partnered research, Hebert, Brandt, Armstead, Adams, and Steck (2009) asserted that "We will never know the real causes of many health disparities until we engage with . . . individuals and communities at highest risk" (p. 1216).

For these reasons, we turned to a community-driven, contextually rich, and action-oriented research approach which expands our understandings of the complex factors that influence health, health outcomes, and quality care—especially for vulnerable populations. Nurse researchers who use CBCAR and engage with communities to determine their most relevant health concerns could show promising inroads for improving health and equalizing health care for all. Additionally, nurse researchers who choose CBCAR to engage all stakeholders in determining organizational factors that influence quality of care could provide valuable guidance for system improvement and organizational change.

■ CBCAR Principles

We draw on the work of Israel, Eng, Schultz, & Parker (2005), Horowitz et al. (2009), and Olshansky (2008) to describe underlying CBCAR principles. **Figure I-2** identifies these principles and illustrates how they play out in the process.

Figure I-2 Community-Based Collaborative Action Research Process

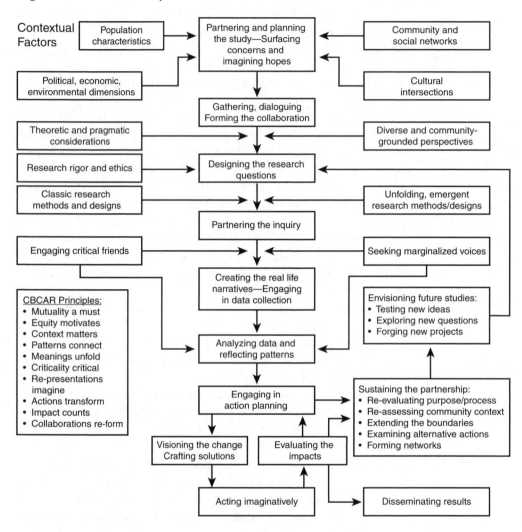

Mutuality, a Must

The CBCAR process is highly relational and conscientiously attends to the creation of equitable, open, trustworthy, collaborative partnerships. Community members and researchers are recognized equitably for their talents and contributions, share in dissemination of results, and mutually benefit from the partnered project. Co-learning and shared capacity-building occur as all partners invest efforts to understand the issues at hand.

Unfortunately, in many indigenous and underserved communities, the very word *research* provokes anxiety and raises expectations of being exploited (Wells & Jones, 2009). Prior (2007) advocated for a decolonizing research agenda that "decentres the focus from the aims of the researcher to the agenda of the people" (p. 165) and upholds the values of spirit and integrity. Prior asserted that research should evoke discourse by "developing meaning or truth through a relationship of trust, reciprocity, and co-operatively evolved methods of research that remain true to the context of the story being presented" (p. 166). For this to happen, a solid, trusting, mutual relationship must first exist. This is where CBCAR begins. All partners come together in a spirit of oneness and solidarity to create relationships that are nonexploitative and enhance the social and emotional lives of all people who participate (Stringer, 2007). Wholeness and mutuality imply equitable relationships rooted in social justice.

Equity Motivates

Equity implies just and fair practices whereas equality often suggests same or similar in value or quantity. Equity can be achieved in treating people equally; however, equity implies even greater responsibility than equality. The fair and just practices associated with equity are strong, underlying values in CBCAR partnerships and projects. Most CBCAR projects aim to improve health by attending to and correcting not only social inequalities but also system inequities or inadequacies that result in health disparities.

Context Matters

Adopting an ecological perspective, CBCAR methodically explores people's histories, cultural paradigms, and sociopolitical and economic realities. Kalipeni and Oppong (1998) underscored the importance of historical depth in our inquiry and presentation of findings. Exploring the history of the current situation can potentially free people from automatically assuming the blame for their predicament. Instead, people's situations are viewed within a sociopolitical ecology with multiple intersecting and catalytic factors that influence health. CBCAR uncovers, explores, and addresses these contextual factors from multiple vantage points. Community strengths along with challenges are acknowledged as CBCAR builds on existing assets—especially during action planning—to correct system deficiencies that interfere with health.

Patterns Connect

Central to the CBCAR process is inquiry that reveals patterns of the whole. We start to appreciate how systems and structures that are often objectified and placed at a distance are really ours and illustrate spaces that we share with each other and with the earth and air that surround us. Patterns can be seen through epidemiological and demographic data along with people's narrative histories, everyday experiences, and reflective meaning making. CBCAR partners seek all data that elicit deeper and wider understandings about interactional patterns that shape the situation being studied.

Meanings Unfold

Similar to other constructivist paradigms, CBCAR is a fluid and iterative process that unfolds gradually to create unique and cyclical pathways. Even if a traditional, quantitative research design fits into a CBCAR project, it becomes part of a larger, iterative process that unfolds as more becomes known and informs subsequent phases. As partnerships develop and sustain themselves over time, projects may unfold in stages. For example, early in a partnership when less is known about a topic, an inductive, exploratory process is used to co-learn variables. As the partnership matures and more becomes known, CBCAR partners might call upon a more fixed, deductive design to test effectiveness of a community-developed program or intervention (Olshansky, 2008). The key is to allow the unfolding meanings within the CBCAR process to inform each phase and then, accordingly, shift the CBCAR course in a scientifically rigorous yet flexible manner.

Criticality Critical

As increasingly diverse views and voices are engaged in the CBCAR process, the pattern of the whole is perceived in more detail. We often do not see the world as it is, but rather as we are. When we engage in authentic dialogue with people very different from ourselves, we are able to see the world more fully. Prior (2007) pointed out that many Indigenous cultural paradigms have been marginalized by perspectives from the Western world. CBCAR uncovers currents of meaning within the local context and avoids collating them into similarities.

Sagor (1993) encouraged research partners to identify and invite *critical friends* into the research process. Rather than fracturing the project, diversity strengthens CBCAR. Wells and Jones (2009) suggested that research partners' openness to "diverse perspectives, even when focusing on design and methods" is important and "part of the rigor of partnered research" (p. 321). The key challenge is to work effectively within diversity. This requires research partners to develop several process-oriented skills—some of which are listed in **Box I-1**. These processes encourage researchers to view people's differences as assets and capitalize on those as diverse knowledge and action ideas continually coexist within the CBCAR process.

Re-presentations Imagine

Once the pattern of the issue under study has been identified, it is presented to the wider community for critique and amplification of meaning. Language is of utmost importance whenever people's narratives are summarized. Since language is often used to serve people who hold power, the language we use in

---

Box I-1 Process Skills

CBCAR is both process and relationship oriented. The following skills are developed throughout this book:

- Critical thinking skills related to ethical and scientific research practices
- Analytical skills for understanding the dynamic and complex contexts within which the planning of action-oriented research with culturally diverse groups takes place
- Reflexive thinking skills that expand nurse researchers' awareness of their own beliefs, assumptions, and values and how they influence the inquiry process
- Reflective thinking skills that loosen boundaries and see new combinations
- Collaborative inquiry skills for working effectively with others toward raising pressing and pertinent questions, planning shared pathways, and achieving common goals
- Leadership skills that allow nurses to participate more effectively in healthcare decision making
- Relational skills for establishing effective and productive partnerships with vulnerable populations, health professionals, and other primary healthcare stakeholders
- Innovative thinking skills that imagine new possibilities
- Ethical thinking skills that bring human rights and social justice into all interactions
- Positive thinking skills that continually acknowledge community strengths and assets while still working to address problems and barriers

---

talking about the research process and findings should be collaboratively and carefully analyzed so it can be understood by all audiences. Once we see the construction of reality in more than just the dominant worldview, new possibilities can be created (Reason & Bradbury, 2001). Through dialogue, multiple worldviews are shared and understood; life becomes richer and more fulfilling for all. Ricoeur (1991) asserted that narratives of real-life experiences result in practical knowledge. Gadamer (1979/1981) agreed and suggested that practical knowledge possesses unique opportunities and stated, "It [practical knowledge] is capable of contributing in a special way to the broadening of our human experiences, our self-knowledge, and our horizon" (p. 110).

Actions Transform

Failed community initiatives can often be attributed to narrow vision, imported knowledge, or vested interests. CBCAR widens our vision, produces knowledge from inside communities, and balances the interests of multiple stakeholders. Interweaving knowledge production and pragmatic action, CBCAR investigates various perspectives on what has been done and what is missing. In collaborative analysis and knowledge production, we often find new avenues for informed action. CBCAR recognizes that the wisest ideas for health or system improvements often emerge from what Dr. Paul Farmer (2005) called collaboratively bearing witness to the suffering of others and sharing compassion and solidarity with those in need. These "ways of knowing" (Farmer, p. 27) accompanied by actions that make systems work effectively for all by diminishing unjust hardships, alleviating health disparities, and advancing human health and flourishing are what matters most in CBCAR.

Impact Counts

In CBCAR, measuring impact is both a necessity and a challenge. Constructive social or organizational change in whatever form it takes has relatively few measures that apply to underserved populations. Additionally, community members, community-based organizations, and academic researchers may have different viewpoints on desired outcomes and outcome measures (Scarinci, Johnson, Hardy, Marron, & Partridge, 2009). Moreover, many evaluation research methods call for predetermined outcomes, whereas CBCAR evaluation outcomes usually emerge from the process itself. However difficult, participatory planning for impact evaluation is an important component of CBCAR.

Collaborations Re-form

Fluidity and sustainability are key concepts in CBCAR projects. Partnerships are fluid as different teams may form within the project over time. A formal research team comprised of community representatives and academic researchers usually forms to initiate the project, but as the project progresses, new people may become engaged in subteams that form for data collection, analysis, or presentation. Stability is provided by including a few members from the original research team on each subteam that forms. Generally, engaging additional community members contributes to project sustainability. Furthermore, as learning occurs in CBCAR projects, new partnerships often re-form around related projects or new initiatives so partnerships, while fluid, are sustained.

■ CBCAR Process

Diagramming steps in a dynamic process often simplifies it to the point of losing its natural flow and unique emergence. However, diagrams can be valuable learning tools, so we captured the CBCAR process that was initially depicted in Figure I-1 and inserted more steps into each phase in Figure I-2. This way, readers have a better grasp of the whole—of course, knowing that the whole can never really be pictured, only experienced. Therefore, we do not intend Figure I-2 to be prescriptive. Rather we see it as a map that may guide readers as they initiate their CBCAR projects. As we iterate many times in this book, CBCAR partners find their own unique pathways while still drawing on common principles. We created the figure to provide readers with an outline meant to guide, not prescribe. Concepts in the visual depiction form the basis for book chapters and are explained throughout the book.

■ Overview of the Book

How readers choose to enter this book depends on their learning styles, unique talents, and research intents. We have written this book in the form of an unfolding story; however, some readers may want to jump into the methods chapters (4, 5, 6, & 7) before reading our stories of CBCAR (Chapters 1 & 2). Others might prefer to start by reading how we wove theoretical threads from nursing and other disciplines to create a nursing approach to CBCAR (Chapter 3).

When planning the book, we decided to apply two educational approaches—narrative pedagogy (Brown & Rodney, 2007; Dahlberg, Ekebergh, & Ironside, 2003; Ironside, 2003; Young, 2007) and Ausubel's Advanced Organizer Model (Joyce, Weil, & Calhoun, 2003). By starting with our own CBCAR stories and incorporating story into the research ethics chapter, we hope to engage readers in the whole-brain exercise of learning a process while feeling the experience. We appeal to the left hemisphere by presenting the research framework and its theoretical foundations within our stories. Appealing to the right hemisphere, we use the stories to draw readers into the affective experience of being transformed by others in the research process. Structuring the CBCAR landscape, these stories become the advance organizer that prepares students to learn subsequent steps. Chapter 1 describes Margaret's introduction to CBCAR as she engaged with her own multicultural community to identify and address health barriers for women and girls of color. She examines the history and nature of action research and brings to that process the nursing perspective of collaboration. Furthermore, applying the unitary participatory paradigm, she describes her research journey with young men who were incarcerated for murder. Her unique nursing perspective provides new ground from which to examine community patterns that unfold from listening to the narratives of individual lives. Margaret's description of partnering with others to develop deeper understandings about community patterns introduces readers to the CBCAR process as it unfolded in her experiences.

In Chapter 2, Carol narrates her experience of using action research in her dissertation project. Wanting to avoid research that sat on a shelf, she engaged with an international nongovernmental organization, the American Refugee Committee, whose mission is to restore productive and healthy lives for people displaced by conflicts and disasters. Statistics from a Rwanda refugee camp indicated that women were suffering disproportionately. Maternal mortality, sexual violence, and HIV infection were taking their toll. However, rather than importing a particular research topic, Carol describes how she first engaged with refugee women in a project to formulate the issues that were important to their lives. She then describes her dissertation journey with this community and the ongoing process of using research data to develop community-based programs. We hope that these narrative descriptions of our research stories in Chapters 1 and 2 will inspire readers to engage with communities and embark on their own CBCAR projects.

Chapter 3 introduces the intricately woven threads that strengthen the CBCAR process. Viewing health within a unitary-transformative paradigm and from a sociological perspective, we see the world as intricately interconnected and relational. Therefore, we apply research procedures to gain the widest possible view of the issue at hand—most usually qualitative and emergent—although we also use quantitative analysis and traditional research designs when needed to better understand health and interaction patterns. Incorporating pragmatic planning into the CBCAR approach, we draw on the tenets of action science to embolden research toward its transformative potential. Throughout the chapter we recognize and celebrate nurses' ways of being in partnership with persons and communities to improve health, well-being, and quality care. With this in mind, we draw on nurses' ethical obligations to treat all human beings equally, with dignity and human rights in mind. Toward that end, we present a rich and colorful theoretical kaleidoscope that challenges readers to think differently about the world and nurses' place in it.

Subsequently, we develop topics related to the practical and technical aspects of CBCAR. As such, throughout each of these chapters, we emphasize research ethics, scientific rigor and process flexibility, and critical self-awareness. Chapter 4 examines the process of creating, entering, and working fluidly in a collaborative research space with others who have similar interests, concerns, and hopes. We use frank descriptions from our own experiences and those of others to illustrate both benefits and challenges of establishing partnerships. Part of forming a research partnership is having a vision of CBCAR's subsequent steps and scope of work; consequently this chapter also overviews the research planning process by anticipating the steps that follow. Collaborative decision making is emphasized, and we offer guidelines on how teams might evaluate their partnering and collaborative processes.

In Chapter 5, we describe entering research settings and collaboratively planning data collection. To ease team planning, we provide three mapping options that data collection teams might use when strategizing their data collection. We emphasize the centrality of qualitative strategies in developing deeper and wider understandings about participants' situations. Ethics and scientific rigor in data collection are also stressed. We then describe observation, interviews, focus groups, and participatory data collection. Sample data collection tools are provided. We acknowledge the circling that occurs between data collection and analysis; however, for clarity's sake, we separate data collection from data analysis in the book. Chapter 6 explores two qualitative data analysis pathways—traditional and emergent, although we also recognize that these pathways might overlap. We once again emphasize the importance of critical self-awareness (reflexivity) and describe activities that facilitate effective teamwork during data analysis. Turning our attention to data, we describe the processes of absorbing, coding, comparing, sorting, and displaying data as techniques to qualitatively analyze meaning and construct patterns of the whole. We conclude the chapter with ideas on reflecting the patterns back to the community and engaging in dialogue about expanded meanings and future action.

In Chapter 7, we examine ways to harness people's collective energies and creative imaginings for designing pragmatically ideal action plans. Beyond simply learning from research and describing practice implications as occurs in many research designs, CBCAR pushes partnerships to continue the research process and design ways to implement the practical implications. A variety of action evaluation techniques are included. Finally, we discuss issues related to dissemination of what has been learned in the CBCAR process.

Chapter 8 is written by Dr. Anita Ho, a philosopher who is on faculty at the Centre for Applied Ethics at the University of British Columbia and the Director of Ethics Services for Providence Health Care where she provides ethics education, policy review, and clinical ethics consultation. Anita is also associate chair and ethicist for the Behavioural Research Ethics Board at the University of British Columbia. Her valuable insights into the complexity of research ethics, especially as it pertains to CBCAR, provides fascinating material for dialogue on the meaning of epistemic inclusion and exclusion, vulnerability, paternalism, protection, and power dynamics in research ethics. Anita also introduces readers to the idea of relational ethics in CBCAR projects and suggests how it might play out in research settings. Threaded throughout Anita's exploration of research ethics is the story of a young Sudanese woman whose dual positions of vulnerability and autonomy raise very real questions about what researchers' ongoing ethical responsibilities to participants actually mean.

Applying for grant money to fund CBCAR projects is the subject of Chapter 9. Because more funding agencies are specifically seeking community-partnered research (Horowitz et al., 2009; Leykum et al., 2009), this topic is becoming increasingly important. Securing funds for partnership and research development in CBCAR projects provides opportunities for deeper partnership commitment and wider community impact. Twelve principles for writing grant proposals are presented and illustrated in a sample NIH-funded CBCAR project. We provide a sample self-evaluation matrix that will assist readers to assess how well their own grant applications adhere to CBCAR principles.

Chapter 10 draws this book to a close by describing the transformative potential of and unfolding futures for CBCAR in health care. Not only highlighting its current status as a research "approach whose time has come" (Horowitz et al., 2009, p. 2640), we push boundaries and imagine new avenues for CBCAR. We also direct readers' attention toward developing their own stories and implementing their own research ideas. We offer a CBCAR idea worksheet that readers might initiate as they examine issues that concern them—in their work settings, the communities they live in, or virtual communities that might form in practice-based research networks.

We hope that the book inspires nurses, who already have many critical collaborative skills, to initiate partnerships with others and design a CBCAR project to improve health outcomes and healthcare quality. Much like the nursing process, CBCAR assesses, analyzes, plans, implements, and evaluates issues of concern. And much like the day-to-day world of nursing, CBCAR is driven by relationships that give it nourishment and deep meaning. Different mechanisms and tools are used in the nursing and research processes, but the overall goal of improving health and well-being for everyone we touch is the same. Spirited nurses who care deeply about health disparities, inadequate healthcare systems, and unjust social structures are encouraged to start thinking about their own potential as action researchers. We offer you this book in the spirit of a whispered dream.

■ References

Brown, H., & Rodney, P. (2007). Beyond case studies in practice education: Creating capacity for ethical knowledge through story and narrative. In L. Young & B. Paterson (Eds.), *Teaching nursing: Developing a student-centered learning environment* (pp. 141–163). Philadelphia, PA: Lippincott, Williams, & Wilkins.

Commission on Social Determinants of Health. (2008). *Closing the gap in a generation: Health equity on the social determinants of health.* Retrieved from http://whqlibdoc.who.int/publications/2008/9789241563703_eng.pdf

Dahlberg, K., Ekebergh, M., & Ironside, P. (2003). Converging conversatons from phenomenological pedagogies. In N. Diekelmann (Ed.), *Teaching the practitioners of care: New pedagogies for the health professions.* Madison, WI: University of Wisconsin Press.

De Negri Filho, A. (2008). A human rights approach to quality of life and health: Applications to public health programming. *Health and Human Rights, 10,* 1–9.

Gadamer, H. (F. G. Lawrence, Trans.). (1979/1981). *Reason in the age of science.* Cambridge, MA: Massachusetts Institute of Technology.

Falk Rafael, A. R. (2005). Speaking truth to power: Nursing's legacy and moral imperative. *Adances in Nursing Science, 28,* 212–223.

Farmer, P. (2005). *Pathologies of power: Health, human rights, and the new war on the poor.* Berkeley, CA: University of California.

Haines, A., Kuruvilla, S., & Borchert, M. (2004). Bridging the implementation gap between knowledge and action for health. *Bulletin of the World Health Organization, 82,* 724–732.

Hebert, J., Brandt, H., Armstead, C., Adams, S., & Steck, S. (2009). Interdisciplinary, translational, and community-based participatory research: Finding a common language to improve cancer research. *Cancer Epidemiological Biomarkers and Prevention, 18,* 1213–1217.

Horowitz, C., Robinson, M., & Seifer, S. (2009). Community-based participatory research from the margin to the mainstream: Are researchers prepared? *Circulation, 119,* 2633–2642.

Ironside, P. (2003). New pedagogies for teaching thinking: The lived experiences of students and teachers enacting narrative pedagogy. *Journal of Nursing Edcuation, 42,* 509–516.

Israel, B., Eng, E., Schultz, A., & Parker, E. (2005). Introduction to methods in community-based participatory research for health. In B. Israel, E. Eng, A. Schulz, & E. Parker (Eds.), *Methods in community-based participatory research for health* (pp. 3–26). San Francisco, CA: Jossey-Bass.

Joyce, B., Weil, M., & Calhoun, E. (2003). *Models of teaching.* Boston, MA: Allyn & Bacon.

Kalipeni, E., & Oppong, J. (1998). The refugee crisis in Africa and implications for health and disease: A political ecology approach. *Social Science & Medicine, 46,* 1637–1653.

Leykum, L., Pugh, J., Lanham, H., Harmon, J., & McDaniel, R. (2009). Implementation research design: Integrating participatory action research into randomized clinical trials. *Implementation Science, 4,* 69–76. doi:10.1186/1748-5908-4-69

Lincoln, Y., & Guba, E. (2000). Paradigmatic controversies, contradictions, and emerging confluences. In N. Denzin & Y. Lincoln (Eds.), *Handbook of qualitative research* (pp. 163–188). Thousand Oaks, CA: Sage.

Marmot, M. (2007). Achieving health equity: From root causes to fair outcomes. *Lancet, 370,* 1153–1163.

Olshansky, E. (2008). The use of community-based participatory research to understand and work with vulnerable populations. In M. de Chesnay & B. Anderson (Eds.), *Caring for the vulnerable: Perspectives in nursing theory, practice, and research* (pp. 269–275). Sudbury, MA: Jones and Bartlett.

Prior, D. (2007). Decolonizing research: A shift toward reconciliation. *Nursing Inquiry, 14,* 162–168.

Reason, P., & Bradbury, H. (2001). Introduction: Inquiry and participation in search of a world worthy of human aspiration. In P. Reason & H. Bradbury (Eds.), *Handbook of action research: Participative inquiry & practice.* London, UK: Sage.

Ricoeur, P. (1991). Life in quest of narrative. In D. Wood (Ed.), *On Paul Ricoeur: Narrative and interpretation* (pp. 20–33). New York, NY: Routledge.

Sagor, R. (1993). *How to conduct collaborative action research.* Alexandria, VA: Association for Supervision and Curriculum Development.

Sanders, D., Labonte, R., Baum, F., & Chopra, M. (2004). Making research matter: A civil society perspective on health research. *Bulletin of the World Health Organization, 82,* 757–763.

Scarinci, I., Johnson, R., Hardy, C., Marron, J., & Partridge, E. (2009). Planning and implementation of a participatory evaluation strategy: A viable approach in the evaluation of a community-based participatory program addressing cancer disparities. *Evaluation and Program Planning, 32,* 221–228.

Seifer, S., & Sisco, S. (2006). Mining the challenges of CBPR for improvements in urban health. *Journal of Urban Health, 83,* 981–984.

Semenza, J., & Maty, S. (2007). Acting upon the macrosocial environment to improve health: A framework for intervention. In S. Galea (Ed.), *Macrosocial determinants of population health* (pp. 443–461). New York, NY: Springer.

Stringer, E. (2007). *Action research.* Los Angeles, CA: Sage.

Wells, K., & Jones, L. (2009). "Research" in community-partnered, participatory research. *JAMA, 302,* 320–321.

Woolf, S. (2008). The meaning of translational research and why it matters. *JAMA, 299,* 211–213.

Yamin, A. (2008). Will we take suffering seriously? Reflections on what applying a human rights framework to health means and why we should care. *Health and Human Rights, 10,* 1–19.

Young, L. (2007). Story-based learning: Blending content and process to learn nursing. In L. Young & B. Paterson (Eds.), *Teaching nursing: Developing a student-centered learning environment* (pp. 164–188). Philadelphia, PA: Lippincott, Williams, & Wilkins.

Chapter 1

Methodology Unfolding

Margaret Dexheimer Pharris

*B*ooks, career paths, and most everyone and everything important in our lives have a way of presenting themselves at the right time. They cannot always be planned, but rather, they show up through some set of circumstances. We may or may not be ready for all they have to teach us. If we are awake and aware, we are able to take notice and engage with them in a meaningful way, and we are transformed. If not, perhaps they will cycle around again—or perhaps it is a missed opportunity—others will arise.

Take a moment, put this book down, and think about the most important people and events in your life—how did these relationships and experiences unfold? Actually, take more than a moment; get some paper and a pencil, and jot down your insights about the unfolding pattern of meaningful events and people in your life (a process of pattern recognition described in Newman, 1994). Do not limit yourself to words; let the pattern flow on paper as it has in your life.

As you examine the unfolding pattern of your life, chances are good that you will recognize that many of your most cherished relationships and experiences were not planned in advance; they came to you, and the essence of who you are evolved with and through them. This chapter, this entire book,

1

is about something that came to us and that we co-created with a whole host of people. It was birthed and attended to by many people in many places. I offer you a written account of what I have witnessed and experienced as a scholar interested in engaging with others to assure that health, human rights, and dignity are nurtured in the lives of all people. I trust you will take it further.

As I tell students, the most important text is that which arises within you while you are reading; pay attention to your insights as you critically read. Do not just take what is written as a recipe. See it rather as a springboard from which you will take the ideas further, or leap forth in a new direction more perfectly suited for the contexts in which you are working and living. We anticipate that your work will be even richer than ours.

In February of 2003, while on a writing spree in New Zealand with Drs. Merian Litchfield and Helga Jónsdóttir, I had the good fortune of meeting Dr. Alice Fieldhouse, a nurse educator and leader in her 10th decade of life. Leaning now and then on a cane, this spry nurse leader walked determinedly along the sun-, salt-, and wind-kissed wharf of Wellington toward the coffee shop to meet us. As we sipped our coffee, I asked Dr. Fieldhouse what advice she had for me as a younger nurse educator. She looked deeply into my eyes and said, "Teach in such a way that your students are on your shoulders and can see further down the horizon than you can." And so it is. We engage with texts and with mentors in such a way that we are boosted up to look a little further along the horizon to see new possibilities for more meaningful action. It is in this spirit that I tell the following story about how our community-based collaborative action research (CBCAR) process came to be.

■ The Birth of Community-Based Collaborative Action Research

It was the spring of 2001. I was a new faculty member at St. Catherine University (then named the College of St. Catherine), and I was given course release time to develop a research proposal. Serendipitously, I had been invited to a neighbor's home for tea, and she had also invited the community health initiatives director for the neighborhood health center. They wanted to apply for an Office of Women's Health grant to establish a National Community Center of Excellence in Women's Health in our multi-ethnic, predominantly African-American inner-city neighborhood—North Minneapolis. They needed an academic partner and faculty members with PhDs to collaborate on the grant. The funding was a long shot—the Office of Women's Health only intended to fund four centers in the entire United States, but we felt that the neighborhood deserved the chance since it had some of the worst racial health disparities in the state. As it turned out, the Dean of the School of Health, Dr. Margaret McLaughlin, had been the director of an Academic Center of Excellence in Women's Health in Pennsylvania; she was very interested in the partnership, not only because of her commitment to women's health, but also for the opportunity to connect the college to communities of color in a meaningful way. It was a good fit for St. Catherine's mission and values. We eagerly responded and offered our expertise.

One of the grant requirements was that a community-based action research process be in place to identify and address barriers to health for women and girls of color. As I wrote that section of the grant, I pondered what it meant to be truly community based and to what extent we, as the academic partner, were going to, or even *should* do, to assure that the action component be carried out. An initial literature search on community-based action research yielded terms such as *participatory action research, collaborative action research,* and *community-based participatory research,* as well as several others. I wondered what the specific differences were between these concepts and which, if any, we should embrace. I immersed myself in the literature and interviewed researchers whose work involved engagement with communities. What I learned filled me with excitement about the possibilities; yet, I was left with questions about what approach would be the best fit for our community. I was particularly interested in how action research might be used to address health inequalities. Delving into the action research literature, I found a rich history and many possible pathways.

Exploring the History and Nature of Action Research

In my exploration of the literature on action research, I found that action research was developed to bring about meaningful social change. The term *action research* is often attributed to social psychologist Kurt Lewin who proposed in the 1940s that workers should be actively engaged in determining what makes for best working conditions and productivity; that the sole goal of action research is not publication, but rather meaningful social change (Lewin, 1948); and, that theory and practice should be joined in a symbiotic relationship to one another (Holter & Schwartz-Barcott, 1993). Applying action research to a variety of social situations, McTaggart (1996) pointed out that rather than being a template, procedure, or method, action research is a potent *process* involving "a series of commitments to observe and problematize through practice a series of principles for conducting social enquiry" (p. 248). The process of action research engages a group of people in identifying issues of central concern to them, asking critical questions about the history and context of the issues, exploring how best to gather and analyze data to address the issues of concern, and creating action plans to improve their situation (McTaggart, 1996). In the 1980s, nurses began capitalizing on the potential of action research to improve clinical practice (Badger, 2000; Holter & Schwartz-Barcott, 1993). Action research has been appreciated by nurses for the way in which it closes the gap between theory and practice (Rolfe, 1996).

Participatory Action Research

Addressing the need for emancipation, Hall (1997) pointed out that during the 1970s, people throughout Africa and Latin America questioned the wisdom of dominant research methodologies because of their colonizing nature—researchers coming in from the outside, researching the experience of "the other," and taking the findings to the north for publication. From the southern hemisphere came a call for increased participation of and democracy for people involved in the situations being researched, so they could create their own transformative action-oriented knowledge. In Tanzania, researchers developed and called for "participatory research" (Hall, 1997). During the same time period in Colombia, Orlando Fals Borda (1995) was applying a method he developed of *investigación acción participativa* (participatory action research), which prompted researchers to join people suffering injustices to not only investigate the injustices, but also to uncover and name the structures that permit and perpetuate the injustices. This process resulted in the discovery of ways to rechannel collective energies toward courses of action that bring about justice and equality. Fals Borda drew attention to the importance of avoiding intellectual imperialism by aligning academic knowledge to become complementary and reciprocal with popular knowledge (Fals Borda & Rahman, 1991).

Following this vein of work, Smith (1997a) presented a process of *participatory action-research* that involved a group of people collectively entering "into a living process, examining their reality by asking penetrating questions, mulling over assumptions related to their everyday problems and circumstances, deliberating alternatives for change, and taking meaningful actions" (p. 173). Smith pointed out that the prevailing scientific method was problematic because of the monopolistic way in which knowledge was defined. Citing the work of Ekins (1992), Smith (1997b) stated, "Those holding this world view [scientism], certain of its successful achievements in prediction and manipulation of the physical environment, continue to devalue the 'ideas, experiences and accumulated wisdom of the majority of humankind'" (p. 5). Embracing this new convention of research, Freire (1997) pointed out, "When people are the masters of inquiry—the owners of the questions under study—their research becomes a means of taking risks, of expelling visible and invisible oppressors, and of producing actions for transformation" (p. xi).

Calls for participatory action research from various parts of the world stressed the importance of research concerns *arising from* and *being defined by* people within communities or practice settings where transformation is needed. Furthermore, participatory action researchers suggested that decolonizing research methods must attend to social networking, critically analyze whose issues are being served, and uncover and correct unequal power dynamics (Young, 2006).

Collaborative Action Research

The word *participate* generally means to take part or share in, while *collaborate* implies that parties are working jointly (Pearsall & Trumble, 2002). Collaboration implies a full and equal partnership, whereas participation could be partial. Sagor (1992) presented a model of *collaborative action research* that involves people with common interests working together to investigate issues of concern and devise actions to improve their situation. Sagor's model was originally developed for teachers who sought to improve teaching/learning processes. Sagor proposed the following five steps:

- Problem formulation—which includes reflective interviewing, analytic discourse, and graphic representation to formulate the problem statement
- Data collection—which aims to view the problem through triangulated sources of data
- Data analysis—which involves identifying themes, interrogating the data through use of a matrix, and forming and presenting new conclusions through a revised graphic representation
- Reporting of results—with the aim of engaging a wider network in making sense of what has been found
- Action planning—to determine how to initiate and evaluate the needed changes that have been identified

The steps are then repeated such that continuous cycling occurs. Sagor encouraged collaborative action researchers to invite critical friends who, without a stake in the process, can honestly and boldly critique the project. Like other action researchers, Sagor cautioned against using this as a prescriptive methodology, pointing out, "At its core, the process values empowerment, initiative, and experimentation" (p. 75).

Community-Based Participatory Research

Although action researchers generally embraced wide participation and social transformation as a goal, community-based researchers in the 1990s generated a related process that they termed *community-based participatory research* (CBPR). Israel, Eng, Schultz, & Parker (2005) conducted an extensive review of the CBPR literature. Their analysis identified the following nine key principles of CBPR:

- Acknowledgement of community as a unit of identity
- Commitment to building on strengths and resources within the community
- Facilitation of collaborative, equitable partnership in all phases of research, involving an empowering and power-sharing process that attends to social inequalities
- Fostering of colearning and capacity building among all partners
- Integration and achievement of a balance between knowledge generation and intervention for the mutual benefit of all partners
- A focus on the local relevance of public health problems and on ecological perspectives that attend to the multiple determinants of health
- Involvement of systems development using a cyclical and iterative process
- Dissemination of results to all partners and involving them in wider dissemination of results
- Involvement in a long-term process and commitment to sustainability

In CBPR, the collaborative aspect of relationships between partners throughout the research process is essential, signifying equal involvement between partners who each share their unique strengths.

Having a basic understanding of the philosophical thought and assumptions underlying participatory action research, collaborative action research, and community-based participatory research, I continued my exploration of the literature to more fully understand the nature and possible limitations of action research and determine how it might best be applied to address health inequalities in North Minneapolis.

Action Research: A Verb

Minkler and Wallerstein (2003) referred to CBPR and other participatory approaches, not as methods, but as *orientations* to research, which blur the line between researcher and those researched and build the capacities of both. Emphasizing the emancipatory nature of action research, Reason and Bradbury (2001) stated that the approach "starts with everyday experience and is concerned with the development of living knowledge, in many ways the process of inquiry is as important as specific outcomes." Furthermore, they claimed that action research is "a living, evolving process of coming to know rooted in everyday experience; it is a verb rather than a noun" (p. 2).

If action research is a verb, how then do action researchers define their inquiry process? Beyond the core principles of participatory action research, collaborative action research, and community-based participatory research identified in the literature, no set design for action research exists. Instead, the design of an action research project is determined by the research question, which is framed by the people involved in the process; the methods used to collect and analyze data unfold from the nature of the research problem and the community in which it is situated (Badger, 2000).

In addition to who defines the research agenda, there are varied opinions about the role of the professional researcher, ranging from being a person who comes into the situation to facilitate change with and for participants around a pre-identified issue, to being a person who comes into the situation in a spirit of collaboration with those affected—bringing to the relationship specific knowledge about data gathering and analysis and ethical protections for both participants and processes (Badger, 2000). The research methods experts may be members of the community or practice environment where the action research is taking place. Whether research team members are from the academy or are members of the community, or both, their role needs to be clearly identified and the power dynamics analyzed on an ongoing basis. Identifying at the outset of the project who will be responsible for what is ideal; reassessing and renegotiating this as the need arises are also important. It is also helpful for team members to dialogue upfront about their self-interests in the topic and what they hope to gain from the process.

Critique of Action Research

Critics of action research claim that it represents a process similar to problem solving, professional development, quality assurance cycles, or reflective practice—all processes that would be rejected by traditional science because they do not produce results that are generalizable to other situations. Critics also raise ethical concerns that collaboration may mask subtle exploitation (Badger, 2000). Conscientious action researchers commit themselves to bold conversation with partners and critics to uncover any coercive dynamics in the research process. They also do not aim for generalizability of findings, knowing that the aim of this research process is to improve the situation for those affected by the issue being researched in the location it is being researched. Findings from other parts of the country or world may not fit the local context. Although findings might provoke insights for people in other communities or organizations, it is more likely that the *process* is generalizable, even though modifications and adaptations to the process are almost always necessary. Conscientious action researchers also recognize that addressing inequalities is most often a long and arduous process.

In addressing the pessimism surrounding the potency of the participatory action research process, McTaggart (1996) pointed out that social advantage is reluctantly surrendered, and disadvantage is persistently difficult to redress. He stated, "Most injustice is sustained deliberately, systematically and hegemonically by longstanding social practices which promote advantage as well as disadvantage" (p. 241). McTaggart called for vitalizing more complex networks of participants to do this important work in a manner that is generous, tolerant, and strategic. In the process, all participants usually experience some degree of transformation and emancipation. McTaggart embraced emancipation, not so much as an end product to strive for, but as a process, with participants constantly asking whether the situation at hand is improving and if so, for whom?

Grounding the CBCAR Process Within the Local Context

After reviewing the literature on the types, strengths, and limitations of action research, our challenge in North Minneapolis was to define the action research process upon which we were embarking. The philosophical values underpinning the participatory action research literature were certainly attractive and applicable for our situation. We had some of the worst health disparities in the state, and had one of the greatest concentrations of social service agencies as well. Meanwhile, health and wealth were not increasing in North Minneapolis. Initiatives to improve our health and well-being were defined in response to funding bodies who issued requests for grant proposals that changed every few years with the interests of the funders. Agencies were revising their strategic plans based on the mandates of funding agencies rather than based on the needs of the community. What seemed most important to us was that our research agenda be defined by people from the community; we knew that the wisdom for health resided with them.

Tentatively defining the process for the grant application was one step—we stated we would reverse the flow of the research question from being university-defined and controlled to being community-defined and controlled. Drawing on the work of Sagor (1992), we described a five-step cyclical process of problem formulation, data collection, data analysis, reporting results, and action planning, which we presented as our action framework. The more important step would be redefining the research process with community partners if the grant was funded, which it was.

Identifying CBCAR's Theoretical Underpinnings

At the time that I entered into the grant-writing process, my research, practice, teaching, and way of being in the world were firmly situated in a unitary participatory paradigm (Heron & Reason, 1997; Newman, 1994). This paradigm includes the positivist paradigm, yet moves beyond simply examining cause and effect relationships. For example, when researchers operating within a positivist paradigm use a randomized controlled study to conclude that a medication is less effective in a given population, researchers operating within a unitary participatory perspective can enter the situation to engage with people from that population, perhaps at their request. They would see the positivist study as one pattern—one piece of information— and then collaboratively engage with people within the population to see the situation with a wider lens. Perhaps there is a history of distrust of the medical establishment due to well-documented abuses, or perhaps the population is disproportionately low-income and the medication is very costly, so people are rationing it and thus watering down its effect; or, it may be both factors along with several others. Once this knowledge situated in the community is uncovered, and if it is important to the health and well-being of the people within the population, a dialogue between all stakeholders—people within the population, healthcare providers, academics, insurers, and even pharmaceutical companies—can shed light on how to better conceptualize and organize healthcare services within the community. To provide a more concrete and real-life example, I will describe research I conducted in the mid-1990s that led me into the unitary participatory way of doing research. This work provided insight into how the unitary participatory research paradigm might engage communities in an emancipatory process.

Beginning in the late 1980s, the youth homicide rate in our community began to multiply. I was asked to join a team of people within the health department that represented some of the finest minds in the community from several disciplines. We pored over statistics on arrest, booking, presentencing, and economic assistance for adolescents who were convicted of murder. However, when finished, we could only conclude that youth do not murder on Tuesday nights and that they usually used guns—we knew precious little about the lives of these young people who had murdered. A new approach to understanding this issue was needed. My research up until that time had been largely quantitative. I realized that to fully understand the mystery of why so many teens were suddenly grasping guns and killing others, we would have to listen to the youth incarcerated for murder. I jumped research paradigms and drew on the work of nurse theorist, Dr. Margaret Newman (1979, 1986, 1990,

1994, 2008). This work was not conceptualized within an action research framework. It did, however, give rise to a new way of conceptualizing action research. Understanding a community problem within its context and fully comprehending the whole is more likely to happen when unitary data collection and analysis methods are employed.

To understand the pattern of increasing youth homicide, I invited teenage boys incarcerated for murder to become co-investigators with me (Pharris, 2002). Following a protocol outlined by Newman (1994) I asked only one question: "Tell me about the most meaningful people and events in your life." I expected a 20-page narrative for each youth; the shortest narrative was 200 pages. Each week I returned to the prison with the evolving narrative and diagram of the important people, events, and transformation points in their lives, and we talked until they could hold up the diagram and say, "This is everything that is meaningful in my life."

Upon comparing the common patterns of the teens' lives, what became visible was not simply a common pattern of troubled youth, but rather our pattern as community. I shared the study findings with people from 16 different youth-serving agencies and groups to see if the findings resonated with their experience, and to dialogue about what actions were called for. In the dialogue, people realized what they could do differently on a very concrete level to alter the pattern of youth homicide in our community. We all saw ourselves in the pattern that arose in the young men's stories. Once unitary data are collected, the identified patterns can be presented to the wider community to envision meaningful actions to address the problem being researched.

As I listened long enough to the young men in this study, I literally entered into four of their stories. For example, one young man described being 8 years old when his mother received a call from the hospital to come right away—that her brother had been shot and was in critical condition. The young man recounted going with his mother to the hospital emergency room and choked up as he described the moment that the charge nurse said to his mother, "I am so sorry, we did everything we could, but we could not save your brother's life." He recalled his deep sadness, which pulled him down and was suddenly complicated and engulfed by a larger wave of fear and concern for his mother as she collapsed into the nurse's arms. As I listened to him tell this very tragic and frightening story, I had been seeing the scene of his mother and the nurse through his eyes, his perspective, and could feel his terror, but when he mentioned his uncle's name and described his mother collapsing, I suddenly shifted to the other side of the scene. The scene came up from the recesses of *my own* memory where I could feel the weight of his mother in my arms as the two of us sank to the floor; warm tears saturated my scrubs and as the minutes passed, took on a clinging chill. I had been the charge nurse in the trauma center emergency room that night. I have a peripheral recollection of the drooping shoulders and wide watery frightened eyes of the children silently staring at the woman in my arms. What troubles me to this day is that I do not remember having helped those children process their uncle's death. I believe I was solely focused on their mother; I talked about what she needed to do to move through her grief so that she could do what needed to be done in the next few days. I know now, the deep impact such experiences have on young children and that as nurses we can help them and the adults who care for them learn how to begin the grieving process. Our care can interrupt the cycle of violence and alter the trajectory of young lives. When I presented the common patterns and the stories of youth convicted of murder to people in the community who care for young people at risk for violence, our ensuing dialogue about the meaning of this pattern helped each of us see how we are essential aspects of the whole and how we might alter what we do and thus alter youth homicide in our community.

Consistent with the theories of Bohm (1980) and Newman, this research process showed that we can delve into the lives of individuals to see the pattern of the community as a whole, including our place in it. In engaging people in dialogue about community patterns and their meaning, actions for optimal community health become visible. The essential aspects of Newman's theory of health are the focus on identifying patterns of interactions and energy flow, engaging in dialogue about the meaning of the patterns identified, and envisioning actions and transformation.

Freire (1970/1999) saw transformation as the intended outcome of our reflection and action upon the world, and called this process of reflection, action, and transformation *praxis*. Newman (1990) refers to her research methodology as *research as praxis*, in which research, practice, and theory are reflexively engaged as one expanding and evolving whole. Each aspect of this undivided whole informs the others. Freire (1970/1999), who envisioned knowledge development as participatory and arising from the people most affected by the issue at hand, defined praxis as "reflection and action upon the world in order to transform it" (p. 33). Similarly, in my experience with Newman's theory, the intention to come in from the outside and *empower* and *change* society is not consistent with a unitary participatory paradigm because it assumes that power is not already situated within the community and that the community needs to be acted upon. It is important to note that the relational process of interpreting meaning and engaging seemingly opposing views in dialogue is associated with profound transformation; however, it is not transformation that is predefined or aimed for, but rather a transformation that is constructed from within the research process. The most powerful actions arise out of community dialogue about the meanings of patterns identified. The unitary participatory theoretical perspective acknowledges that the knowledge needed to address identified problems resides within the community. Action researchers can trust that what should arise from the community will arise, that power is already present, and that the answers to identified problems will become clear through exploration and dialogue, as will necessary actions to remedy the situation. Researchers do not need to assume total responsibility for instigating or controlling those actions (Jónsdóttir, Litchfield, & Pharris, 2003; Litchfield, 1999).

Drawing on these theoretical underpinnings, when designing our research plan in North Minneapolis we realized the importance of entering into equal relationships that focus on dialogue to uncover the meaning of historical and emerging patterns within the community. We knew that wherever we entered in, if we concentrated on deepening and expanding the circle of dialogue and engaged people in identifying meaningful patterns in the community, insights into action would arise. We were aware that our action research process would be uniquely shaped because of its roots in a unitary participatory paradigm.

Learning by Doing

Once the grant was funded, our first task was to expand the circle of dialogue to identify the focus of our first research project. The newly hired Coordinator of the Community Center of Excellence in Women's Health (CCOEWH), Dr. Paulette Sankofa, and I expanded our search and critique of the action research literature to discern a process that would engage community women in identifying the barriers to health for women and girls of color in North Minneapolis, which was the research focus of the CCOEWH. With her rich scholarly background in critical pedagogy, Dr. Sankofa brought Paulo Freire's (1970/1990, 1997, 1998) influence, which infused our work with a critical consciousness that constantly sought to examine the nature of the myriad relationships we had. Freire (1998) calls researchers to embrace a restless curiosity. Critical consciousness and restless curiosity moved us toward uncovering what was hidden in the health disparities statistics in our community. We decided that I would invite two or three graduate nursing students to work with us, and Paulette and her staff would begin identifying the organizations and places in the community where women and girls gathered so that we could invite women representing all aspects of the community into the research process.

I entered the first year graduate nursing research class with my colleagues to explain to the students the kind of research we each were involved in so they could select an advisor based on goodness of fit with their research interests. I explained that I was involved in a research *process*, not just a *project* and that if the students wanted to study a specific research topic, this was not the project for them. On the other hand, if they wanted to partner with women from a community to engage in dialogue to identify and address the greatest barriers to health for women and girls of color, this would be a good project for them. The caveat, I told them, was that they may be spending a year exploring transportation or childcare access as barriers to health. I stressed that the community gets to decide the research question. I left the class doubtful that anyone would be interested. However, by the time I reached my office door, two breathless adult nurse practitioner graduate students, Linda Amaikwu-Rushing and Krista Ollom, were already there, excitedly proclaiming, "Dr. Pharris, we want to work with you!" We all smiled, knowing we were about to embark on a very meaningful and interesting journey. Another graduate student, Debra Fitzgerald, a pediatric nurse practitioner student, joined the team shortly thereafter.

Paulette, Linda, Krista, Deb, and I immersed ourselves in the literature to explore ways in which we could best facilitate women from the community to identify the research question and sources of data for our first cycle of action research. We affirmed that we would follow Margaret Newman's (1994) hermeneutic-dialectic mode of inquiry that involves a continual process of dialogic engagement centered on what is meaningful to community members—listening, attending to patterns, reflecting, and trusting that transformation would ensue as the community comes to understand itself and its capacity to act more fully. This process was consistent with Freire's (1970/1990, 1998) model of emancipatory education, which involves listening; engaging in participatory dialogue; envisioning action and change; and acting, reflecting on action, and acting again with new insights. We concluded that we needed to create our own hybrid research methodology, which would include:

■ Creating a trusting and meaningful bond between the community and the research team
■ Committing all members of the collaboration to periodically assess for power inequalities in our relationships and our processes
■ Engaging the community to define the research question
■ Drawing on academic knowledge of research methods

- Seeking out and embracing critical friends who could challenge our process
- Collecting data in partnership
- Engaging the community to determine action steps and dissemination venues

Since we wanted to signal an equal partnership and full engagement in the process, we decided that the word *collaboration* was more fitting than *participation*, even though we fully embraced the values coming from the participatory action research literature. We decided to name the process we were developing *community-based collaborative action research* (CBCAR), which we defined for the community as a community-driven systematic inquiry, conducted collaboratively between those affected by the issue being studied and those skilled in research methodologies, for purposes of education and taking action on effecting change. We saw CBCAR as combining the insight of the community into its own situation with the research skills of college faculty and students in a dialogic collaboration in which knowledge, skills, and insights are exchanged, and transformation becomes a possibility for all those involved. As a social action process, CBCAR assumes that knowledge is related to power and that power is related to change.

In determining the logistics of how to begin, we were influenced by Sagor's (1992) process for formulating the problem to be studied. Sagor outlined a process of reflective interviewing where small groupings of people identify an issue of concern, which in our case would involve women's health. The issue should be something we could influence, and be something that the women care deeply about. The next step is analytic discourse, which is similar to a group interview through which circle sharing goes on until everyone in the small group feels they have articulated everything they know about the subject, and the group feels they have a full grasp of what they know about the issue at hand. The process then moves from the left to the right brain as the group develops a graphic representation of all of the relevant factors, variables, and contexts related to the identified issue. The group then interrogates itself to identify how they know what they know, what assumptions are being made, who is affected, and what permits and perpetuates the problem. Out of this interrogation, the problem statement is formulated, and at least three possible sources of data to gain more information are identified.

The other concept we drew from Sagor's (1992) work was that of a critical friend. We extended the concept to include someone who was not necessarily already a friend, but to stretch our reach beyond our immediate network to identify people who could challenge the credibility and rigor of our research process and the integrity of our relationships. Consistent with Newman's (1994) dialectic process, we felt that we would be able to see what was there more clearly if we engaged different perspectives. We did not shy away from people who were critical, but rather saw them as potential critical friends, who could improve the rigor of our process. Some critical friends we sought out, others came to us. We were not surprised that some unanticipated critical friends attended our first women's advisory council meeting.

In addition to the challenge of critical friends, we looked to Lather's (1991) descriptions of validity in emancipatory research. In order to check for limited vision or vision altered by the passion of the research team, Lather recommends (1) *triangulation* to cross-check information and strengthen the trustworthiness of the data; (2) enhancement of *construct validity* by systematically asking critical questions at every step so that representative knowledge can be constructed; (3) return of data to participants for analysis and interpretation to increase the credibility of findings and thus assure *face validity*; and (4) assurance of *catalytic validity*—a process that orients, focuses, and energizes participants so that transformation can be a reality. We worked to assure catalytic validity by weaving research results into a spoken-word narrative, which we used to engage the larger community in a dialogue about potential action steps. Reliability—assuring that the measure used in a study can be used in another setting to produce similar results—is not appropriate since the entire research process is constructed by those involved, and thus is unique to the local setting. It could be concluded that the *process* is a reliable process for engaging communities in understanding and transforming their own situation.

The CCOEWH staff identified 50 organizations where women gather in the community and invited representatives from each organization to come to a 4-hour Saturday morning meeting to identify the barriers to health for women and girls of color and begin an action research process. We expected around 10 women to show up; however, 50 women exuberantly flowed through the doors of the health center conference room on that early April morning in 2002. To randomly create diverse small groups, a floral plant with a unique symbol around its base was placed in the middle of each table, and the same symbols were alternated on the name tags, which were stacked so that people who came together would be sitting at different tables. The demographics of the women represented the demographics of the community. A hum of excited engagement radiated throughout the room. After a centering reflection and welcome, the women began working in their table groups to interview one another and articulate all that they knew about health and its barriers for women and girls of color. Spirited dialogues sprang up at the tables. When we reconvened at lunchtime to share our findings, the women stated they needed another Saturday morning to truly discern and describe the most pressing barrier for us to examine in our action research.

A few weeks later, 65 women and girls arrived—mostly African American, and also Hmong American, Mexican American, American Indian, Lao American, and European American women. We broke down into eight groups, and when we reconvened, each of the eight groups identified *racism* as the major barrier to health for women and girls of color. We decided to explore the experience of racism, health, and well-being for women and girls of color in North Minneapolis and reengaged the small groups to identify numerous places within the community where we might be able to gather data. We decided to focus on interviewing women and teens who represented the diverse aspects of the community, but also to include a few groups of healthcare providers. Specifically, the women wanted to explore how women and girls identified health, how they defined racism, what they saw to be the interplay between the two, what negative experiences they had had that they attributed to race/racism, what positive experiences they had had that they attributed to race/ethnicity/culture, and how they envisioned a community healthcare system at its best. These became our research questions. During planning sessions, the data collection team decided to also ask healthcare professionals to describe how race affected their care of patients. The research questions lent themselves to a phenomenological qualitative data collection method, using focus groups and individual interviews. Women from the community were recruited to join the research team.

The first task of the research team was to engage critical friends to challenge and thus strengthen our process. We sought methodological critique, which helped us see that we should avoid the word "racism" in any recruitment information and rather, refer to the interplay of race, health, and well-being so that we would not be accused of only involving women who were comfortable talking about and able to identify racism. We sought theoretical critique. Dr. Margaret Newman, whose theory informed our work, met with us. We decided that CBCAR was a fitting image in that like a taxi or cab car, the university researchers are driving the car in that they know the methodological streets to take, but they are at the service of the community, who is telling them where they want to go. Dr. Newman mentioned that she saw the theory as the headlights that helped everyone clearly see (and thus understand the meaning of) what was in front of them.

Since the word *research* was not warmly received in the community, particularly by African Americans who were well aware of the history in the United States of repeated victimization of African Americans by medical research (Washington, 2006), Paulette Sankofa and I went on a community radio and cable television program, hosted at a local restaurant with about 50 people in attendance, to talk about what we were planning to do with and through this research. We were looking for community-based critical friends. The hard questions we expected came; people grilled us on our intent and our process. One woman was particularly and persistently critical—we approached her afterwards and asked her to stay in contact with us as a critical friend; we needed her critical eye and questions. Throughout this research process, we found that as our relationships developed, critical friends became good friends, and we needed to stretch out even further beyond our circle of comfort to seek new critical friends. It became a continual process of extended networking.

We also tried to stretch our reach by identifying diverse groups through which to recruit participants for the focus groups. Once we had Institutional Review Board approval, and we had conducted training sessions on data collection and focus group facilitation using a circle process, we formed data collection teams. Women from academia partnered with women from the community who had volunteered at the advisory council meeting to conduct focus group and individual interviews to listen to the experiences of women in North Minneapolis. One team went to the streets to reach women who were unconnected to formal organizations, and another team recruited women in the clinic waiting room. We organized focus groups of teens, block club leaders, women from various African-American and Spanish-speaking churches, women from community organizations, African immigrant women, Hmong women, Lao women, Native-American women, women who were being prostituted, women from the local mosque, and healthcare providers—always assuring that the focus group leader was able to relate well with the group. We listened widely and intently, audiotaping and transcribing each session. The women who participated came from all walks of life and varied in age and religious affiliation. We wanted as complete a pattern of the community as possible.

After nearly a year of data collection, and after all of the data had been transcribed, the academic partners and CCOEWH coordinator convened to analyze the data—we assumed that since those of us from academia had the training in data analysis, we should be responsible for analyzing the data. When we began the data analysis process, each of us at once came to a collective insight—who are *we* to analyze these data? We realized that the women and girls from the community needed to be part of the data analysis process; they would be able to see much more depth and complexity than we ever could. We stripped the data of identifiers—color coding each transcript by ethnicity or age or social group—and invited women from the advisory board to help analyze the data. For example, African-American women analyzed the data from the groups of African-American women, Latina women the Latina data, and teens analyzed the teen data. Each woman on the data analysis team received the color coded data prior to the analysis session and was asked to carefully read each narrative once for comprehension of the whole and at least one more time to identify significant themes and quotes. The narratives had a wide right margin for notes. When the groups got together, they each determined their own process. We had sticky notes, markers, scissors, tape, and large sheets of paper for the groups to work with. Each group determined significant themes and quotes. In this process, we saw so much more than academics alone could begin to identify and understand. *Community involvement in data analysis was added as an essential element of our CBCAR process.*

The next challenge involved discerning how to reflect the data back to the community—should we use PowerPoint presentations, charts, graphs. . . ? Based on our theoretical underpinnings, we firmly believed that the necessary action steps would arise from engaged dialogue about what was meaningful in the patterns we were seeing. The question was, how do we present the pattern of these rich data in an engaging way? We could and did present colorful pie charts that depicted data from a brief demographic sheet we had each woman complete, listing age, "race," source of health care/healing, diagnosed "diseases" and whether or not she saw herself as healthy. The pie charts demonstrated that half of the women who had at least two diagnosed diseases, such as diabetes and heart disease, described themselves as healthy. In addition, half of the women who had no medical or mental health problems stated they were not healthy. This pattern reinforced Newman's theory (1994) that health is more than the absence of disease. In fact, the women in this action research study described relational and spiritual connectedness as being essential aspects of health. We suddenly realized that perhaps our community was much healthier than the State Department of Health measures had captured with *their* definitions of health. Perhaps *we* were the healthiest community and people in the suburbs were the *least* healthy! We began to revel in our strengths, while not losing sight of the very real need to improve physical and mental health in the community. When we engaged in dialogue about the meaning of the pattern we were seeing, we began to see ourselves in a new light that enhanced our capabilities.

Although the data from the demographic sheets could be displayed in graphic format, we determined that to do justice to the women's powerful stories in the taped narratives, we needed to leave the stories as whole as possible. Mrs. Nothando Zulu, Director of the Black Storytellers' Alliance, and I spent 2 days weaving together the stories that the data analysis teams marked as most salient and representative of the identified themes. From this process, Mrs. Zulu created a narrative that could be performed by women who demographically represent the community. This multicultural spoken-word narrative was performed for the women's advisory council of the CCOEWH, on community radio and television, and in various community forums, always asking what was missing from the narrative to better represent the listeners' experience, and what needed to happen to create a healthier community. The dramatic narrative of women's stories resonated with people in the community, and insights into action arose in each dialogue. We discovered that art is an effective way to present research findings and engage people holistically; it provokes a response that improves vision for community health. We decided to add using art to reflect research findings back to the community as a potentially powerful aspect of the CBCAR and community health process.

When the narrative was performed for the 70 women at the women's advisory council meeting, they determined two action steps. Because young women in the study only saw racism as interpersonal and were not able to identify the systemic and cultural manifestations of racism, and thus were not able to defend themselves from internalizing it, the women decided it was important to engage young women with older women to learn how to identify, critique, and not internalize racism. We developed *Let's Talk About Race* forums so that adolescents could learn from their Elders how to deal with and not internalize everyday racism, and how to protect and nourish their health. This project was funded by the Women's Foundation of Minnesota, the General Mills Foundation, and the Archie D. and Bertha H. Walker Foundation. An evaluation of two series of pilot forums resulted in publication of a curriculum guide,

Racism and how it affects your health: A curriculum guide for people who care about African-American adolescent females and their health, and DVDs, which have been distributed widely—in the state, nation, and several other countries experiencing threats to healthy identity development for youth of color (Ellis & Pharris, 2007).

The second action step was to produce a DVD of the narrative on women's experiences of health, well-being, and racism to stimulate community dialogue and educate healthcare professionals, teachers, and others; 250 copies were made and distributed, and it has been made available as an online stream at: http://minerva.stkate.edu/womenhealth.nsf. When the DVD is shown within the community, participants are asked what they would change in the spoken-word narrative to better reflect their experience and what insights they have related to community actions to improve the health of women and girls.

We had agreed up-front that the community would drive the dissemination decision-making process. The women's advisory council determined that rather than publishing our findings in a national or international journal, we needed to get the findings into the hands of physicians in Minnesota— they were the main audience for what we learned. For that reason, the findings were published in *Minnesota Medicine* (Amaikwu-Rushing, Fitzgerald, Wilson, Smith, Irwin, & Pharris, 2005) and a monograph of the research process, findings, and implication was published and disseminated by NorthPoint Health & Wellness Center (Pharris, Amaikwu-Rushing, Fitzgerald, Ollom, Sankofa, McMorris et al., 2004). We found that writing for publication was something that few community members were interested in; yet, seeking ways to share writing tasks is vitally important, as is deconstructing the dynamics when writing is left to or seized by academic partners.

The process of dialoguing about the findings from this research and discerning appropriate actions created ripples of transformation throughout the community, health center, and university settings. In addition to the forums for teens, there have been myriad changes in the health center—from installing privacy curtains in the exam rooms for patient comfort in situations where the provider does not speak the patient's language and an interpreter is needed—to quality assurance data being looked at by "race" wherever possible—to the health center staff reflecting (looking like) the patient population all the way to the board of directors and CEO. Identifying and taking steps to eliminate racism in all of its forms has been woven through various courses in the University's nursing department and is the focus of two new graduate level courses that aim to give nurse practitioners and nurse educators the knowledge and skills needed to take leadership in creating inclusive practice environments and dismantling racism in systems and structures. A book has been written to help make nursing education environments more inclusive (Bosher & Pharris, 2008).

New research questions have been identified, and additional cycles of action research have been completed to better understand disparities for youth and for women with diabetes (see for example Yang, Xiong, Vang, & Pharris, 2009). Our experience has shown us that to understand the whole of the community and its health patterns, gathering data that are not particulate in nature is best. Additionally, the fewer questions asked, the better. Although demographic data and survey questions provide a general overview of the community, people's narratives about their lives and experiences, when appreciated across participants, provide a clearer lens to see and understand community health contextually.

■ Lessons Learned: Revising the CBCAR Process

In addition to learning that narratives yield rich data for understanding community health patterns, our CBCAR experience has given us a useful framework from which to work. We learned the importance of forming a strong relationship between academic researchers and community members and creating a process by which power dynamics, self-interests, and assumptions are periodically and systematically assessed and analyzed. We learned that the process by which the research question is defined is extremely important and must invoke a commitment to creating the time and space in which even the quietest of voices can be heard. This process cannot be rushed, and great effort should be exerted to include and hear various perspectives on the issue, so that patterns can be most fully understood. We learned that data collection methods will be dictated by the question at hand and that triangulation of sources is desired for a fuller view of the situation. At this point, research partners trained in the academy need to interrogate what they know from their professional training and what they are hearing from the community about data collection. Serious self-reflection and communal critique to interrogate decisions are important at this step. We learned that critical friends are invaluable and that the circle of critique has to be continually widened as critical friends become good friends.

We also learned that academic researchers have the responsibility to protect privacy and uphold ethical principles dictated by university Institutional Review Boards, that community views of ethical action also need to be elicited and engaged in the process whenever possible, and that once identifiers have been stripped from the data, more valid results are seen when the people affected help to analyze the data. We learned that data analysis provides insight into the pattern of health and that the pattern is best reflected back to the larger community in the form of art. Art helps people grasp the pattern on a holistic level so that holistic actions can be envisioned.

We learned that presenting findings is not an end, but rather a means to generate dialogue among those involved so that the meaning of the findings can be more fully understood. When all of the people who are part of the pattern of health—from those who suffer to those who are benefiting from the systems that perpetuate the suffering—are involved in the dialogue, the ripples of transformation will be wider, more enduring, and more able to address root causes. CBCAR collaborators strive to erase boundaries so that the circle can be widened to involve all people who are connected to the issue. Through the dialogue, creative actions arise to address the issue at hand. We learned that when actions are determined, an evaluation plan should be put in place to identify specifically how we will know that good has been done when the action is completed. We learned that emancipation is indeed a long journey that brings meaningful liberation all along the way and that CBCAR is a cyclical process through which new questions and insights constantly arise.

Let us now travel across the ocean for another view of how CBCAR might be envisioned in a very different community, and then we will take a more in-depth look at theoretical and methodological underpinnings.

■ References

Amaikwu-Rushing, L., Fitzgerald, D., Wilson, C., Smith, K., Irwin, D., & Pharris, M. D. (2005, Feb). Health, well-being and racism. *Minnesota Medicine, 28–31,* 41.

Badger, T. G. (2000). Action research, change and methodological rigor. *Journal of Nursing Management, 8*(4), 201–207.

Bohm, D. (1980). *Wholeness and the implicate order.* London, UK: Routledge & Kegan Paul.

Bosher, S. D., & Pharris, M. D. (Eds.) (2008). *Transforming nursing education: The culturally inclusive environment.* New York, NY: Springer.

Ellis, C., & Pharris, M. D. (2007). *Racism and how it affects our health: A curriculum guide for people who care about African-American female adolescents and their health.* St. Paul, MN: College of St. Catherine.

Fals Borda, O. (1995, April). *Research for social justice: Some North-South convergences.* Plenary address at the Southern Sociological Society Meeting, Atlanta, GA.

Fals Borda, O., & Rahman, M. A. (1991). *Action and knowledge: Breaking the monopoly with participatory action research.* New York, NY: Apex.

Freire, P. (1970/1990). *Pedagogy of the oppressed.* New York, NY: Continuum Publishing.

Freire, P. (1997). Foreword. In S. E. Smith, D. G. Willms, & N.A. Johnson (Eds.), *Nurtured by knowledge: Learning to do participatory action-research* (pp. xi–xii). New York, NY: Apex.

Freire, P. (1998). *Pedagogy of freedom: Ethics, democracy, and civic courage.* Lanham, MD: Rowman & Littlefield.

Hall, B. (1997). Preface. In S. E. Smith, D. G. Willms, & N.A. Johnson (Eds.), *Nurtured by knowledge: Learning to do participatory action-research* (pp. xiii–xv). New York, NY: Apex.

Heron, J., & Reason, P. (1997). A participatory inquiry paradigm. *Qualitative Inquiry, 3*(3), 274–294.

Holter, I., & Schwartz-Barcott, D. (1993). Action research: What is it? *Journal of Advanced Nursing, 18,* 296–304.

Israel, B. A., Eng, E., Schulz, A. J., & Parker, E. A. (Eds.). (2005). *Methods in community-based participatory research for health.* San Francisco, CA: Jossey-Bass.

Jónsdóttir, H., Litchfield, M., & Pharris, M. D. (2003). Partnership in practice. *Research and Theory for Nursing Practice, 17*(3), 1–9.

Lather, P. (1991). *Getting smart: Feminist research and pedagogy within the postmodern.* New York, NY: Routledge.

Lewin, K. (1948). *Resolving social conflicts: Selected papers on group dynamics.* G. W. Lewin (Ed.). New York, NY: Harper & Row.

Litchfield, M. (1999). Practice wisdom. *Advances in Nursing Science, 22*(2), 62–73.

McTaggart, R. (1996). Issues for participatory action researchers. In O. Zuber-Skerritt (Ed.), *New directions in action research.* London, UK: Falmer Press.

Minkler, M., & Wallerstein, N. (2003). Introduction to community-based participatory research. In M. Minkler, & N. Wallerstein (Eds.), *Community-based participatory research for health* (pp. 3–26). San Francisco, CA: Jossey-Bass.

Newman, M. A. (1979). *Theory development in nursing.* Philadelphia, PA: F. A. Davis.

Newman, M. A. (1986). *Health as expanding consciousness.* St. Louis, MO: Mosby.

Newman, M. A. (1990). Newman's theory of health as praxis. *Nursing Science Quarterly, 3,* 37–41.

Newman, M. A. (1994). *Health as expanding consciousness* (2nd ed.). Sudbury, MA: Jones and Bartlett.

Newman, M. A. (2008). *Transforming presence: The difference nursing makes.* Philadelphia, PA: F. A. Davis.

Pearsall, J., & Trumble, B. (2002). *Oxford English reference dictionary* (2nd ed.). Revised. Oxford, UK: Oxford University Press.

Pharris, M. D. (2002). Coming to know ourselves as community through a nursing partnership with adolescents convicted of murder. *Advances in Nursing Science, 24*(3), 21–42.

Pharris, M. D., Amaikwu-Rushing, L., Fitzgerald, D., Ollom, K., Sankofa, P., & McMorris, C. et al. (2004). *Health, well-being, and racism: The experience of women and girls of color in North Minneapolis.* Minneapolis, MN: Community Center of Excellence in Women's Health.

Reason, P., & Bradbury, H. (2001). Introduction: Inquiry and participation in search of a world worthy of human aspiration. In P. Reason & H. Bradbury (Eds.), *Handbook of action research: Participatory inquiry & practice* (pp. 1–14). London, UK: Sage.

Rolfe, G. (1996). Going to extremes: Action research, grounded practice, and the theory–practice gap in nursing. *Journal of Advanced Nursing, 24*(6), 1315–1320.

Sagor, R. (1992). *How to conduct collaborative action research.* Alexandria, VA: Association for Supervision and Curriculum Development.

Smith, S. E. (1997a). Deepening participatory action-research. In S. E. Smith, D. G. Willms, & N. A. Johnson (Eds.), *Nurtured by knowledge: Learning to do participatory action-research* (pp. 173–263). New York, NY: Apex.

Smith, S. E. (1997b). Participatory action-research within the global context. In S. E. Smith, D. G. Willms, & N. A. Johnson (Eds.), *Nurtured by knowledge: Learning to do participatory action-research* (pp. 1–6). New York, NY: Apex.

Washington, H.A. (2006). *Medical apartheid: The dark history of medical experimentation on Black Americans from colonial times to the present.* New York, NY: Harlem Moon.

Yang, A., Xiong, D., Vang, E., & Pharris, M. D. (2009). Hmong American women living with diabetes. *Journal of Nursing Scholarship, 41*(2), 139–148.

Young, L. (2006). Participatory action research (PAR): A research strategy for nursing? *Western Journal of Nursing Research, 28*(5), 499–504.

Chapter 2

CBCAR: Insights Developing

Carol Pillsbury Pavlish

My journey with community-based collaborative action research (CBCAR) began at the bedside. As an oncology nurse in a fast-paced university setting, I met three young African immigrant women who were diagnosed with cancer and subsequently learned that they were HIV positive. Over the course of several weeks, one of the women shared her story of escaping war in her homeland and seeking shelter in a refugee camp where she was sexually assaulted by soldiers. As a white, middle-class, North American nursing instructor who taught at a women's college, I was a naïve foreigner to this woman's experience but also knew that to help students provide quality nursing care, I needed to grasp an element of her difficult journey. After listening to her story, I read extensively about women's health and violence risks in conflict settings around the world, and deeply contemplated the differences that separated us and the common goals that connected us. Slowly, over the course of several months, my worldview on health and well-being gradually unraveled and reshaped. Extending beyond a view of health as biological, psychological, and spiritual processes in a lived body, I learned to also honor health as a human experience that represents a lived and relational being within a particular social, political, economic, and environmental context. That shift in perspective also shifted my viewpoints on research.

Enlightened and transformed by my experience with these three young women, I returned to graduate school to pursue education in international health and community and organization development. Approaching dissertation planning, I sought to implement a research practice that mirrored my view of bedside and community-side nursing—that is, not over, or in front of, or instead of—but rather at the side of. In this chapter, I detail a community-based project that guided the selection and direction of my dissertation. Hoping to improve refugee women's health and well-being, I volunteered my research services to the American Refugee Committee (ARC), an international nongovernmental organization that works in several postconflict settings around the world. In the sections that follow, I first explain theoretical background in community development and action research and then describe the project partnership with ARC. Finally, I detail the community setting before describing the collaborative action research and development process that evolved.

■ Community Development

Straying from the typical definition of community development as economic prosperity and industrial progress, Bhattacharyya (1995) proposed a new definition of community development that is both "distinctive and universal" (p. 60). Community is defined as *solidarity*, which refers to "a shared identity and a code for conduct, both deep enough that a rupture in them entails affective consequences for the members" (p. 61). Development refers to *agency*, which means the "capacity of people to order their world, that is, the capacity to create, reproduce, change, and live according to their own meaning systems, including the power to define themselves as opposed to being defined by others" (p. 61). At that time, viewing development as "agency" contrasted sharply with mainstream Western development practices, which usually consisted of outside forces entering communities and imposing change. Three overlapping principles pertained to Bhattacharyya's more expansive concept of community development. *Self-help* is predicated on the belief that people are capable and should be allowed to solve their own problems. *Felt needs* implies the capacity of people to define their own concerns, and *participation* refers to the intentional, active inclusion of community members in the development process. These three principles effectively guide the practice of community development anywhere in the world (Bhattacharyya, 1995).

When viewed as agents in community development, community members become active in producing knowledge to guide social change. Kamata (2000) described locally-based knowledge as "historically constituted [emic] knowledge instrumental in the long-term adaptation of human groups to the biophysical environment" (p. 55). Community-based knowledge represents the practical, traditional, and often tacit wisdom of local residents, including socioeconomically marginalized groups. In criticizing traditional ways of conducting Western research and planning Western development projects in low-income countries, Sillitoe (1998) offered many examples of how expensive research and community projects imposed in a top-down fashion have collapsed. For example, when charging into social systems with project initiatives, planners who introduce their own (etic) knowledge systems into communities often ignore locally-based (emic) wisdom, and community residents usually view this lack of respect as "offensive interference" (Sillitoe, 1998, p. 226). Therefore, researchers and program planners need to acknowledge the significance of local knowledge and incorporate local wisdom into planning community health and development projects.

■ Community Action Research and Learning

Gibbons et al. (2000) distinguished between Mode 1 and Mode 2 knowledge production. Mode 1 represents the traditional, discipline-specific way of producing knowledge, for example, the scientific method. Claiming that Mode 2 expands beyond Mode 1, the authors asserted, "Mode 2 knowledge is created in broader, transdisciplinary social and economic contexts" (p. 1).

Complex, interrelated, heterogeneous, and messy contexts are the production and application landscapes for Mode 2 knowledge. Spreading the responsibility of knowledge production to nontraditional work, space, and time dimensions, Mode 2 stimulates deeper understanding of people's life experiences through interactive analyses that occur within rather than separate from their contexts.

Community action research is an example of Mode 2 knowledge production. Producing practical knowledge that is important to people's everyday experiences, community action research aims to create more equitable and sustainable relationships within community systems and structures and increase people's well-being (Reason & Bradbury, 2001). Researching social, cultural, economic, and other contextual factors that impact people's lives contributes important knowledge for professionals who are interested in planning community improvements. In describing a community empowerment approach to health education, Israel, Checkoway, Schulz, and Zimmerman (1994) claimed that prior to implementing community health and development programs, professionals must learn about community members' stressful life events, daily hassles, and chronic hardships. Creating programs based on that information is more likely to succeed than those planned without this contextualized knowledge.

Another benefit of community action research is that learning occurs within the research process. Brookfield (1993) asserted, "If people had a chance to give voice to what moves and hurts them, they would soon show that they were well aware of the real nature of their problems and of ways to deal with these" (p. 234). Freire (1993) claimed that action research intertwines learning, personal empowerment, and social transformation. Within action research, learning becomes a process of "conscientization" which begins at the "least-aware stage" where nothing is questioned, fatalism is prominent, and external forces are seen to be in charge. Midway through the learning process, people begin to acknowledge they have some control over their lives and commence to question existing circumstances. The final phase is "conscientizacao" where people understand the contextual factors that impact their reality and become more active in constructing a different, more just reality (Freire, 1993, p. 109). Similarly, Senge and Scharmer (2006) described action research as the formation of learning communities within and between organizations where a diverse group of people form knowledge-creating systems through collaborative research and capacity building. These interactive, knowledge-creating systems produce changes required for organizational development and knowledge innovation. Nonaka, Konno, and Toyama (2001) suggested that successful organizations deliberately create time and space for their workers to share perspectives, analyze problems, and co-create solutions. As a form of action research, this process relies on collective reflections to create organizational change. Community and organization development professionals who implement action research view people within communities and organizations as active agents in the processes of social change.

■ Participatory Research

Participatory research, a particular type of community action research, is an "alternative to research determined by the dominant group and aims to produce knowledge from the perspective of marginalized, deprived, and oppressed groups of people and classes and in so doing aims to transform social realities" through better and more appropriate program planning (de Koning & Martin, 1996, p. 14). Henderson (1995) claimed that participatory research "involves a mutually educative encounter between researcher and researched that generates both data and theory" (p. 62). Additionally, King, Henderson, and Stein (2001) discussed this paradigm shift in research from principle-based reasoning toward a relationship-focused approach that emphasizes "relationships, interactions, power, responsibility, and contextual and historical considerations" in examining particular issues (p. 5). The authors asserted that, "Many researchers—including feminist researchers, new paradigm researchers, and participatory action researchers—include the empowerment of research subjects as an ethical imperative" (King et al., p. 9).

Discussing the World Health Organization's definition of health promotion as the "process of enabling individuals and communities to increase control over the determinants of health," Wallerstein (1992) asserted that participatory action research and planning leads to stronger communities and personal and political efficacy (p. 198). For example, describing women living in a village in India, Joyappa and Martin (1996) offered one example of how participatory research changed a community. Responding to a dowry-related murder of a local woman, the women of the village met, identified the major social and political issues contributing to the death (e.g., lack of access to health care, lack of educational opportunities for women and girls, lack of political power, and acceptance of violence), confronted the patriarchy's opposition, hosted an all-village assembly, opened a high school for girls, and organized free healthcare camps. This incident offers powerful testimony to how social transformation can result from community women's active participation in community development and transformation.

Based on a strong commitment to social justice, participatory research has become increasingly significant in the field of health care (Israel, Schultz, Parker & Becker, 1998). De Koning and Martin (1996) suggested two reasons for this growing popularity. First, the biomedical interpretation of poor health, supported by studies conducted in laboratories, in many cases differs from the understanding embedded in local culture and history. Secondly, many cultural, historical, socioeconomic, and political factors that are difficult to measure have a crucial influence on the outcomes of health interventions. The authors claimed that health professionals "cannot ignore these factors and pretend that the world outside the laboratory is the same as inside" (de Koning & Martin, 1996, p. 1).

The theoretical threads of community health and development, community learning and action research, and participatory research wove into a community-based collaborative action research project in preparation for my dissertation. I turn next to the international organization with which I worked.

■ Project Partnership

Operating primarily in the Middle East, Asia, and Africa, the American Refugee Committee works with local community partners in several countries to provide opportunities and technical assistance to persons displaced by conflict or disaster. After providing postcrisis, emergency relief, ARC helps displaced people and their host communities rebuild healthy and dignified lives and regain secure and self-sufficient livelihoods. Their programs are primarily focused on promoting safe motherhood, preventing violence against women, managing healthcare clinics, and providing work opportunities.

With critical science and participatory research methods in mind, I asked ARC to select a particular site where I could implement a collaborative research approach. ARC subsequently selected a refugee camp located in northern Rwanda where I partnered with local ARC community health workers to plan a community assessment project that opened dialogue with refugee women to learn about their health concerns. The primary goal was to seek contextualized data that could inform the expansion of ARC's health programs for women.

Two primary assumptions guided the planning of the community assessment project to determine my dissertation topic. First, I assumed that political structures often silence women's voices. Therefore, refugee women's health experiences were rarely represented in research or planning activities. Furthermore, contextualized knowledge about women's health experiences was also rare. Most international agencies pursued large-scale, cross-national, generalizable data, which, while important, has limited utility for planning contextualized health programs. I assumed that situated understandings would contribute to practical program planning and therefore, viewed refugee women's perspectives as a valuable source of knowledge.

Second, ARC believes that to be successful in a region, their workers must uncover community-based knowledge that is practical, traditional, and often tacit. Locally-based knowledge is historically-situated, emic knowledge and should include information from socially marginalized groups (Kamata, 2000). Working through local partners and constituencies, ARC uses a participatory approach to assess the type of programs and services local people and communities need to rebuild healthy and productive lives. ARC bases its relationships with displaced and host communities on mutual respect and meaningful exchange of knowledge and values. Additionally,

ARC deliberately incorporates emic and tacit knowledge of the most vulnerable populations into program planning and implementation. ARC's belief in the significance of local knowledge obligated us to incorporate local wisdom into this research and development project.

■ Background on Research Setting

Rwanda is often recognized as the country of one thousand hills. One of those hills is the site of the refugee camp that is located near Rwanda's northern border, approximately one mile from a small town. Operated by the United Nations High Commissioner for Refugees (UNHCR) and the American Refugee Committee (ARC), the refugee camp was established as a result of the civil wars in Rwanda and the Democratic Republic of Congo (DRC). As the most densely populated country in Africa, Rwanda emerged from Belgian colonial rule in 1961 with limited land and many disputes over land rights (Gourevitch, 1998; Kane, 1995). Partly as a result of colonization and postcolonial power disputes, in 1994, Rwanda became the site of the most devastating genocide in world history (Ward, 2002). Rwandan rebel forces killed an estimated 750,000 to 1,000,000 Rwandan Tutsi and Hutu moderates (Ward, 2002). The massive genocide created a million Rwandan refugees who fled into bordering countries. When an aggressive army composed primarily of exiled Tutsis advanced on Kigali and defeated the Hutu rebels, the war concluded. However, fearing retribution, the Hutu rebels fled into surrounding countries, including Rwanda's neighbor to the north, the DRC. Angry and still violent, Rwandan rebels proceeded to create terror among many DRC citizens who, in turn, fled into Rwanda and have settled into refugee camp along the Rwandan border (Ward, 2002).

Refugee camp residents receive assistance from UNHCR and two nongovernmental organizations—staff members of Jesuit Relief Services (JRS) who provide free primary and secondary education, and African staff members of ARC who provide health care. Approximately 11,000–12,000 DRC citizens resided in the camp at the time of this project in

2002–2003. Sporadic fighting along the Rwanda and DRC border continues, with a recent report identifying several warring rebel forces working against UN peacekeepers and the Congolese army (British Broadcasting Company, 2009). According to a report in the *New York Times*, 100,000 Congolese civilians were displaced by fighting when rebel forces executed 150 civilians (Gettleman & MacFarquhar, 2008). As a result, the number of Congolese refugees in Rwanda has increased dramatically and required expansion of one camp and establishment of another camp.

A Snapshot: Sights and Sounds of the Refugee Camp

Green plastic tents that can be seen from the highway into town blanket an entire hill. Camp residents (some seeking temporary work, others carrying items from the village market) move freely between the camp and town. The two dirt roads that enter the camp are very dusty in the dry season, and very muddy and slippery during the rainy season. An occasional delivery truck enters the camp; otherwise all transport is on foot, and refugees are often observed walking along the road to and from town.

Men meet frequently in small gatherings along the road or sit in front of the community center to converse with one another. Occasionally, men repair tented structures that have been damaged by weather or age. Busy with various tasks, women are seen working all day throughout the camp. Women, in addition to carrying babies on their backs, also gather the necessary household supplies such as firewood delivered by UNHCR, food, or the water available in two areas of the camp. Women can also be seen washing laundry at the water areas and hanging clothes to dry along the barbed wire fences that encircle some of the camp sections. Women are also seen tending smoky fires that struggle under small, open, but covered shelters. Children can be seen running and playing throughout the camp. The only toys were balls made from various materials strung together. However, children of all ages delighted in throwing and chasing the homemade balls. Small children wear only shirts; school children wear their school uniforms—blue dresses for girls and tan shirts and shorts for boys. Adolescent girls tend to gather in small groups to talk; adolescent boys are often seen playing various sports on the cemented basketball court.

The living shelters are arranged in uneven rows that are tiered along and encircle the hill. Most of the family shelters are made of plastic sheets spread over wooden structures constructed from tree branches. A few family shelters are more permanent and made from cemented clay. The family shelters (approximately 8 × 10 feet) are very small and close together. Each family shelter houses at least one, and sometimes two, families. Most people spend their days outdoors and seek shelter only during rain or at night. On the fringes of the camp, larger plastic tents are constructed. These tents house several families; new families arrive twice a week and are sheltered in the larger, tented structures for sometimes several months before family shelters become available.

Generally, people talk very quietly. The sounds in the camp are sounds of work—repairs being completed on structures, laundry being cleaned, small meetings occurring, meals being prepared, people gathering in lines when delivery trucks arrive, and children playing on their way to and from the camp school. Because the camp rests on a hill, vehicles that traverse the roads into the camp are always noticed. Vans carrying familiar Rwandans who staff the camp hospital and clinic arrive consistently. Strangers are quickly noted, and polite curiosity is often displayed. The sights and sound of the camp are very consistent; every weekday seems to be similar. People seem to appreciate the predictability of the days but also enjoy the opportunity for a break in the routine that accompanies new projects.

■ Phase 1: Community Assessment Process

Even though ARC headquarters had communicated about the project with their field staff, and the field staff had offered preliminary approval, I still needed to establish relationships inside the camp in order to proceed. The Camp Manager invited me to a meeting with camp political leaders, who included the Camp President, Vice-President, Advisory Council, and section chiefs. During this meeting, we discussed possible ways to assess women's health; their primary advice was to conduct an assessment in all 13 sections of the camp and communicate with section chiefs as the project proceeded. Camp leaders also suggested meetings with the camp physician and nurses as well as the women's leader, social advisor, and headmistress for the camp school. During subsequent meetings with these camp officials, I queried their perspectives on women's health and sought their advice on ways to access information from a wide variety of women. Each official approved the project and provided valuable guidance.

Collaborative Planning

Once the project was approved, I met with 13 Congolese refugee women who were employed by ARC as community health workers. Since I am not fluent in the Kinyarwanda language, I contacted a local translation service and subsequently contracted with Emily, a Rwandan woman who is fluent in English, Kinyarwanda, French, and Swahili, as my interpreter. Having been a refugee herself during the Rwanda genocide in 1994, Emily was particularly sensitive to and interested in refugee women's situations. We stayed on the edge of town near the refugee camp during the project. Emily was present at all meetings with camp officials and community health workers. During our initial meeting with the refugee women who worked as community health workers in the camp, Emily and I learned about their work—the daily routines as well as the challenges and the opportunities. Assigned to different subsections of the camp, health workers' responsibilities included health education and counseling, early detection of illnesses, and community health surveillance. Expressing concern about projects that never seemed to produce results for women, the community health workers were curious about my work and the project's intent. Genuinely sharing information, deliberately seeking honest perspectives, and responsively listening to concerns were essential components of this working partnership. The health workers' willingness to engage in the process was critical to the project's success.

After receiving approval from all stakeholders, the community health workers, Emily, and I considered ways to assess and analyze refugee women's perspectives on their health situations.

After much discussion, we decided that conducting focus groups was most conducive to our intent to reach all camp sections and as many women as possible within our allotted time frame.

Subsequently, the community health workers, Emily, and I met in the refugee camp for a week-long session on the best ways to facilitate focus groups in the Congolese tradition. We exchanged information on the skills of question writing, probing for depth, and encouraging equal participation among focus group members. During our planning sessions, the community health workers wrote 12 focus group questions in Kinyarwanda, which were used consistently by all health workers during all focus groups (see **Box 2-1**). Furthermore, we created an interview template that arranged the questions according to a framework provided by Krueger and Casey (2000). Based on years of experience conducting human science research with focus groups, Krueger and Casey recommended sequencing of questions according to warm-up, transition, key, and summarizing questions. Therefore, the community health workers and I structured their focus group questions accordingly.

Because community health workers identified that probing for depth was difficult for them, we also constructed and practiced probing questions, such as, "Can you tell me more about that?" and, "What do you mean by that?" All questions were written in the Kinyarwanda language for health workers to use as a guide to enhance consistency among all focus group sessions. Topics such as how to handle conflict, how to encourage women to discuss sensitive topics, and how to preserve confidentiality were also emphasized in these working sessions.

Data Collection

Six two-person, health worker teams were established with one person ready to substitute in case of an unforeseen absence. Each team was composed of a facilitator who asked the questions and probed for depth and a note taker who recorded the session in writing. All teams conducted focus group sessions on three separate mornings in each subsection of the refugee camp with a total of 100 refugee women participating. I did not attend any of the focus group sessions since the community health workers thought Emily and I could be a distraction to the focus group process.

Box 2-1   Focus Group Questions

Warm-Up Questions
1. What are your ages and the number of children you have?
2. How is life in this community—for the women who live here?

Transition Questions
3. After getting married, how do you think life changes?
4. What do you think is the difference between delivering your baby in the hospital and delivering your baby in the home?
5. What do you think prevents mothers from bringing their children in for vaccinations?

Key Questions
6. What kinds of problems do you have in your day?
7. What kind of work do you do everyday and how does that affect your health?
8. What kinds of illnesses do you have frequently, and why do you think the illnesses happen?
9. What factors affect women's health in this community?
10. What will you do in the future to take care of your health?
11. What hopes do you have for your future?

Summarizing Question
12. Of all the things we talked about today, what is the most important to you?

Pavlish, C. (2005a). Refugee women's health: Collaborative inquiry with refugee women in Rwanda. *Health Care for Women International, 26,* 880–896.

After compiling but prior to analyzing data, the health workers, Emily, and I examined the characteristics of the focus group participants. All focus group participants were originally from the Democratic Republic of Congo (DRC) where they had been living in small villages. Tending to cows and goats and raising crops to market in nearby cities sustained their livelihoods. The women left the DRC with their families when militant rebels invaded their land and threatened to kill them. UNHCR established a refugee camp close to the DRC border. However, in 1997 families were moved from that site because militants penetrated security and massacred numerous camp residents. Subsequently, refugees were moved to their present location in Rwanda. Most of the women who participated in the focus groups had been living in this refugee camp for at least 5 years. Participants ranged in age from 18–45 years, and all women cared for at least 1–8 children. Some of the women also reported caring for younger siblings and refugee orphans. Many of the women were married, some were widowed, and others had never been married.

Shared Data Analysis

Each afternoon, Emily and I met with the community health workers to systematically review question-by-question the focus group data that had been gathered in morning focus group sessions. Copious notes were taken, and then large English and Kinyarwanda language transect charts were constructed (transecting questions with each focus group's responses) to aid in the visual depiction of all the data. Miles and Huberman (1994) asserted that visually displaying qualitative data in an organized, systematic assembly facilitates analysis, conclusion drawing, and action planning.

All focus group teams reported that women expressed significant interest in their health and the health of their families. Focus group participants said they enjoyed the focus group sessions and appreciated the efforts of the community health workers to listen to participants' perspectives and concerns. Although many political leaders warned us that women were "shy" and might not discuss their concerns, we learned that when offered the opportunity, women were not only very interested in health but also very forthright about their concerns.

Once all the focus groups had been held and all data compiled into transect charts, the community health workers, Emily, and I met to review all data and construct prevalent themes emerging from the transect charts and focus group session notes. The data analysis process was very difficult because our data was cumbersome, we were crossing languages, and the health workers claimed they had never previously examined data for themes. We started by devising themes within each question but quickly abandoned that process when the community health workers stated they could not see themes—only responses. However, health workers asserted they could examine responses and see lessons. Therefore, we constructed conceptual maps with women's health in the center and the lessons we learned from focus group participants surrounding the center. We started with many lessons that we learned affected women's health, and then kept abstracting to larger lessons. Five major lessons emerged at the conclusion of data analysis (see **Table 2-1**). The lessons were interrelated and tightly woven into two major concepts—women's voices and women's struggles (Pavlish, 2005a).

Table 2-1   Refugee Women's Health Concerns

Data themes	Specific health concerns
Health effects of poverty	Being poor leads to forced choices such as selling food to purchase other essentials, prostitution, broken relationships, forced early marriage.
Struggle to survive	Being refugees away from homeland stability and productivity leads to human stagnation, chronic sadness, and dependence on others.
Overburden of daily work	Securing and preparing food and water, finding and carrying wood, caring for children, washing clothes, and managing daily household tasks leads to many physical ailments and psychosocial disruption.
Ambivalence about reproductive decisions	Loving children, distrusting medical birth control methods, feeling social pressure to be mothers, and yet wanting control over reproduction leads to confusion and mental distress. Silence about these issues leads to anxiety and loneliness.
Lack of freedom to express themselves	Expressing loyalty to husbands and yet sometimes constrained and hurt by their relationships leads to sadness, loneliness, physical injuries, and family trouble.

Pavlish, C. (2005a). Refugee women's health: Collaborative inquiry with refugee women in Rwanda. *Health Care for Women International, 26,* 880–896.

■ Phase 1: Community Development Planning

Based on community assessment findings and community health workers' interpretations, the following conclusions about women's health in the refugee camp seemed warranted. First, although reproductive health was a primary concern for participants, women perceived health as broader than the physical health concerns regarding reproduction. Stagnation, mental distress, and gender relationship concerns were reported to have many health effects for women. Therefore, assessment findings offered support for expanding the women's health agenda beyond reproductive health. Planning health programs to address the social, economic, and political contexts for refugee women was initiated.

Second, many of the specific health issues identified by focus group participants pertained to the issues of women's social status and gender relationships mediated within the DRC cultural context. Methods to create social structures that support better health outcomes for women seemed necessary. However, community health workers warned that improving social and cultural conditions to promote and support women's health must emerge from within the refugee community. Oduyoye (2002) asserted that, in Africa, the key to social change is inclusion. ARC reaffirmed its commitment to utilize participatory approaches to analyze social practices that negatively impact women's health. Opportunities to open dialogue about how to create social change were planned.

Third, most health concerns expressed by focus group participants occur in the context of women's daily lives. Therefore, improving the quality of women's daily lives seemed necessary to improve women's health. For example, every focus group reported how poverty affects women's health and daily lives. Participants asserted that poor nutrition, poor living conditions, prostitution, fear, and sadness frequently resulted from poverty. Most focus group participants expressed eagerness for income generation strategies as a means to improve women's health and well-being. By offering women more than just financial gain, income generation projects seemed to also provide the basis for building new lives, creating new social structures, providing supportive networks, and enhancing women's social status.

Expanding refugee women's health agenda, changing social norms, and improving refugee women's daily lives were the primary health and development challenges that resulted from this community assessment project. New community-based health programs designed to address women's concerns were developed in collaboration with both male and female community health workers at the camp. Income generation projects, educational programs, and skills training were developed to improve women's health outcomes. However, before planning participatory workshops to examine social norms on gender roles and relationships, community health workers suggested that we learn more about the gendered experience in daily lives. In addition, advising that women's health experiences are best understood in the context of men's experiences, these female health workers recommended that we interview both refugee men and women. Therefore, I planned a narrative research study for my dissertation to examine refugee women's and men's perspectives of their lives.

■ Phase 2: Dissertation Research—Studying Lives

After collaborating with refugee women to plan and conduct the women's health assessment in Phase I, the dissertation phase seemed very lonely. Emily continued to provide very valuable guidance in working with participants; however, fewer voices in data analysis seemed to restrain the research. Nevertheless, dissertation criteria at that time required independent work, and therefore, planning, conducting, and writing this narrative research was deemed my responsibility. After briefly explaining the study, I describe the manner in which community residents were included in the process.

Narratives contain people's perceptions and, often, their own interpretations of meaning derived from lived realities (Polkinghorne, 1988; Riessman, 1993; Vaz, 1997). Even though subjectivity is often deeply distrusted in many sciences, subjective descriptions are highly valued in narrative research because they are rooted in time, place, and personal experience.

Details about persons' experiences yield certain truths about people's socially-located lives and identities (Lawler, 2002). By studying narratives of refugees' lives, I aimed to develop deeper understandings of the cultural and social context in which women's health experiences occur. This understanding was beneficial to the process of planning context-specific programs to improve women's health and development opportunities.

ARC representatives selected two Congolese community health workers to recruit potential research participants. Using purposeful rather than convenience sampling, I asked recruiters to select potential participants from various categories, such as frequent visitors to the health clinic and marginalized groups in the camp. Emily and I conducted at least two and sometimes three in-depth interviews with 14 refugee women and 15 refugee men.

We first elicited narrative by asking participants to describe memories and anecdotes about significant events and people in their past and present lives, as well as stories about their ordinary days. Given the freedom to choose their own topics and anecdotes, all participants chose primarily to describe their present situations. During follow-up interviews, we explored topics from their first interview in greater depth. In the data analysis phase I worked alone to separate text by gender and conduct systematic, inductive, across-case data analysis. Mapping data such as women's relationships (see **Figure 2-1**) stimu-

Figure 2-1 Web of Women's Relationships in an East African Refugee Camp

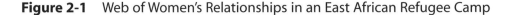
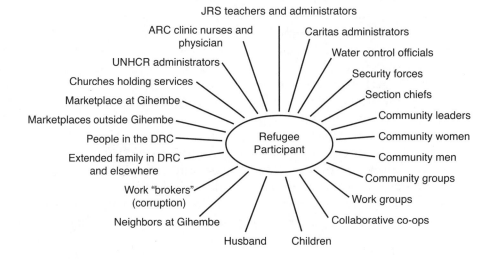

lated analytic questions, which then guided my return to the data for evidence of women's agency and power dynamics (Pavlish, 2005b). Creating matrices such as women's responses to relationship conflicts (see **Table 2-2**) was another useful method for digging more deeply into data. After creating and

Table 2-2 Researcher-Identified Conflicts and Participant Responses

ID#	Conflicts	Responses
1	Neighbor asks for two bowls of rice in return	No choice—give her two bowls back
	Husbands and wives	Women forced to make money to keep husbands
	Women and girls pressured into too much sex	Men go from one woman to next
2	None reported	Live day-by-day-by-day
3	Section chief asks for favors	Not give him anything (respects herself; not have anything to give)
4	Internal conflict–grief vs responsibilities	Anguish, sadness
5	Husband about infidelity, sex, AIDS	Tried to resist, anger
	Community about how they treat her	Sadness
6	Husband took money, abused her	Went to Congo police
	Congo police told her to handle own family problems	Stayed with husband longer, but fearful
7	Husband raped her	Went with him to Congo
	Social pressure on family chief	Works hard but can't always do it
	Social pressure on adolescent girls	Voices concern for adolescent girls
8	Brother-in-law raped her	Confused, seeking guidance and assistance
	Sister—imagined conflict	
9	Male section chief refused to do repairs	Frustrated, persisted in seeking repairs
	Corrupt leaders give jobs to those who pay	Discusses their behavior
10	Section chief about shelter repairs	Persists in asking
11	Internal conflict—ambiguity about husbands	Avoids new marriage because of her observations
12	Husband about infidelity	Confronts him
	Woman asking for husband	Confronts and fights her
13	Corrupt political system	Describes examples
	Healthcare system	Voices concerns
14	UNHCR not offering nutritious food	Wants to run a market
	Rebels took husband, possessions, and land	Very sad

Table 2-3   Prevalent Themes in Refugees' Narratives

Themes in women's narratives	Leaving the good life behind
	Worrying about their daughters
	Feeling ambivalent about marriage
	Lacking hope in the future
Themes in men's narratives	Leaving the good life behind
	Having no peace in the heart
	Fearing the future

Pavlish, C. (2007). Narrative inquiry into life experiences of refugee women and men. *International Nursing Review, 54,* 28–34.

analyzing multiple matrices and figures and identifying major content categories in the gendered text, I sorted content categories into themes within each gender (see **Table 2-3**). Attempting to remain as descriptive as possible, I utilized sections of participants' narratives to verify the themes.

■ Phase 2: Evidence-Based Community Development

Deeper understandings about refugees' daily lives provided ARC with information about gendered experiences. One of the most significant findings was that every woman's story contained a component of gender-based violence. Sexual violence, exploitation, discrimination, intimate partner violence, and forced early marriages were most prevalent. Female participants directly connected violence to their health and described sadness as well as physical harm.

After sharing preliminary data analysis with female and male community health workers at the camp and receiving verification of themes, the community health workers, Emily, and I collaboratively planned participatory exercises to open dialogue with community members about gender relationships, gender-based violence, health, and HIV infection. ARC also initiated mental health counseling and expanded their gender-based violence program to include more prevention methods and enhance the counseling program. In addition, women advocates were established within each camp section.

■ Conclusion

Looking back, I realize that community-based collaborative action research was a learned process, and people who lived in the refugee camp were my teachers. Although not a prospectively-planned path, the process that evolved illuminated a methodology that has guided me in several subsequent projects. For example, because improving women's health in this refugee camp required change in the social norms and structures that impact women, a community-based collaborative action research project on human rights and gender practices was initiated.

Lincoln (1998) described a research paradigm shift from "understanding to action" (p. 18). Describing an urgent need for participatory and action-oriented research, Lincoln cited three emergent reasons:

■ Continuing and widening disparities
■ Increasingly scarce resources
■ Growing awareness that social change is not successful without the active participation of those who are most impacted

Reason and Bradbury (2001) described the primary purpose of participatory action research as producing practical knowledge that increases individual and community well-being. Cultural, historical, socioeconomic, and political factors have a crucial impact on people's health and, while difficult to measure, these factors are an essential component of people's health experiences and thus must be considered in action research processes. The deeper and contextualized understandings that resulted from this community-based collaborative action research project with refugee women provided evidence for changing some camp policies, practices, and programs.

However, in addition to changing context, this phased and collaborative research process transformed me in three significant ways. First, I now believe that community-based, collaborative, and action-oriented inquiry is a strikingly valuable and valid research endeavor. Researching life experiences reveals useful, contextual information for practitioners to apply when working to improve people's lives. Nestled in life experiences are human fears, hopes, regrets, injustices, successes, ideas, innovations, values, plans, resilience, and frailties. When planning change to improve human conditions, researchers and practitioners benefit from deeper understandings about life experiences. Changed lives potentially unfold from studying lives.

Second, I now believe that recognizing human similarities is just as important as respecting differences. Throughout data collection in this research process, I focused primarily on the vast differences between participants and me. Our contexts, daily struggles, opportunities, and historical pasts distanced us. However, as I listened to their narratives, I learned that we also share commonalities. Our shared experiences of motherhood and deep love for our children united us. Our concern for other women connected us. Our commitment to providing good lives for our families joined us. Our joys and pains in struggling with relationships also united us. In our human efforts to understand one another without claiming to be the other, we recognized the similarities as well as the differences.

Third, my perspective about health also shifted. Instead of simply defining health in a holistic manner, I would now expand the definition to describe health as a dynamic and multifactored ecological experience. Health is more than just physical, mental, and spiritual well-being. Health is more than an individual, family, or community experience. Health occurs in the context of the daily experience—in the context of our collectivity, work, gender, environment, culture, relationships, politics, economics, social norms, history, faith, and daily lives. I now believe that health and well-being are about the web—and not just the spiders—which means that we must all accept some responsibility for each other and the conditions in which we live. In addition, as human beings who are unique and yet share some commonalities with all other human beings, we need to care about and accept responsibility for the web, for the type of web we weave together.

■ References

Bhattacharyya, J. (1995). Solidarity and agency: Rethinking community development. *Human Organization, 54,* 60–69.

British Broadcasting Company News. (2009). Rwanda arrests Congo rebel leader. Retrieved from http://news.bbc.co.uk/2/hi/africa/7846339.stm

Brookfield, S. (1993). Self-directed learning, political clarity, and the critical practice of adult education. *Adult Education Quarterly, 43,* 227–242.

De Koning, K., & Martin, M. (1996). Participatory research in health: Setting the context. In K. de Koning, & M. Martin (Eds.), *Participatory research in health: Issues and experiences.* (pp. 1–18). London, UK: Redwood Books.

Freire, P. (1993). *Pedagogy of the oppressed.* New York, NY: Continuum.

Gettleman, J., & MacFarquhar, N. (October 29, 2008). U.N. blocked from pulling workers out of Congo. *New York Times.*

Gibbons, M., Limoges, C., Nowotny, H., Scwartzman, S., Scott, P., & Trow, M. (2000). *New production of knowledge: Dynamics of science and research in contemporary societies.* London, UK: Sage.

Gourevitch, P. (1998). *We wish to inform you that tomorrow we will be killed with our families.* New York, NY: Farrar, Straus and Giroux.

Henderson, D. (1995). Consciousness raising in participatory research: Method and methodology for emancipatory nursing inquiry. *Advances in Nursing Science, 17,* 58–69.

Israel, B., Checkoway, B., Schultz, A., & Zimmerman, M. (1994). Health education and community empowerment: Conceptualizing and measuring perceptions of individual, organizational and community control. *Health Education Quarterly, 21,* 149–170.

Israel, B., Schultz, A., Parker, E., & Becker, A. (1998). Review of community-based research: Assessing partnership approaches to improve public health. *Annual Review for Public Health, 19,* 173–202.

Joyappa, V., & Martin, D. (1996). Exploring alternative research epistemologies for adult education: Participatory research, feminist research, and feminist participatory research. *Adult Education Quarterly, 47,* 1–14.

Kamata, Y. (2000). Indigenous knowledge, cultural empowerment and alternatives. *Contributions to Nepalese Studies, 27,* 51–70.

Kane, H. (1995). *The hour of departure: Forces that create refugees and migrants.* Washington, DC: Worldwatch Institute.

King, N., Henderson, G., & Stein, J. (2001). Relationships in research: A new paradigm. In N. King (Ed.), *Beyond regulations: Ethics in human relationships in research* (pp. 1–17). Chapel Hill, NC: University of North Carolina Press.

Krueger, R., & Casey, M. (2000). *Focus groups: A practical guide for applied research.* Thousand Oaks, CA: Sage.

Lawler, S. (2002). Narrative in social research. In T. May (Ed.), *Qualitative research in action* (pp. 242–258). Thousand Oaks, CA: Sage.

Lincoln, Y. (1998). From understanding to action: New imperatives, new criteria, new methods for interpretive researchers. *Theory and Research in Social Education, 26,* 12–29.

Miles, M., & Huberman, A. (1994). *Qualitative data analysis.* Thousand Oaks, CA: Sage.

Nonaka, I., Konno, N., & Toyama, R. (2001). Emergence of "ba": A conceptual framework for the continuous self-transcending process of knowledge creation. In I. Nonaka, & T. Nishiguchi (Eds.), *Knowledge emergence: Social, technical and evolutionary dimensions of knowledge creation* (pp. 13–29). New York, NY: Oxford.

Oduyoye, M. A. (2002). *Daughters of Anowa: African women and patriarchy.* Maryknoll, NY: Orbis Books.

Pavlish, C. (2005a). Refugee women's health: Collaborative inquiry with refugee women in Rwanda. *Health Care for Women International, 26,* 880–896.

Pavlish, C. (2005b). Action responses of Congolese refugee women. *Journal of Nursing Scholarship, 37,* 10–17.

Pavlish, C. (2007). Narrative inquiry into life experiences of refugee women and men. *International Nursing Review, 54,* 28–34.

Polkinghorne, D. (1988). *Narrative knowing and the human sciences.* Albany, NY: State University of New York Press.

Reason, P., & Bradbury, H. (2001). Inquiry and participation in search of a world worthy of aspiration. In P. Reason, & H. Bradbury (Eds.), *Handbook of action research* (pp. 1–14). Thousand Oaks, CA: Sage.

Riessman, C. K. (1993). *Narrative analysis.* Newbury Park, CA: Sage.

Senge, P., & Scharmer, C. (2006). Community action research: Learning as a community of practitioners, consultants and researchers. In P. Reason, & H. Bradbury (Eds.), *Handbook of action research.* Thousand Oaks, CA: Sage.

Sillitoe, P. (1998). The development of indigenous knowledge: A new applied anthropology. *Current Anthropology, 39,* 223–253.

Vaz, K. M. (1997). Social conformity and social resistance: Women's perspectives on "women's place." In K. M. Vaz (Ed.), *Oral narrative research with black women* (pp. 223–249). Thousand Oaks, CA: Sage.

Wallerstein, N. (1992). Powerlessness, empowerment, and health: Implications for health promotion programs. *American Journal of Health Promotion. 6,* 197–205.

Ward, J. (2002). *If not now, when?: Addressing gender-based violence in refugee, internally displaced, and post-conflict settings.* New York, NY: The Reproductive Health Consortium.

Chapter 3

Theoretical Foundations of CBCAR

Theory provides roots to ground practitioners of a discipline. Although the tree above the roots may bend with winds of changing trends, although it may be grafted with branches from other trees and evolve in a new variety, theory that is nourished by practice is a living and growing entity that provides support for practice while dynamically defining the characteristics and parameters of practice. Falk-Rafael (2005, p. 39)

*F*or organic and dynamic systems to thrive through the winds of change, they must have strong roots. Coursing through the roots of community-based collaborative action research (CBCAR) are interwoven sources of inspiration and guidance from practice-informed theory grounded in: (1) social justice and human rights (Boutain, 2008; Chambers, 2003; De Negri Filho, 2008; Seifer & Gottlieb, 2010; Sen, 2004, 2005; UN Department of Economic and Social Affairs, 2006; Wilkenson & Pickett, 2009; WHO, 2002; Yamin, 2008); (2) the unitary-transformative and participatory paradigms (Cowling, 1999, 2007; Heron & Reason, 1997; Newman, 1994, 2008; Reason 1998; Skolimowski, 1994); and (3) action science (Argyris,

1993; Argyris & Schön, 1978; Fals-Borda & Rahman, 1991; Freire, 1970/2001; Reason & Brandbury, 2001, 2008; Smith, Wilms & Johnson, 1997; Stringer, 2007; Whitehead, 1989, 2009). Combined, these three theoretical root systems provide the DNA that guides the development of CBCAR nursing knowledge to focus on the pattern of the whole, while exploring the meaning of issues from the perspective of the people most affected, so that new possibilities of health and community well-being can be envisioned (Pharris, 2005). Its theoretical roots make CBCAR resilient and strong, enabling it to address health inequities and adapt to any context. The seeds of CBCAR can sprout and thrive across practice settings, country boundaries, and cultures. CBCAR grows in such a way that it is uniquely shaped by the people involved, by local culture, and by sociopolitical history; it is shaped by the entire environment in which it is rooted. An ecological perspective is essential in tending to a healthy CBCAR process.

The CBCAR approach flows from several assumptions (see **Box 3-1**). A foundational assumption is that the world is an undivided whole, in which we are all intimately connected as one. Health is manifest in the patterns of interactions between people and their environments. Nurses' sense of common humanity and professional ethical stance compel them to work for social justice and human rights wherever inequalities exist; this work is an enspiriting relational process. When working with people, nurses understand that individuals and communities have the best insight into their own situations. When nurses enter into partnership with individuals and communities to dialogue about what is meaningful in terms of health, patterns emerge and new insights into action are envisioned. Change is seen as emergent and transformational; it is not predetermined or prescribed.

In this chapter, we present an overview of the theoretical sources that inform CBCAR. Specifically, we will outline pertinent theories articulated by nursing, health, and social science scholars. These theoretical sources serve as the root system of a CBCAR approach to addressing health inequalities and creating healthier communities and systems of health. In this chapter, we do not document the historical development of action and par-

---

Box 3-1 Assumptions of CBCAR

- All living things are part of one unitary participatory whole.
- Change is transformational and unpredictable.
- People and communities have the best insight into their own situations.
- For nurses, social justice is a mandate to identify and address inequalities and threats to human rights, freedoms, and capabilities.
- The purpose of research is to address inequalities and promote human flourishing.
- Nurses enter into partnership with communities to understand patterns of health.
- Pattern reflects the dynamic interaction of people with their environments.
- Pattern recognition organizes meaning.
- Dialogue centered on meaning gives rise to unforeseen learning and action potential.

---

ticipatory research approaches, so as not to repeat information that can be found in previous chapters. Rather, we present a composite of pertinent theoretical thought from various strong voices. It is our hope that you, the reader, will pay attention to what resonates within you as particularly important—this is DNA that will give shape to your work.

■ Theoretical Roots of CBCAR

Social Justice and Assurance of Human Rights

The International Council of Nurses' (2006) *Code of Ethics for Nurses* states that in addition to promoting and restoring health, preventing illness, and alleviating suffering, respect for and protection of human rights is inherent in nursing. Nurses are guided by national and international codes of ethics to be a strong voice at the policy level to assure the health and well-being of the entire population. In addition to nurses' responsibilities to individuals, nurses have obligations to society and the environment. The code states the following:

> The nurse shares with society the responsibility for initiating and supporting action to meet the health and social needs of the public, in particular those of vulnerable populations. The nurse also shares responsibility to sustain and protect the natural environment from depletion, pollution, degradation and destruction. (p. 2)

Nursing, by its very nature and commitment to protection and promotion of health, particularly for the vulnerable[1] places nurses in a position of perpetually responding to the pressing needs before them, yet there is a mandate to take a more ecological approach to assuring the health of the population. In a proactive and socially responsible manner, CBCAR affords nurses the space and relational capacity to engage in meaningful dialogue with the people and communities they serve in order to determine what they need to live healthy, whole lives, and what social structures must be changed so that all humans can flourish on a protected and preserved planet. CBCAR utilizes a wide ecological lens to uncover inequities and the absence of basic human rights and addresses them. This moves nurses away from a solely needs-based stance toward a rights-based stance, and thus more closely aligns nurses with their ethical commitments. Nurses continue to respond to needs, but in the context of a much wider view of solutions that assure and promote human rights and equity.

Advocacy, which has always been a central tenet of nursing, is redefined in the CBCAR process in a manner that is consistent with its explication by several nurse scholars. Calling nurses beyond a paternalistic view of advocacy, Spenceley, Reutter, and Allen (2006) presented the work of Fowler (1989), suggesting that as advocates, nurses protect human rights, preserve values, defend personhood, and champion social justice (p. 181). In order to carry out these mandates, nurses must be educated and qualified in these areas. The ICN code of ethics instructs nurse educators to weave into the curriculum the concepts of "human rights, equity, justice, and solidarity as the basis for access to care" (p. 5). To assure that these conditions are met, nurses will need to engage with others at the social policy level where goals of nursing advocacy can be fulfilled (Spenceley et al., 2006). CBCAR is a vehicle to fulfill this mandate.

In CBCAR, nursing advocacy involves an authentic, engaged presence with others so that the meaning of vulnerability and the context that shapes it can be fully explicated, with patients/communities directing the way to move through the situation at hand. This is consistent with Gadow's (1980) description of advocacy as an authentic interrelationship of nurse and client, present to one another as whole people clarifying what the patient wants to do to move through the given situation. Nursing since its inception in many forms around the world has been shaped by its response to human need in times of infirmity, injury, birth, and death.

Questions about inequalities; obligation to care for those who are suffering, injured, vulnerable, or infirmed; and ownership and distributions of resources have always been part of the human discourse. This discourse has given rise to the concept of social justice. Many people confuse social justice with distributive justice (an equitable distribution of benefits and burdens), commutative/market justice (a fair exchange of money for goods), retributive justice (punishment for problematic actions), restorative or compensatory justice (restoring to people what they lost by being harmed by another) (Grace, 2009, p. 25). Social justice contains aspects of each of these types of justice, yet reaches further to assert the responsibility of each person to be concerned about the common good of all—particularly those who are suffering—and to analyze who benefits and who is harmed by discrimination, oppression, inequalities, and environmental exploitation. As a core value of nursing, social justice mandates that nurses collaborate with others to change systems that undermine the health and well-being of populations (Bekemeier & Butterfield, 2005). In explicating the urgent role of social justice in what nurses do, Drevdahl, Kneipp, Canales, and Dorcy (2001) asked, "What would happen if we treated people in poverty as if they were drowning? As if they were having a myocardial infarction?" (p. 28). The immediacy with which nurses respond to human suffering is a hallmark of the profession. In this sense, social justice is a virtue that makes human flourishing possible (Miller, 2009). Social justice is as much about responsibility as it is about rights. Social justice asks: *What does one generation owe to the next and to the preceding generation* (Miller, 2009)? *What are the reciprocal responsibilities we have to each other? To what extent are we interested in and willing to extend ourselves for the sake of the common good?*

Social justice is the force that keeps a free market economy fair. To that end, the United Nations (UN) Department of Economic and Social Affairs, in its 2006 document *Social Justice in an Open World,* asserted that "power comes with the obligation of service" (p. 8). This UN document, which was written in response to growing inequalities among countries, frames economic justice as an essential aspect of social justice and points to the fact that social justice extends to the environment in the following manner:

> Social justice may be broadly understood as the fair and compassionate distribution of the fruits of economic growth; however, it is necessary to attach some important qualifiers to this statement. Currently, maximizing growth appears to be the primary objective, but it is also essential to ensure that growth is sustainable, that the integrity of the natural environment is respected, that the use of non-renewable resources is rationalized, and that future generations are able to enjoy a beautiful and hospitable earth. The conception of social justice must integrate these dimensions, starting with the right of all human beings to benefit from a safe and pleasant environment; this entails the fair distribution among countries and social groups of the cost of protecting the environment and of developing safe technologies for production and safe products for consumption. (p. 7)

Strong and coherent social and economic policies are the marker of a just nation. With its focus on transformational change, CBCAR can be a vehicle for promoting good governance. On this theme, Seifer and Gottlieb (2010) pointed to the power of community-academic participatory research partnerships to create social justice and transform institutions and the way they operate. These authors stated:

> Creating social justice involves changing inequitable systems, policies, cultures, and values, and fundamentally redefining how we understand community, health, science, knowledge, and evidence. This demands that we challenge and change the assumptions, systems, policies, culture, and values of the everyday organizations in which we work as well as the major institutions that shape and govern us. (p. 1)

Not all nurses can clearly define how social justice, as a core nursing concept, informs their practice or how it shapes their role in society. In a thorough review of social justice in the nursing literature, Doris Boutain (2008) pointed out that nurses often fail to see that a professional mandate to promote social justice involves actively changing institutions and social relationships to promote equity and providing health care as a moral obligation to a citizenry for whom health care is a basic human right (p. 42). Boutain called nurses to a multifocal approach to social justice so that systems of advantage and disadvantage can be brought to light and dismantled. Boutain stated:

> Social justice asserts that vulnerable persons should be protected from harm and promoted to achieve full status in society. The dynamics of being perceived as privileged or vulnerable would require exploration. Particularly relevant would be an investigation of how nurses themselves are influenced by privilege as they espouse their role as social justice advocates. One question becomes focal: can nurses really promote a social justice agenda when that promotion will result in the critique and dismantlement of their own advantage?
>
> Social justice critique means, for example, that one must recognize the social factors that construe persons as privileged and/or vulnerable at different points in time. A social justice agenda necessitates transforming systems that promote subordination or disadvantage in the long term and the immediate conditions that limit self-actualization in the short term. (p. 45)

To this end, Boutain pointed to the work of Iris Marion Young (1990) who describes oppression as having five faces: exploitation, marginalization, powerlessness, cultural imperialism, and violence. Describing the experience of powerlessness, Young explained the oppressive impact of *professionalism*—with its authority, sense of self, and status—all of which the powerless are lacking. Professionalism upholds mental work over manual work, being self-directive over being told what to do, and being middle class over working class—implying a different way of dressing, acting, and eating, as well as living in a different place and manner. Of course, "race"[2] and gender mediate how professionalism is experienced and received (Young, 1990). Professionals—nurses certainly included—are generally well meaning, with a desire *to help* others. When *service* is provided in a system of distributive justice (versus social justice), the service is often provided to someone who is already marginalized, and the person providing the service (the privileged professional) remains in a position of power, which further adds to the powerlessness of the person in need (Boutain, 2008). Professionalism upholds class structure and places a divide between working and middle class people. Analyzing the flow of money, it is easy to see that it is professionals and their communities who benefit economically from such exchanges.[3] Money flows from the marginalized to those already privileged. Social justice for nurses involves persistent self-reflection to ponder whether we are working from a position of privilege or a stance of solidarity, and repeatedly asking the questions: *Who is benefiting here and how?* and *What can I alter in my practice to better ameliorate the inequalities I am uncovering?*

Boutain (2008) built on the work of Holland (1983) to provide a framework for embodying a social justice practice. This framework helps nurses understand and counter the antecedents, processes, and outcomes of injustice with a three-pronged approach consisting of social justice awareness, amelioration, and transformation. The first, social awareness, entails exploring our mental conceptions of others as vulnerable or privileged, as well as exploring which systems of oppression and domination create and perpetuate these categorizations in the culture and in our minds. Boutain encouraged nurses to do self-interviews and to talk with and get to know people in each category to fully understand their experiences. She also recommends literature searches, taking in media sources, and reading books to become more aware of the historical origins of vulnerability and privilege, as well as the social structures that perpetuate them. The second, amelioration, involves taking action to ease suffering and to respond to immediate needs. The third, transformation, is aimed at the policy level. Transformation seeks to change unjust social structures that foster inequalities (Boutain, 2008). When nurses partner with people and communities experiencing inequalities in a CBCAR process, transformation is the result of the research partnership.

Nussbaum (2000) also offered fertile thought for research and development with vulnerable populations. Focusing on human dignity, Nussbaum's capabilities approach offers a feminist political philosophy that underscores the importance of viewing all human beings as ends rather than as means toward ends. Nussbaum's philosophical perspective arose from work with many women living in poverty around the world, primarily in India, and therefore, offers researchers a context that is global in nature. Focusing on life qualities, social progress, and human capabilities (such as being able to live to an old age, enjoying bodily integrity, having control over one's environment), Nussbaum created a thought-filled perspective that expands the responsibility of research beyond measurement toward construction of social norms that allow even the most vulnerable community members to realize their capabilities and flourish. Amartya Sen (2005), while hesitating to embrace a universal list of human capabilities, pointed out that the capabilities framework promotes public reasoning through "transparent valuational scrutiny of individual advantage and adversity" (p. 157). The very dialogue about the freedom or capability to meet one's nutritional needs, to be well sheltered, to move about, or to receive adequate health care provokes an analysis of social position, personal ability, and the extent to which local public policy promotes human capabilities.

Human capabilities are more likely to flourish in societies where human rights are clearly defined and protected within the community context. Human rights are generally categorized into first and second generation rights (Nickel, 2007; Pavlish & Ho, 2009a; Sen, 2004; UN, 1948, 1966). First generation human rights are aimed at the legislative level, directing governments to assure that they and their citizens refrain from actions that would violate human dignity and security, and that they assure certain freedoms such as freedom of speech and freedom of religion. Second generation human rights are aimed at social and economic well-being through the assurance of access to education, an adequate standard of living, and health care. Human rights are correlated with good governance (Pavlish & Ho, 2009a) and impeded by weak governments and economic structures (Pavlish & Ho, 2009b). It is not just governments, however, that have the power to promote human rights.

In their work with displaced people in Southern Sudan, Pavlish and Ho (2009b) found human rights to be promoted by community cohesion, responsibility, connectedness, and economic opportunity (p. 290). They cited An-Na'im and Hammond (2002) to point out that human rights values of justice and individual dignity predated the arrival of Europeans to the continent of Africa and that the assurance of human rights needs to be reconceptualized as "a common struggle for social justice and resistance to oppression" (An-Na'im & Hammond, 2002, p. 19). The work of Pavlish and Ho called for proactive engagement of nurses with people and populations to address the oppressive social structures behind human rights violations. A human rights approach is enhanced by community engagement; it also strengthens community engagement (London, 2007). When people in communities investigate and analyze the social determinants of diseases and injuries and engage in social discourse on the ethical aspects of health as a human right, they lay the groundwork for restructuring social policy and action to ensure equity in quality of life (De Negri Fihlo, 2008; London, 2008). Meaningful protection of human rights goes far beyond enacting international and national legal declarations to involve relational engagement with people who are marginalized and/or impoverished, with the end result of changing social structures and thus promoting human flourishing, social justice, and community within the local context. In this manner, CBCAR is driven by human rights theory.

Amartya Sen (2004) proposed that while many people embrace the general concept of human rights, they often exclude economic and social rights, such as entitlement to subsistence and health care, from the list of protected human rights. Sen frames human rights as not just "legal commands," but more importantly as "ethical demands" that propel action by those who are in the position to secure the underlying freedoms that shape human rights; he asserted that a theory of human rights must be freed from the confines of the "juridical model in which it is frequently incarcerated" (p. 319). Sen promotes an interactive process of unobstructed dialogue across boundaries to more fully understand differing points of view of human rights. Through such a dialogue, each person gains insight into effective actions. Every person has an obligation to give reasonable consideration to actions that assure the freedoms and capabilities of others (2004). We must begin by taking people's suffering seriously and in so doing, our approaches to health and human rights are transformed (Yamin, 2008).

Dr. Paul Farmer (2008), medical anthropologist and founder of Partners in Health, called people concerned about health and human rights into a "virtuous social cycle" involving pragmatic solidarity with poor and marginalized people to redress and reverse the historic flow of resources from poor communities to wealthy ones. The transfer of resources includes not only natural resources of the land, but also human labor, payment for *professional* services, acceptance of government subsidized aid and aid workers, and interest payments on loans—in all of these instances, money goes from those who have little to those who have much. Farmer (2004) gave these conditions the label of *structural violence* and calls for justice at the structural level. Basic social and economic rights become a possibility for people who are suffering when academics move from studies that only describe health inequalities to praxis (reflection and action) that addresses health inequalities in partnership with those who are suffering.

Efforts to identify human rights violations and address health inequalities are best directed by those who are experiencing the violations and inequalities. This involves nurses being present, being in relationship, and listening attentively. Pavlish and Ho (2009c) demonstrated the importance of attending to definitions of human rights that arise from engaged listening to the perspective of those most in need of human rights protection. Drawing on the work of Musimbi Kanyoro's African perspective of feminist hermeneutics (meaning making), they wrote: "Possessing a voice, but not being heard represents 'choked silence' and advances marginalization, which exponentially contributes to vulnerability" (2009c, p. 154). Similarly, Farmer (2008) challenged the concept of the "voiceless poor" pointing out that the poor have a voice and are able to use it—the question is one of proximity to and action with those who are able to hear and have the resources to make a difference. Farmer stated, "The best science (that is, the knowledge that most effectively meets essential needs related to the health of human populations) springs from and is guided by an activist commitment to work with disadvantaged communities in realizing their economic and social rights" (p. 13). While the 1948 United Nations Universal Declaration of Human Right was unquestionably the most important move in the last century for promoting global human rights activities, there has not been widespread legalization or institutional enforcement of these rights. Much is left to be done in the realm of monitoring, public recognition, activism, and social construction to advance human rights, freedoms, and capabilities (Sen, 2004). CBCAR holds the potential to effectively address these issues.

The Nature of Change

Change arises spontaneously on the horizon when dialogue opens the space for new meanings and insights. CBCAR draws on Gadamer's theory of the fusion of horizons. The horizon refers to the "range of vision that includes everything that can be seen from a particular vantage point" (Gadamer, 1965/1988, p. 269). Gadamer asserted that through dialogue, researchers and community members expand and fuse horizons and "part from one another as changed beings. The individual perspectives with which they entered upon the discussion have been transformed, and so they are transformed themselves" (Gadamer, 1979/1981, p. 110).

Dialogue focused on meaning is central to the theory of Newman (1979, 1994, 1999, 2008), who built on the theoretical work of quantum physicists, David Bohm (1980) and Ilya Prigogine (1976), to see health as a constantly evolving pattern of interactions with the environment. The role of the researcher is to partner with people and/or communities to identify what is meaningful in terms of health, and attend to recognizing and understanding the unfolding patterns of interaction with the environment. The major intent is not to come in and fix a problem with outside knowledge. There is no value judgment in this theoretical perspective; everything is understood in the context of environmental and interpersonal interactions and the meanings they hold. As the meaning of patterns in the lives of individuals, families, organizations, and/or communities is recognized, the road to optimal health and well-being becomes visible. Through this evolving process, existing social realities are critiqued and new ones are created. Inequalities are addressed in a meaningful way. Change in which health flourishes comes from within; it is not inflicted from the outside. It is a co-participatory rather than an interventionist process. Newman's theory has been applied and tested across a wide array of practice settings in various countries (Endo, Miyahara, Suzuki, & Ohmasa, 2005; Jónsdóttir, 1998; Litchfield, 1999; Pharris 2002; Picard & Jones, 2005; Yang, Xiong, Vang, & Pharris, 2009). These studies from various country settings have shown that change is only fully seen and comprehended in retrospect—it is not predetermined or prescribed. Transformations in health and well-being are a result of the process of recognizing pattern and meaning. A new vision for practice is constructed in the process.

■ What You See Depends Upon Where You Stand

Emancipatory Knowing

Nurses throughout the world are intimately involved in theory development to improve practice and promote human flourishing (Salas, 2005). In 1960 Chinn and Kramer assumed the scientific view of truth in their first book on theory development. Mentors challenged them to realize that traditional science left out essential aspects of nursing practice; yet, they observed that nurse scholars who did the kind of work that produces empirical results in controlled studies were more highly esteemed. When they encountered Barbara Carper's (1978) work at the same time that they were studying feminist theory, their world shifted and they came to embrace the four patterns of knowing in nursing proposed by Carper (ethical, aesthetic, personal, and empirical). Jill White's (1995) addition of the sociopolitical pattern was widely accepted, yet Carper and Chinn viewed the sociopolitical as part of the aesthetic pattern of knowing—a deep way of knowing the context. In writing the seventh edition of *Integrated Theory and Knowledge Development in Nursing*, Chinn and Kramer (2008) felt they needed to explicate how patterns of knowing address social change and social justice. Since Carper deduced her four patterns of knowing from a philosophical analysis of the literature of the time, and since the social submissiveness of nurses was still predominant in society, even though social activism was also present in the 1970s, concepts of social activism or social justice did not appear in nursing publications. For this reason, Carper's review of the literature yielded no writings on social activism even though it was a core value of nursing at the time (Chinn, 2008).

Chinn and Kramer (2008) proposed an additional pattern of knowing—emancipatory knowing—which provides a lens that turns a skeptical eye towards all we know and all that we do. Emancipatory knowing constantly raises new challenges and questions to bring about new, broader, and deeper insight. Emancipatory knowing focuses on provocation rather than prescription. It sees injustice and strives to achieve the good of society. "This kind of knowing seeks freedom from institutional and institutionalized social and political contexts that sustain that which is unjust—that perpetuate advantage for some and disadvantage for others" (2008, p. 5). Emancipatory knowing can see wrongs and figure out a way to achieve good. Emancipatory knowing asks four questions:

1. What are the barriers to freedom?
2. What is wrong with this picture?
3. Who benefits?
4. Who is invisible? (Chinn & Kramer, 2008)

Ecological Perspective

Like emancipatory knowing, the ecological model challenges researchers to look at relationships within a broader sociological context. The ecological model is context driven, looking always from the center, where the problem resides, out to the concentric realities that surround it. Sources of health problems and their solutions are conceptualized within a series of concentric circles with the individual in the middle, then the interpersonal, organizational, community, society, and supranational (Kok, Gottlieb, Commers, & Smerecnik, 2008). However, looking at five or six concentric circles does not translate the interactions *between* those levels—the borders between areas are where the most friction is. Within the inquiry of CBCAR, the focus on the whole identifies the varying concentric aspects, which are viewed as a holarchy.[4] More importantly, CBCAR examines the margins between what had previously been seen as distinct and unrelated entities. Groups of people representing various aspects of the community begin to realize that they are responsible for the well-being of the entire community. They come to recognize the space they share, and rather than negotiating relationships and the distribution of goods, rights, and resources across those boundaries covertly, it becomes an overt, transparent process. In CBCAR, negotiations of *who* has a right to *what* are brought to the forefront. The dynamics underlying the distribution of resources become transparent, which is rarely the case for marginalized communities, who must often take the back door approach and hope for the best. Once people realize on a deep level that we are all one ecological system and have responsibility for each other, conversations about who is benefiting and who is suffering, and why, lead to a transparent process of renegotiating how resources will be allocated and in what ways relationships need to be rewoven and transformed.

■ A Unitary Participatory Grasp of the Whole

Views from Nursing and Action Science

The participatory paradigm, or worldview, acknowledges that phenomena are not particulate, and thus cannot be objectively and precisely measured and described as truth. Rather, all knowledge involves our own subjective understanding and participation in constructing a representation of the phenomena we encounter. Heron and Reason (1997) gave the example of encountering the hand of another person with our own hands. As we feel the person's hand, we are also experiencing the reciprocal interaction between the person's hand and our hands. Our intentionality impacts what we experience, as does the other person's receptivity and experience, only part of which we might perceive and be able to represent when we describe the encounter. Objective reality is always shaped by the knower. We are intricately interwoven into the universe we explore (Skolimowski, 1994). Knowledge develops through action, from our experience of the world in which we live. Self-reflexive attention is necessary to develop a critical conscious awareness of the subjective ground on which one is standing and the presuppositions one holds. When we move from critical subjectivity to critical intersubjectivity through dialogue and engagement with others, we come to know the phenomenon under study much more fully (Heron & Reason, 1997).

Action research is seen by Reason and Bradbury (2001) as a verb rather than a noun, and defined as, "a participatory, democratic process concerned with developing practical knowing in the pursuit of worthwhile human purposes, grounded in a participatory worldview" (p. 1). Reason and Bradbury stated that at this moment in history there is a need for a new paradigm, a new way of thinking, a new way of being in the world. They pointed to the fact that as a world community we are heading toward "ecological devastation, human and social fragmentation, and spiritual impoverishment" (p. 4). The purely positivist paradigm is no longer enough; a new worldview is desperately needed (Reason & Bradbury, 2001). To that end, Reason and Bradbury (2001) drew on the work of Lazlo to describe the world as "a whispering pond, a seamless whole in which the parts are constantly in touch with each other. Wherever scientists look and whatever they look at, they see nature acting and evolving not as a collection of independent parts, but as an integrated, interacting, self-consistent, and self-creative whole" (p. 7).

When we think of a unitary participatory universe, we realize that we are part of the evolutionary unfolding of life—

we are not standing outside of the process, but rather are actively engaged in it. We stand at the side of every other living being—not above or below. It makes sense that research informed by this way of looking at reality actively engages us as participants in the emerging process and that we could not prescribe or predict with any degree of certainty what is going to happen. In this research, we remain open to unforeseen possibilities.

Philosopher Henryk Skolimowski (1994) invited us to think of a time in the evolution of life on earth when there was no eye, which is difficult to imagine for those of us who have sight, as we are accustomed to interacting with our world using our eyes to take in visual cues and to appreciate the visual beauty around us. Skolimowski pointed out that since "the first amoebas started to articulate themselves from the original sea of the organic soup," they began "to react to the environment in a deliberate and semiconscious manner" (p. 15) and developed more sophisticated senses to interact with the world. There was an augmentation of consciousness as organisms reacted with the environment in ever more purposeful and knowing ways. Skolimowski queried that if the eye was one of the latent possibilities in evolution, then

> [i]s it reasonable to assume that evolution has exhausted the stock of its possibilities? Or is it more reasonable to suppose that other forms of seeing are in store for us and, if they become part of our natural capacities, we shall be able to reveal through them new aspects of reality? If this happens, then part of the magical will become part of the natural. Perhaps this is the way we should look at evolution—as transposing that which is in the realm of magic into the realm of the natural. Evolution is the unfolding of natural magic.
>
> With new sensitivities we articulate the world in new ways; we elicit new aspects from the world. The power of sensitivities is the power of co-creation. No aspect of reality imposes itself on us with an irresistible force; we take it in and assimilate it only when we acquire a way of seizing and comprehending it; when we come to possess an appropriate sensitivity that is able to process it for us. (p. 14)

In his book *On Dialogue,* physicist David Bohm (1996) presented a different view of participatory thought. Bohm documents how early human cultures felt that with their thoughts they were in some way participating with what they saw—that while they saw many, many seals, they viewed them as a manifestation of one seal—with one spirit manifesting as many. Cultures that abundantly used participatory thought most likely also used literal thought for practical activities, but the things that mattered deeply involved participatory thought. People were deeply aware of their oneness with each other and with all living things. A particulate view of reality is a more recent and Western way of thinking. Perhaps the closest many people can get to understanding participatory thought is the feeling of oneness and meaningful connectedness after a disaster . . . the way a family pulls together after the sudden death of a loved one, each member intimately feeling the others' unspoken pain . . . the thoughtful connectedness with and between the people of Haiti after the 2010 earthquake . . . the people affected by the December 26, 2004 Indian Ocean earthquake and tsunami . . . the people of the US on September 11, 2001.

As a global community, we are coming to an understanding that we need to find a more sustainable and meaningful way of living on this planet. People in affluent societies are reaching their limit of material consumption—at times drowning in stuff—having to make great efforts to eat less, while over a billion people in the world do not have sufficient food to meet minimal daily requirements. A participatory mind reconnects us as a human family; it connects us with the Earth.

A process is needed to uncover the connection between knowledge and the power to act. Reason and Bradbury (2001) called for a "pedagogy of the privileged" (matching Freire's pedagogy of the oppressed) to engage those who are in positions of power—those who are members of privileged groups. Chinn (2008) stressed that as nurses we are committed to relieving suffering and pain through mutually transformative practice. She critiqued the prescriptive approach to practice that asserts that *we* have the answer and *we* know what is good for others. In participatory practice we are not experts of truth, but rather facilitators creating spaces where others can speak and act on their own behalf. We need to create the space for those we care about to find their own solutions. We must move toward a fruitful sense of dislocation from the center and find ways to constantly challenge and place our own voices in the background so that the previously marginalized voices can move to the center and be heard (2008).

Sorrell (2003) stressed the importance of people from dominant cultures listening in the "thin place" or the place where the natural and sacred worlds merge and where seen and unseen realities share common ground. She cautioned against "benumbment" (para. 7), which is the failure to slow down and create the open space for intimate listening to the suffering of others. Rather, Sorrell (2003) asserted, we must work to hear, understand, and honor the entirety of the experience of marginalized people. It is in this open listening that potential for transformation and action arise. In a call to move from a benumbed material level to an enlivened spirit level, Wilkinson and Pickett (2009) graphically documented the ill effects of inequalities within a country, not only on the poor, but also on the affluent. Generally speaking, people in societies where there is little inequality experience less depression, anxiety, and other psychosocial problems than the affluent in high-inequality countries. As a global community, we are approaching the limit of what economic growth can do for us (2009). It is time for transformation.

Transformative Paradigm

Donna Mertens (2009) proposed a transformative paradigm for research and evaluation that embodies social justice. The axiology (ethical stance) of this paradigm involves respect for cultural norms of interaction and defines beneficence as the promotion of human rights and increase in social justice. The ontology (assumptions about the nature of reality) of Mertens' transformative paradigm rejects cultural relativism and "recognizes the influence of privilege in determining what is real and the consequences of accepting one version of reality over another; multiple realities are shaped by social, political, cultural, economic, ethnic, gender, disability, and other values" (p. 49). The epistemology (assumptions about the nature of knowledge and the relationship of the knower to what is known) recognizes the interactive link between the researcher and participants and sees knowledge as historically and socially situated. It specifically addresses issues of privilege and power. Development of trust is seen as critical. Finally the methodology of Mertens' transformative paradigm includes qualitative methods that are dialogical. Merten's methodology also allows for the use of quantitative and mixed methods. The focus and questions are identified interactively between the researcher and participants. "Methods are adjusted to accommodate cultural complexity; and contextual and historical factors are acknowledged, especially as they relate to discrimination and oppression" (p. 49). Mertens described the characteristics of the transformative paradigm as follows:

- Places central importance on the lives and experiences of communities that are pushed to society's margins
- Analyzes asymmetric power relationships
- Links results of social inquiry to action
- Uses transformative theory to develop program theory and inquiry approach (p. 48)

Mertens' (2009) transformative paradigm has methodological and relational similarities with the unitary-transformative paradigm proposed by Newman, Sime, and Corcoran-Perry in 1991; however, they differ in intent and judgment. In the unitary-transformative paradigm, attention is on recognizing patterns of health and engaging in dialogue about their meaning. The notion and meaning of power differentials and privilege are a construction of the dialogue. Researchers do not enter relationships or situations with any predetermined judgments. Through dialogue, new ways of viewing the world and new insights into action arise. In the unitary-transformative paradigm, the nature of reality is seen as one indivisible whole (unitary), and change is seen as unpredictable and unidirectional, always moving toward a higher level of complexity (transformative). Wholeness is inherent in all living things (Newman, Sime, & Corcoran-Perry, 1991).

The unitary-transformative paradigm includes all theoretical perspectives. Newman (2003) stressed the importance of acknowledging barriers posed by institutional structures and the ideological boundaries arising from globalization, as well as the connectedness of emerging nursing theories. She drew attention to the "boundaries imposed on nursing knowledge by conferences, organizations, and books that separate and isolate nurse theorists of one persuasion from nurse theorists of another, and also, that separate theorists and researchers from practitioners" (2003, p. 241). Newman (2002) described the evolution of nursing theories as a holarchical (rather than hierarchical) progression moving "from emphasis on *physical* care to *interpersonal* process to an *integrative* approach to a *unitary* perspective" with each succeeding level transcending and including the previous ones. In a holarchy, which is a central concept in the unitary-transformative paradigm, each realm is at once whole and yet part of a larger whole. Philosopher Ken Wilber described the evolution of theory in general as moving "from *matter* to *body* to *mind* to *spirit* with each subsequent realm of knowledge transcending and including the realm that preceded it" (Newman, 2002, p. 3).

Newman (2003) suggested that to get rid of the boundaries that keep us from living in wholeness and health, nurses must: (1) stand in the center of their own truth—letting go of externally imposed values so that their own inner voice can emerge, allowing nurses to fulfill their purpose in society; (2) let go of rights and wrongs, a process that enables nurses to be in relationship with others who hold values contrary to their own and thus, support their action potential; and, (3) create a vision of a caring community from which transformation can occur. Newman reminded nurses that transformation often occurs during times of great chaos and disequilibrium—they should not shy away from these circumstances, as it is here where new possibilities break forth (2003). In order to see the evolving pattern of chaos to order, the pattern of the whole must be appreciated over time.

In the process of inquiry, research partners draw on research procedures that provide the widest possible view of the issue at hand—most usually qualitative and emergent. The unitary-transformative perspective involves a process of widening our lenses further and further to see the larger context, the more encompassing whole. With this wide view, we are able to see the interconnectedness—the oneness—of all. We can also see how the pattern evolves over time. Yet, in this unitary participatory mindset, we are not distant, but rather are intimately present. We are able to deeply feel the suffering of others and are moved to address the inequalities, the nature of which becomes more visible as we look at the interconnections of the whole. In order to grasp a view of the whole—understanding the phenomenon under study within the broadest possible context—it is helpful to use data collection strategies that are whole rather than particulate. Broad, open-ended qualitative inquiry is generally the best way to grasp the pattern of the whole. An example of a CBCAR project that used whole methods of inquiry can be found in **Box 3-2**.

Box 3-2 One Community's Experience with CBCAR—
Seeking to View the Whole

Yang and colleagues (2009) provide an example in a CBCAR project that was a follow-up action step of the research presented in Chapter 1. Women in this follow-up action expressed concern about the rapidly rising rate of diabetes in the Hmong community. Physicians in the partnership expressed the view that the women were "noncompliant"—the physicians did not know how to assist their Hmong-American patients. The CBCAR partners (a university–community health center advisory council collaborative) made the decision that in order to see the pattern of the whole, rather than use surveys or questionnaires related to diabetes management, they would attempt to interview Hmong-American women with "uncontrolled diabetes" (HgbA1c levels significantly above 7), asking only one question to capture their life stories as a whole. In individual interviews, Hmong-speaking nurse researchers asked the women to describe the meaningful events in their lives, creating pictorial scrolls of the evolving patterns in each woman's life and going back week after week until the women could say, "Yes, this is everything that is meaningful in my life." The nurse researchers and women attended to the insights that arose during the pattern recognition process. There was a similar pattern for all of the women. They described an active life back in the highlands of Laos, where they frequently broke a sweat as they carried children and large bags of rice and other foods up and down hills. Fresh fruits and vegetables grew all around them, and they were nurtured by a highly interactive and engaged community, which included their extended families. They lived in harmony and close connection with the land. In sharp contrast, the women described their current lives in the United States, where they live inside impermeable homes and are alone all day while their children work. They struggle to speak and understand the language; they are alone and isolated, afraid to go outside. Their children drive them in cars to buy food that is wrapped in plastic; it is not fresh. The nature of their physical, spiritual, and emotional energy intake and energy releases has drastically changed in both quality and quantity. Their life histories included a great deal of trauma, stress, depression, and loss, which seemed to fluctuate with their blood sugar levels. When the women's life stories were compared and contrasted, a clear pattern was seen. The women knew the conventional wisdom related to diet, exercise, and medication to control their diabetes, but this was not enough. Attention needed to be paid to sources of stress and depression and the physical and emotional constraints on their lives. It was only in keeping their stories whole, in looking at the narrative of what was meaningful in their lives and how it unfolded, that a meaningful pattern of the community emerged.

Once the identifiers were stripped from the women's stories, the data analysis team recruited additional Hmong women from the community to help with data presentation for community validation and revision. A Hmong playwright was recruited to weave the distinct stories into a play that would express the common experiences while protecting individual identity. Several other Hmong community members joined the data presentation team to plan a community presentation of the play (performed by two Hmong nursing students) for the larger community of Hmong women with diabetes to see if the findings rang true for them, and if not, what needed to be changed to better reflect their experience. To engage the wider community in the pattern recognition process, the nurse researchers went on Hmong radio and used other sources to invite Hmong American women with diabetes to a dinner where they presented a play based on the interviewed women's stories. After watching the play, the women were asked to reflect on how the play would need to be rewritten to better reflect their lives and what needs to happen in the community so that they can lead healthy and happy lives. Hmong nursing students facilitated dialogue at each of the circular tables. The women in attendance at the dinner wept as they watched the play, asking "Daughters, how did you *know our story?*" During the dialogue, the women clearly expressed what they needed in order to live healthy lives. This process revealed several action steps—insights that might not have arisen had the CBCAR process involved only asking the women about what they did to *manage* their diabetes. Needed change was most visible through capturing the pattern of the whole of the women's lives and engaging the community in a dialogue about the meaning of the pattern of the whole.

Theory guides the nature of research partnerships, the types of research methods used, and how data are presented and disseminated. Findings and methods arise from the CBCAR process; they are not predetermined. CBCAR generates whole representations of living realities. Most theories presented in refereed journals are propositional theories that present clearly defined concepts and the predictive relationships between them. They are general, yet have the precision to explain behavior and make predictions that could apply across many settings (Whitehead, 2009). Whitehead (1989, 2009) used the idea of *living theories* to distinguish the explanations of action research from the general explanations of propositional theory. Rather than using conceptual abstractions of relations between propositions to explain individuals' actions, in living theory "*individuals generate their own explanations* of their educational influences in their own learning. The explanatory principles in living theory explanations are energy-flowing values embodied and expressed in practice" (Whitehead, 2009, p. 87). Action research clarifies and develops values that give meaning and purpose to our lives. Living theories integrate insights from dialectical and propositional theories while retaining "the distinguishing uniqueness of the particular constellation of values, understandings and contextual influences in the life and research of the individual action researcher" (p. 96). Graduate students working with Whitehead create living theses, which often have embedded artwork and links to streaming video that add life to the written text and bridge the gulf between theory and practice (http://www.actionresearch.net).

Calling nurses into a unitary participatory mode of working for social justice, Chinn (Cowling & Chinn, 2001) proposed a "feminist unitary-transformative stance toward injustice." In this stance, nurses would not prescribe what should happen or what people should do, but rather, they would "articulate, and then live, an attitude, one that comes from seeing all of us as part of a political/cultural pattern that addresses the other not as other but as a kindred spirit that seeks to make peace, that is grounded in values of human health and wholeness" (p. 363).

Cowling has proposed that liberation is the goal of the unitary participatory thinker (Cowling & Chinn, 2001). Because the unitary participatory paradigm is relational and ecological, it necessarily permeates organizational and political structures (Cowling, 2007). As the meaning of power dynamics deepens, reorganization ensues. Cowling (2007) stated:

> The political dimension of participatory wholeness asserts the primacy of people's right and ability to be involved in generating knowledge about them that is not fragmenting, alienating, and restricting in the manifestation of their human existence and experience. The notion of participatory, wholeness extends to groups and communities as well as individuals, implying the need to include muted voices and respect the richness and infiniteness of human patterning. From this perspective flows the potential for the fullest exercise of the power of people to produce their own knowledge that serves their purposes. (p. 68)

Reconciling Wholeness: Rising Above Dichotomies

Cowling (1999) advocated that within the unitary-transformative worldview, nurses must attend to transcending the dichotomies of action and theory, sense and soul, stories and numbers, aesthetics and empirics. When nurses break free from the constraints of these dichotomies, what were formerly seen as opposing forces are now seen as two aspects providing rich insight into the pattern of an undivided whole. Influenced by the work of Martha Rogers (1970), Newman (1979, 1986, 1994, 2008) conceptualized health, not as the opposite of illness, but as encompassing both; one can be terminally ill and yet experience health and wholeness. Communities can experience poor physical health outcomes and still flourish in human connectedness, relationship to the land, and spiritual well-being. This wider, contextual view allows nurses to see the whole of people's experiences and to envision a wider repertoire of possible actions for moving forward. Nurses are thus freed from oppositional thinking, which provokes a war-like response to eradicate the undesirable state, often seen as pathology, enemy, or oppressor. Seeing, rather, what is before us as the evolving pattern of people in interaction with their environments, we are able to melt boundaries and the conflicts they represent. Newman (2003) quoted Wilber, who stated, "Each boundary we construct in our experience results in a limitation of our consciousness—a fragmentation, a conflict, a battle" (pp. 240–241).

An example of this was the CBCAR study described in Chapter 1 where women in the community with the poorest official health indicators in the state answered a question about what health meant to them. They defined health as being connected with loved ones and rooted spiritually. With their new collective definition of health, they realized that they were likely the healthiest, not the least healthy community in the state. There was a transformation of self-view, potential, and community pride.

In the unitary-transformative paradigm, "things that we usually consider irreconcilable—the opposites—are like the crest and trough of a single wave; reality is not just in the crest or trough alone, but in the unity of one inseparable activity. Dividing lines (not boundaries) join and unite as well as divide and distinguish. Like light and dark, one cannot exist without the other" (Newman, 2003, p. 241). Ultimate reality is the union of opposites and once we can see reality as such, we are able to embrace all experience equally and unconditionally, openly and lovingly. There is no success without failure, no pleasure without pain, no joy without sorrow, or ugliness without beauty—all opposites are reconciled. Different theories are applicable under different circumstances and at different times. The overarching concern of nurses, whether it be in research, education, or practice, is to help the people, organizations, and communities they work with let go of the artificial boundaries imposed on their lives and to get in touch with a wider, fuller possibility of health in their lives (2003).

Newman (2002) suggested that research in the unitary-transformative perspective shifts from observation of "the other" to "we" knowledge, which implies a mutual collaboration of everyone involved in the inquiry process. Participatory research is a requisite of the unitary-transformative paradigm in which nursing knowledge is developed, because it acknowledges the need for nurses to recognize that they are situated within the pattern as it is unfolding, as opposed to trying to recognize it from an objective stance (Cowling, 2007; Newman,

1997). Participatory research involves an equal partnership between nurses and the people affected by the situation for which knowledge development is sought. Jónsdóttir, Litchfield, and Pharris (2003, 2004) described nursing partnership as being focused on dialogue with individuals, families, and/or communities in a nondirective, caring, and open manner. Relationships are mutually responsive and focus on that which is of concern to the patient (be it family, individual, or community). The direction of the partnership unfolds within the dialogue, which is focused on the meaning of the patient's experiences. Insights gained reveal more useful ways of comprehending and taking action on the health predicament (Jónsdóttir et al., 2003, 2004). Partnership in participatory research is more in line with the philosophical approach of nursing than research that generates a nurse "expert" who *applies* knowledge to patients (Reed, 2008). There are many sources of inspiration for knowledge development within the participatory paradigm—they come from within the discipline of nursing and from various other disciplines. We look to those that complement yet stretch nursing's way of being in the world.

Extending standard scientific epistemology, Heron and Reason (1997) asserted that "living" knowledge consists of participative realities and critical subjectivities regarding four interdependent ways of knowing: experiential, presentational, propositional, and practical. *Experiential* knowing involves face-to-face encounters in which we feel and image the presence of a living being, place, process, or thing. It involves our inner resonance with what we are experiencing and the way in which we perceive and image it. *Presentational* knowing springs forth from experiential knowing and involves the creation and presentation of an aesthetic representation of the meaning of that which we have experienced. *Propositional* knowing is exemplified by the creation of conceptual terms and verbal or written descriptions of what we have experienced and its meaning. Finally, *practical* knowing puts into practice our conceptual understanding of an experience, as demonstrated by skills and competencies (Heron & Reason, 1997). We learn more profoundly about the world in which we live by moving beyond simply articulating knowledge to actively participating in the development of knowledge that enhances the world and all that is in it (Heron, 1996; Heron & Reason, 1997). Similarly, Chinn and Kramer (2008) advocated for a knowledge that is generated within the situation in which it will be applied, and stress that procedures for generating knowledge should not strip away the context that is relevant to nurses and the people affected by the situation at hand.

Adding to the call for nurses to use participatory methods for knowledge development, Reed (2008) proposed that knowledge is produced in context and is seen as partial, interpretive, and always under construction. Theorizers must seek the indigenous knowledge of those intimately involved in the situation being examined. Just as people engaged in liberation struggles need to adapt their strategies to the local culture and climate, so too nursing researchers who are interested in developing knowledge to improve a situation need to be constantly aware of what is unfolding around them and adapt their methods, interactions, and perspectives as they go. This requires a great deal of attentive awareness and dialogue rooted in critical reflection on what the focus of nursing is.

Litchfield and Jónsdóttir (2008) see the knowledge of the discipline of nursing as personal and participatory, evolving through the everyday, moment-to-moment practice of nurses. They proposed that within a participatory paradigm, the focus of nursing practice is the humanness of the health circumstance. Nurses attend to human accounts of what it is like to live with a certain disease or be in a certain predicament. Each human experience is unique due to the history and character of the people involved and the context within which they live. Litchfield and Jónsdóttir pointed out that the views of knowledge from past eras have obscured the humanness in the way people live their lives—the nature of people's experiences, spirituality, sentience (capacity for perceiving, feeling, consciousness), and mystery have not wholly arisen in the measures of previous research methodologies. They stated that a participatory view "does not negate previous ways of thinking, nor even transcends them. Everything just looks different" (p. 85).

When people join together in participatory research and work collaboratively on problems and reflect on their history, they are able to imagine new worlds they can inhabit (Herda, 1999). Herda stated:

> When we are able to reinterpret our past and fuse our hori-
> zons with other cultures and traditions, then we may be ca-
> pable of projecting in a concrete and persuasive manner
> our interest in freedom. It is obvious that simply or solely
> reinterpreting one's past does not erase the oppressive con-
> ditions of many, or does it establish justice in our societies
> and organizations. The process of refiguring the future is
> as critically important. (p. 10)

Within the unitary-transformative participatory paradigm,
the purpose of research is to promote human flourishing, where
flourishing is "construed as an enabling balance within and between people of hierarchy, cooperation, and autonomy" (Heron
& Reason, 1997, p. 287). A participatory worldview "allows us
to join with fellow humans in collaborative forms of inquiry. It
places us back in relation with the living world . . . to be in relation means that we live with the rest of creation as *relatives*,
with all the rights and obligations that implies" (Heron &
Reason, 1997, pp. 175–176). The participatory worldview
places the response to human problems in a wider spiritual context, thus enhancing the resacrilization or reenchantment of the
world (Cowling, 2007; Reason & Bradbury, 2001).

■ Summary—CBCAR: An Emergent Approach on the Scientific Landscape

As depicted in **Figure 3-1**, the CBCAR approach becomes a
bridge between theory and action. A view of the world as a unitary whole, change as unpredictable and transformative, and
research as participatory guides the methods that will be used
in this research approach. Wholeness, connectedness, and pattern are central. Nurses who use the CBCAR approach concen-
trate on developing partnerships. Dialogue informs and
strengthens CBCAR partnerships, which are nondirective,
open, caring, mutually fulfilling, and focused on identifying
community pattern and its meaning. Social justice and human
rights are ethical rudders of the CBCAR process. CBCAR is action oriented; participatory dialogue on the meaning of patterns

Figure 3-1 The CBCAR Approach Bridges Theory and Methods

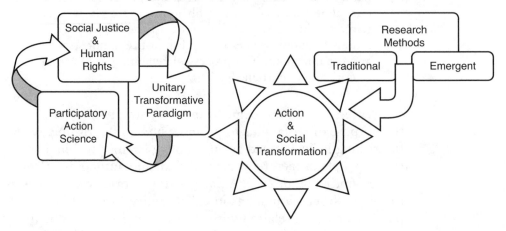

revealed through traditional and emergent research methods give birth to social transformation that reduces inequalities and promotes human flourishing.

CBCAR provides a framework that can be modified and improved upon to fit local sociopolitical, cultural, and historical contexts and give meaning to the transformative work of nurses in partnership with patients, health systems, and communities. It provides guidance without prescription.

We invite you, the reader, to analyze the roots that give life to your work. Do they run deep? What is encoded in their DNA? Will your tree grow strong? What kind of fruits would you like it to bear? This is a time to think about what gives meaning to your work, to your life. What issues are you most passionate about? What do you see as the greatest need to be addressed? There is a well-known quote of theologian Frederick Buechner (1973) in which he describes vocation as "the place where your deep gladness and the world's deep hunger meet" (p. 95). Where is that place for you? If you are not already engaged in a community or professional partnership, who might you partner with to do this work? Think about these questions before you move on to Chapter 4.

We would like to close with a quote from two leading action research scholars, Peter Reason and Hilary Bradbury (2001, p. 2):

Theories which contribute to human emancipation, to the flourishing of community, which help us reflect on our place within the ecology of the planet and contemplate our spiritual purposes, can lead us to different ways of being together, as well as providing important guidance and inspiration for practice.

■ Endnotes

1. Vulnerability reflects the relationship between people/ populations and their environment. Vulnerability can be countered by social policies and practices that are just. For example, a poor person with diabetes and hypertension may be extremely vulnerable in a poor country without a public healthcare system, but not vulnerable in a wealthy country with a strong social support system that assures an adequate income and health care for all. An emergency department nurse is vulnerable to violence and infection, yet structural and organizational changes could reduce the chance of harm. People's freedoms, well-being, and capabilities are shaped to a great extent by the social structures impacting their lives.

2. When the term "race" is used, we place it in quotation marks to indicate that there is no such biological reality. "Race" is a social construct.

3. It is important to realize that many nurses all over the world are not being paid a living wage for the important work that they do. An example is when one of us was giving a keynote speech in Latin America and during the question and answer period a nurse from a rural hospital pointed out that she had not been paid for 4 months because the hospital "ran out of money." Yet, she went to work every day. We also recall sitting together in Durban, South Africa at the International Council of Nurses' 24th Quadrennial Congress during a presentation by nurses from Malawi and Botswana who are part of the Caring for Caregivers network in African countries, where there is a high rate of HIV/AIDS. In this project nurses use their own time and resources to raise chickens and small animals, make and sell food, or plant gardens to

support a system of care for their sister and brother nurses affected by and/or infected with HIV/AIDS. Like the Norwegian Nurses Association, which supports this work, nursing organizations in affluent countries can partner with nursing organizations around the world that are doing extraordinary work in the face of great suffering and inequality.

4. A holarchy is differentiated from a hierarchy in that it does not consist of separate parts that are rank ordered, but rather, it consists of unique aspects that find greater meaning in interaction with the whole. A person in a hierarchy would be in competition with the person above, below, and at the same rank. A person in a holarchy is appreciated for her or his unique contributions, which become greater in interaction with others, thus the entire holarchy grows and improves.

■ References

An-Na'im, A. & Hammond, J. (2002). Cultural transformation and human rights in African societies. In A. An-Na'im (Ed.), *Cultural transformaiton and human rights in Africa* (pp. 13–37). New York, NY: Zed.

Argyris, C. (1993) *Knowledge for action.* San Francisco, CA: Jossey-Bass.

Argyris, C., & Schön, D. A. (1973). *Organizational learning: A theory of action perspective.* Reading, MA: Addison-Wesley.

Bekemeier, B., & Butterfield, P. (2005). Unreconciled inconsistencies: A critical review of the concept of social justice in 3 national nursing documents. *Advances in Nursing Science, 28*(2), 152–162.

Bohm, D. (1980). *Wholeness and the implicate order.* London, UK: Routledge & Kegan Paul.

Bohm, D. (1996). *On dialogue.* London, UK: Routledge.

Boutain, D. M. (2008). Social justice in nursing: A review of the literature. In M. de Chesnay & B. A. Anderson (Eds.), *Caring for the vulnerable: Perspectives in nursing theory, practice, and research* (2nd ed., pp. 39–52). Sudbury, MA: Jones and Bartlett.

Buechner, F. (1973). *Wishful thinking: A theological ABC.* New York, NY: Harper & Row.

Carper, B. A. (1978). Fundamental patterns of knowing in nursing. *Advances in Nursing Science, 1,* 13–23.

Chambers, R. (2003). *Whose reality counts? Putting the first last.* London, UK: ITDG.

Chinn, P. L. (2008). *Scholarship for the good.* Keynote address at the Combined 12th International Philosophy of Nursing Conference and 15th New England Nursing Knowledge Conference, Boston.

Chinn, P. L., & Kramer, M. K. (2008). *Integrated theory and knowledge development in nursing,* (7th ed.). St. Louis, MO: Mosby, Inc.

Cowling, W. R. (1999). A unitary-transformative nursing science: Potentials for transcending dichotomies. *Nursing Science Quarterly, 12*(2), 132–137.

Cowling, W. R. (2007). A unitary participatory vision of nursing knowledge. *Advances in Nursing Science, 30*(1), 61–70.

Cowling, W. R., & Chinn, P. L. (2001). Conversations across paradigms: Unitary-transformative and critical feminist. *Scholarly Inquiry for Nursing Practice, 15*(4), 347–365.

De Negri Filho, A. (2008). A human rights approach to quality of life and health: Applications to public health programming. *Health and human rights 10*(1), 93–101.

Drevdahl, D., Kneipp, S. M., Canales, M. K., & Dorcy, K. S. (2001). Reinvesting in social justice: A capital idea for public health nursing? *Advances in Nursing Science, 24*(2), 19–31.

Endo, E., Miyahara, T., Suzuki, S., & Ohmasa, T. (2005). Partnering of researcher and practicing nurses for transformative nursing. *Nursing Science Quarterly, 18*(2), 138–145.

Falk Rafael, A. R. (2005). Advancing nursing theory through theory-guided practice: the emergence of a critical caring perspective. *Advances in Nursing Science, 28*(1), 38–49.

Fals–Borda, O., & Rahman, M. A. (1991). *Action knowledge: Breaking the monopoly with participatory action-research.* New York, NY: Apex Press.

Farmer, P. (2004). *Pathologies of power: Health, human rights, and the new war against the poor.* Berkeley, CA: University of California Press.

Farmer, P. (2008). Challenging orthodoxies: The road ahead for health and human rights. *Health and Human Rights, 10*(1), 5–19.

Freire, P. (1970/2001). *Pedagogy of the oppressed* (30th Anniversary Edition). New York, NY: Continuum Publishing Company.

Fowler, D. M. (1989). Social advocacy: Ethical issues in critical care. *Heart and Lung, 18*(1), 97–99.

Gadamer, H. (1965/1988). *Truth and method.* New York, NY: Crossroad Publishing Company.

Gadamer, H. (F. G. Lawrence, Trans.). (1979/1981). *Reason in the age of science.* Cambridge, MA: Massachusetts Institute of Technology.

Gadow, S. (1980). Existential advocacy: Philosophical foundation of nursing. In S. F. Springer & S. S. Gadow (Eds.), *Nursing: Images and ideals* (pp. 79–101). New York, NY: Springer.

Grace, P. J. (2009). *Nursing ethics and professional responsibility in advanced practice*. Sudbury, MA: Jones and Bartlett.

Herda, E. A. (1999). *Research conversations and narrative: A critical hermeneutic orientation in participatory inquiry*. Westport, CT: Praeger.

Heron, J., & Reason, P. (1997). A participatory inquiry paradigm. *Qualitative Inquiry, 3*(3), 274–294.

Holland, J. (1983). *Social analysis: Linking faith and justice*. Maryknoll, NY: Orbis Books.

International Council of Nurses. (2006). *The ICN code of ethics for nurses*. Geneva: Author.

Jónsdóttir, H. (1998). Life patterns of people with chronic obstructive pulmonary disease: Isolation and being closed in. *Nursing Science Quarterly, 11*(4), 160–166.

Jónsdóttir, H., Litchfield, M., & Pharris, M. D. (2003). Partnership in practice. *Research and Theory for Nursing Practice, 17*(3), 1–9.

Jónsdóttir, H., Litchfield, M., & Pharris, M. D. (2004). The relational core of nursing practice. *Journal of Advanced Nursing, 47*(3), 241–250.

Kok, G., Gottlieb, N. G., Commers, M., & Smerecnik, C. (2008). The ecological approach in health promotion programs: A decade later. *American Journal of Health Promotion, 22*(6), 437–442.

Litchfield, M. (1999). Practice wisdom. *Advances in Nursing Science, 22*(2), 62–73.

Litchfield, M., & Jónsdóttir, H. A practice discipline that is here and now. *Advances in nursing science, 31*(1), 79–91.

London, L. (2007). Issues of equity are also issues of rights: Lessons from South Africa. *BMC Public Health, 7*, 1–10. doi: 10.1186/1471-2458-7-14

London, L. (2008). What is a human rights-based approach to health and does it matter? *Health and Human Rights, 10*(1), 65–80.

Mertens, D. M. (2009). *Transformative research and evaluation*. New York, NY: The Guildford Press.

Miller, A. (2009). The many faces of social justice. In N. Heitzig, S. Doherty & R. Connors (Eds.), *Global search for justice reader* (pp. 3–18). St. Paul, MN: St. Catherine University.

Newman, M. A. (1979). *Theory development in nursing*. Philadelphia, PA: F. A. Davis.

Newman, M. A. (1986). *Health as expanding consciousness*. St. Louis, MO: Mosby, Inc.

Newman, M. A. (1990). Newman's theory of health as praxis. *Nursing Science Quarterly, 3,* 37–41.

Newman, M. A. (1994). *Health as expanding consciousness* (2nd ed.). Sudbury, MA: Jones & Bartlett.

Newman, M. A. (1997). Experiencing the whole. *Advances in Nursing Science, 20*(1), 34–39.

Newman, M. A. (1999). The rhythm of relating in a paradigm of wholeness. *Image: Journal of Nursing Scholarship, 31*(3), 227–230.

Newman, M. A. (2002). The pattern that connects. *Advances in Nursing Science, 24*(3), 1–7.

Newman, M. A. (2003). A world with no boundaries. *Advances in Nursing Science, 26*(4), 240–245.

Newman, M. A. (2008). *Transforming presence: The difference nursing makes.* Philadelphia, PA: F. A. Davis.

Newman, M. A., Sime, A. M., & Corcoran-Perry, S. A. (1991). The focus of the discipline of nursing. *Advances in Nursing Science, 14*(1), 1–6.

Nickel, J. W. (2007). *Making sense of human rights.* Malden, MA: Blackwell.

Nussbaum, M. (2000). *Women and human development: The capabilities approach.* Cambridge, MA: Cambridge University Press.

Pavlish, C., & Ho, A. (2009a). Displaced persons' perceptions of human rights in Southern Sudan. *International Nursing Review, 56*(4), 416–425.

Pavlish, C., & Ho. A. (2009b). Human rights barriers for displaced persons in Southern Sudan. *Journal of Nursing Scholarship, 41*(3), 284–292.

Pavlish, C., & Ho, A. (2009c). Pathway to social justice: Research on human rights and gender-based violence in a Rwandan refugee camp. *Advances in Nursing Science 32*(2), 144–157.

Pharris, M. D. (2002). Coming to know ourselves as community through a nursing partnership with adolescents convicted of murder. *Advances in Nursing Science, 24*(3), 21–42.

Pharris, M. D. (2005). Engaging with communities in a pattern recognition process. In C. Picard & D. Jones (Eds.), *Giving voice to what we know: Margaret Newman's theory of health as expanding consciousness in research, theory, and practice* (Chapter 8, pp. 83–94). Sudbury, MA: Jones and Bartlett.

Picard, C., & Jones, D. (Eds.). (2005). *Giving voice to what we know: Margaret Newman's theory of health as expanding consciousness in research, theory, and practice.* Sudbury, MA: Jones and Bartlett.

Prigogine, I. (1976). Order through fluctuation: Self-organization and social system. In E. Jantsch & C. H. Waddington (Eds.), *Evolution and consciousness* (pp. 93–133). Reading, MA: Addison–Wesley.

Reason, P. (1998). Three approaches to participatory inquiry. In N. Denzin, & Y. Lincoln (Eds.), *Strategies of qualitative inquiry.* Thousand Oaks, CA: Sage.

Reason, P., & Bradbury, H. (2001). Introduction: Inquiry and participation in search of a world worthy of human aspiration. In P. Reason & H. Bradbury (Eds.), *Handbook of action research: Participative inquiry & practice.* London, UK: Sage.

Reason, P., & Bradbury, H. (2008). Introduction. In P. Reason & H. Bradbury (Eds.), *The SAGE Handbook of action research: Participative inquiry & practice* (2nd ed.). London, UK: Sage.

Reed, P. G. (2008). Practitioner as theorist: A reprise. *Nursing Science Quarterly, 2*(4), 315–321.

Rogers, M. E. (1970). *An introduction to the theoretical nature of nursing.* Philadelphia, PA: F. A. Davis.

Salas, A. S. (2005). Toward a North-South dialogue: Revisiting nursing theory (from the South). *Advances in Nursing Science, 28*(1), 17–24.

Seifer, S. D., & Gottlieb, B. (2010). Transformation through partnerships. *Progress in Community Health Partnerships: Research, Education, and Action, 4*(1), 1–3.

Sen, A. (2004). Elements of a theory of human rights. *Philosophy & Public Affairs, 32*(4), 315–356.

Sen, A. (2005). Human rights and capabilities. *Journal of human development, 6*(2), 151–166.

Skolimowski, H. (1994). *The participatory mind. A new theory of knowledge and of the universe.* London, UK: Penguin Books.

Smith, S., Wilms, D., & Johnson, N. (1997). *Nurtured by knowledge: Learning to do participatory action-research.* New York, NY: The Apex Press.

Sorrell, J. (2003). The ethics of diversity: A call for intimate listening in thin places. *Online Journal of Issues in Nursing.* Retrieved from http://www.nursingworld.org/ojin/ethicol/ethics_13.htm

Spenceley, S. M., Reutter, L., & Allen, M. N. (2006). The road less traveled: Nursing advocacy at the policy level. *Policy, Politics, & Nursing Practice, 7*(3), 180–194.

Stringer, E. T. (2007). *Action research* (3rd ed.). Los Angeles, CA: Sage.

United Nations (1948) *Universal declaration of human rights.* Retrieved from http://www.un.org/overview/rights.html

United Nations (1966) *International covenant on civil and political rights*. Retrieved from http://www.ohchr.org/englis/law/ccpr.htm

United Nations Department of Economic and Social Affairs. (2006). *Social justice in an open world: The role of the United Nations.* New York, NY: United Nations.

White, J. (1995). Patterns of knowing: Review, critique, and update. *Advances in Nursing Science, 17*(4), 73–86.

Whitehead, J. (1989). Creating a living educational theory from questions of the kind, "How do I improve my practice?" *Cambridge Journal of Education, 19*(1), 49–52.

Whitehead, J. (2009). Generating living theory and understanding in action research studies. *Action Research, 7*(1), 85–99.

Wilkinson, R., & Pickett, K. (2009). *The spirit level: Why more equal societies almost always do better.* London, UK: Allen Lane.

World Health Organization (WHO). (2002). *25 questions and answers on health & human rights.* Geneva, Switzerland: Author.

Yamin, A. E. (2008). Will we take suffering seriously? Reflections on what applying a human rights framework to health means and why we should care. *Health and Human Rights, 10*(1), 45–63.

Yang, A., Xiong, D., Vang, E., & Pharris, M. D. (2009). Hmong American women with diabetes. *Journal of Nursing Scholarship, 41*(2), 139–148.

Young, I. M. (1990). Five faces of oppression. In I. M. Young, *Justice and the politics of difference* (pp. 39–65). Princeton, NJ: Princeton University Press.

Chapter 4

Partnering and Planning the Research Process

A friend of ours loved walking in the woods by her home. She lived in the inner city, yet was close to an expansive stretch of woods surrounding two lakes. As the path wound through the west end of one of the lakes, there was a mystical transformation in the environment; that portion of the woods was full of black poplar trees that gently swayed with the wind. Our friend loved the way the leaves rustled with the wind, like a gentle, peaceful wind chime that soothed the soul. Every time we walked through that section of the woods, she expressed her opinion that to have the sound of rustling poplar leaves outside your bedroom window would make for the most peaceful night's sleep. For her 50th birthday, several friends bought a black poplar tree for her to plant outside her bedroom window—it was received as "the best gift *ever*!" Excitedly, our friend ran for a shovel, dug a big hole, and gleefully plopped the tree right beneath her bedroom window, where there was just the appropriate mix of sunlight for a black poplar tree. Unfortunately, our friend gave no thought to preparing the soil to create the best possible environment for the roots to take hold so the tree could receive needed nourishment, and within a year, the little black poplar tree was nothing more than a lifeless stick protruding from the ground. And so it is with community-based collaborative action research (CBCAR); you need to carefully plan your project so that its roots will take hold, and it will grow strong and bear fruit. The best CBCAR projects are thoughtfully planned and diligently researched, with ample time allotted to developing appropriate relationships within the environment and careful tending to that which sustains project growth.

■ Surfacing Concerns and Imagining Hopes

A CBCAR project may arise out of an already existing organizational partnership, or it may arise as one person's idea, such as a university student, or from the work of a small group of people, such as a practice group, who seek partners to explore how to address a barrier to health and well-being or how to transform a system to improve service. The essential element of this research approach is a partnership between people in a community (where barriers to health and/or well-being are a concern) and research scholars, usually from academic institutions, departments of health, or nongovernmental organizations (NGOs). When we use the term "community" in this book, we are referring to any grouping of people, not just to people in a common geographical area. Community could be an interdisciplinary care team; people living and working in a refugee camp; a community health center board of directors, staff, and patients; a small town; or the staff of an inpatient unit. Community is where people are connected, whether by common purpose or by location. CBCAR begins to take root when a concern is expressed, a hope is articulated, and people come together.

■ Gathering, Dialoguing, Forming the Collaboration

When a concern arises, the first task is to carefully consider who should be invited to help shape the CBCAR process that will explore solutions to the concern. For an already existing collaborative, the question is one of expanding the partnerships to address the particular topic of concern. For others, this stage involves pulling together a collaborative that will eventually become a community advisory group for the proposed project, and possibly for an ongoing collaborative partnership aimed at improving health and well-being.

The first step is to consider who is most centrally affected by the issue at hand. We refer to this group as the critical reference group (Genet, 2009). The next step is to think about who within this group is at the margins and therefore is not being heard. The organizing leaders stretch their reach and best attention toward that margin. For example, for a person or collaborative concerned about industrial exposure to undocumented workers, the first step is to create a safe environment to come together with people who are undocumented to explore the issue from their perspective and to identify how their voices could safely be a part of the project. Attention at this phase is on the following:

- Listening attentively to more fully understand the issue from the perspective of the people most at risk
- Entering into a trusting relationship
- Discerning what sort of collaboration will be of most benefit in addressing this concern

Establishing a trustworthy relationship and process takes great care and time and involves many personal meetings. **Box 4-1** outlines a set of guidelines for relationships in CBCAR.

Issues of who can and who cannot be visible might arise and necessitate inviting other concerned individuals and organizations into the collaborative to best address the issue at hand. In the above example involving undocumented workers with hazardous industrial exposures, someone from the State Department of Health's Occupational Health Division, local policy makers, and representatives from local foundations might be good partners to invite into the collaborative partnership. Through hearing the stories of the workers and through the relational processes of CBCAR, they will be educated and moved to take action.

Box 4-1 Guidelines for Relationships in CBCAR

Relationships in CBCAR are:

1. Mindful of each person's human dignity and uphold their pride
2. Equal, not hierarchical
3. Caringly honest, tactful, and sensitive
4. Able to respectfully stay with conflict, knowing it has something to teach
5. Eager and able to address inequalities, assumptions, and biases
6. Cooperative, not competitive
7. Loving and joyful

In some situations, the critical reference group may not be able to fully voice their own concerns. For example, if the critical reference group is people with advanced Alzheimer's disease, it will be essential to invite caregivers and family members of people with Alzheimer's into the partnership. Deciding who will be invited in as partners needs to be carefully considered. It helps to make a visual diagram—perhaps a large sheet of butcher paper on a wall to map out all of the people and groups of people—formal and informal—who have a stake in the issue, along with the interconnections among them. This will provide a visual representation of the current pattern of connections in the community (from the perspective of the organizers). If the organizers focus on the people with the most lines drawn to them and invite only these people to an initial meeting, chances are that they will have a group of people who are overly busy and who are unlikely to imagine new possibilities beyond where the community is already at with the issue. When pulling together the collaborative, it is important to consider the following questions: Who is affected to the greatest extent? Who might have a unique and valuable insight? Who else might be concerned about this topic? Who has the power to make structural changes to improve this situation? How can a relationship be woven together with the people who have been identified?

Who is the best person to initiate the contact? A snowballing process is used to form relationships with possible collaborators. One person is identified, and that person is asked if she or he knows of someone else who might be interested in the project or knows of other people who would be interested, who are affected by the issue, or who might have a different perspective on the issue (Stringer, 2007). This organizational effort is like preparing the ground to plant a tree. The groundwork is essential; it takes research, time, and substantial, persistent, and sustained effort.

This is the time to intentionally and conscientiously move from *I*, to *we*. It is always tempting to simply complete the tasks at hand on one's own, sometimes in the name of responsibility, often in the interest of *just getting the task done*. CBCAR is a collaborative effort; its transformative power arises from the central collective that moves together through all major decisions. It is the responsibility of the original organizing leader(s) to "build and establish collaborative relationships through mutual understanding of expectations, clear communication, empathy and continual dialogue" (Chiu, 2006, p. 192). Being strongly knit together from the very beginning is essential. The more diverse the threads of the collaborative, the richer and stronger it will be, but diverse threads must be carefully gathered; they rarely present themselves together.

To ensure that all necessary voices are at the table, it helps to redraw the pattern of all the people and organizations that are centrally and peripherally involved in the issue, using concentric circles, with those who are most affected by the issue in the center of the diagram. Attention is paid to forming a collaborative where all of the voices can be heard, which means consideration must be paid to whose presence would silence the voices at the center. CBCAR strives for full inclusion of the most marginalized voices and protection from ill effects (see Chapter 8 by Dr. Anita Ho for an in-depth analysis of this ethical issue). All attempts must be made to honor and protect the safety of the vulnerable while doing the hard work of clearing the road for their story and wisdom to make its way to the minds, hearts, and paradigmatic views of the people with the power to change the structures that impact and impinge on vulnerable lives.

To assure that there is equity of voice, Wright, Roche, Von Unger, Block, and Gardner (2010) recommended that community-based collaborations strive for "co-learning and reciprocal transfer of expertise by all partners," "shared decision-making power," and "mutual ownership of the processes and products of the research enterprise" (p. 116). To reach this co-responsible stance requires reflection on which principles and values will guide the research partnership. Focusing on the ethics of community-based participatory research, Schaffer (2009) analyzed how virtue ethics might apply to the work of university researchers and came to the following conclusions:

> The virtues of compassion and humility foster inclusiveness and integration of community perspectives in research collaboration. Courage requires researchers to step out of the research safety-net to listen to community member voices and wisdom and share power in research decisions. Honesty requires researchers to communicate realistic expectations for research outcomes, share all findings with the community, and consider community perspectives in research dissemination. Systematic involvement of the community in all steps of the research process represents the virtue of practical reasoning. From a justice perspective, [community-based participatory research] aims to restore communities rather than take from them. (p. 83)

In CBCAR, findings are co-discovered within the partnership and dissemination is determined collaboratively. CBCAR also entails dialogue to uncover and declare co-responsibility of each partner to the other(s). In the initial phases of a project, it is important to talk about what ethical principles, values, and commitments guide the work. This is an ongoing topic of dialogue, which is revisited as new members join CBCAR teams—it may actually even guide who is sought out to join CBCAR efforts. In the initial phase of the organizing process, it is important to determine what other groups or interests should be represented at the table.

In the long run, it is helpful to invite into the collaborative policy makers and leaders of organizations that can make a difference; that is, if they are willing to adopt a nondirective stance and allow more vulnerable voices to assume center stage. For example, in a study involving patients from a community clinic who were struggling with health problems exacerbated by poverty and social stresses, the medical director of the clinic participated on the community advisory group. As a member of this group, he helped to formulate the research question; he was also a member of one of the data analysis teams. The medical director consciously reflected on his role in the group and the fact that whatever he knew from years of medical school and practice was not sufficient to address the issue in the community he served. He also reflected on the potential power differential between himself and patients and community members in the group. He had a certain type of insider knowledge (medical), and they had a different type of insider knowledge (lived experience and knowledge of the community context). All those involved might subconsciously act out of the cultural norm of deferring to the knowledge of "the doctor." The medical director made a concerted effort to be a listener; he reined in his natural tendency to offer a medical opinion, making a special effort to first think about whether it was necessary to the group process. He found a more authentic way of being present to the group and gained great knowledge and insight into the lives of his patients and how best to care for them. He came to understand the trajectory of the disease process and the forces that most strongly impact it in a whole new light. The learning was definitely mutual—a two-way street. The CBCAR process is transformational for all involved.

When deciding who to invite into the partnership, it is important to consider the effect new partners might have on the strength of each partner's voice and to create a process by which everyone is heard, particularly the critical reference group—those who are most impacted by the issue of concern. Additionally, inviting in policy makers and representatives from larger organizations provides a more overarching view of the community and may help steer the group to potential funding streams.

Being inclusive at the very beginning of the partnership is essential, as is "being open and honest, being able to listen well, and being able to directly address and speak frankly about contentious but important issues, such as power differentials, racism, and financial decisions" (Seifer, 2006, p. 993). When all partners are able to reveal their interests and motivations for working on the project, fuller understandings ensue. People work best together when they know each other's stories. To reach this deep level of sharing, the original organizers attend mostly to the process of creating a healthy environment for dialogue, trusting that the people present will be able to unearth the needed direction for the project.

Beginning each meeting with an inspirational reflection, perhaps by a trusted spiritually-centered elder or other member of the community, takes the participants to the emotive and creative space that gives birth to transformation. Planning the initial meetings is an act of midwifery, where the organizers create a safe and nurturing space and attend to calling out the power of the participants to give birth to their own unique process and project. Circular seating works best. The physical space where initial meetings take place speaks loudly to all participants; insightful organizers choose and create the space for these early meetings very carefully, attending to accessibility and the comfort of all so that true dialogue can take place.

Learning to Dialogue

CBCAR projects will be more successful in their efforts and enjoy healthier processes if they learn early on how to *dialogue* rather than simply *discuss*. Over the past 3 decades, democratic dialogue has been at the core of action research projects, particularly those aimed at workplace process improvement (Phillips, 2004). Consistent with the theoretical roots of CBCAR, when people come together to discern the nature of the issue at hand, what is to be done about it, and who should do what, it is essential that the process create a space where all voices can be heard and meaning can be expressed and understood from multiple perspectives. CBCAR projects take shape through dialogue; careful attention to shaping the dialogue process can create that space from which meaningful actions emerge. Scharmer (2009) encouraged deep listening and dialogue, describing the process as connecting with the "mind, heart, and will wide open" (p. 394). In this process, participants are able to "suspend judgment and connect to wonder" and think and see together (2009, p. 133). Guba and Lincoln (1989) proposed a hermeneutic-dialectic process, or meaning-making dialogue, that fully engages people as equal and active participants in creating their own reality—a process with the potential to "unleash energy, stimulate creativity, instill pride, build commitment, prompt the taking of responsibility, and evoke a sense of investment and ownership" (p. 227).

Theoretical physicist David Bohm (1992, 1996) taught that dialogue, when done well, leads to transformation of individual and collective consciousness. According to Bohm (1992), dialogue involves meaning flowing through, between, and among the whole group leading to the emergence of a new understanding. Bohm differentiated dialogue from discussion, which has the same root as percussion and concussion, indicating beating something, perhaps breaking it apart. Discussion becomes a cradle for fragmentary thought. Dialogue, on the other hand, involves a slower pace in which participants are alert to nuances and connections. To differentiate the two, Bohm gave the example of a watch that has been smashed into pieces. The pieces are very different from the parts that went into the making of the watch—parts that had an integral relationship in making up a functional whole (Nichol, 1996). Dialogue nurtures a view of our place in an interconnected, living, functional whole. Discussion is like a ping-pong game where participants attempt to make points. In dialogue, everyone wins. Another analogy Bohm (1992) used to teach this concept is that of light. Ordinary light is incoherent and goes in all directions; a laser on the other hand is a convergence of light waves all going in the same direction and thus building up strength as a unified whole. Dialogue involves a common tacit group awareness that suspends impulses, opinions, judgments, and assumptions, leading to fellowship, friendship, participation, and sharing (Bohm, 1990).

Engaging in dialogue involves openness to a new way of seeing the world and engaging possibilities for action; dialogue is concerned with meaning as collectively expressed and understood. Dialogue brings to light previously unseen biases, assumptions, and structural and cultural barriers. Our thoughts are shaped by our unique experience of the world. "Dialogue is a way of observing, collectively, how hidden values and intentions can control our behavior, and how unnoticed cultural differences can clash without our realizing what is occurring" (Bohm, Factor, & Garret, 1991, para. 3).

Bohm (1992) asserted that dialogues should be initiated for a reason and begin with a facilitator explaining what dialogue is, how it works, and what it means (as explained above). There is no fixed agenda or set outcome; the outcome emerges from the dialogue. There is not a leader per se, rather one or two experienced facilitators who work themselves out of the position as the dialogue unfolds. They may point out when the group seems to have reached a sticking point, but otherwise are equal members of the group. The length of the dialogue is agreed upon at the outset—usually about 2 hours. Someone is asked to keep and call time. Optimal dialogues have representatives from various subcultures of the larger community (1992). The diversity helps to reveal unnamed cultural systems and ideologies that govern the way we unknowingly think and act. Bohm, Factor, and Garrett (1991) pointed out that:

> Each listener is able to reflect back to each speaker, and to the rest of the group, a view of some of the assumptions and unspoken implications of what is being expressed along with that which is being avoided. It creates the opportunity for each participant to examine the preconceptions, prejudices and the characteristic patterns that lie behind his or her thoughts, opinions, beliefs and feelings, along with the roles he or she tends to habitually play. And it offers an opportunity to share these insights. (para. 12)

When CBCAR projects create dialogue processes where divergent viewpoints can be critically considered, new ways of viewing the world and new possibilities for community action emerge within the collective consciousness of the group. Kristiansen and Bloch-Paulsen (2004) defined dialogue as "an exploratory conversation in which the partners jointly strive to achieve a better understanding or to become wiser together. It is characterized by sharing, daring, and caring" (p. 373). Sharing implies the willingness to share knowledge with the group. Group members "dare" when they expose assumptions to be questioned and analyzed. Finally, "caring means that the exploratory mood is based on an honest and forthright intent toward others" (p. 373).

Dialogues are mutual learning processes through which all participants' views and realities are transformed (Widdershoven, 2001). The dialogue begins in an open manner and facilitates the involvement of all participants in identifying the research topic and the voices that are missing within the partnership to inform the CBCAR process. This open dialogue process gives clarity to the direction the CBCAR project is taking and helps identify missing voices for the community advisory group.

Formalizing the Partnership: Creating Memorandums of Understanding

Before exploring how to form a community advisory group and organize the research teams, we want to pause to address those CBCAR efforts that involve partnerships between formal organizations. In the excitement of coming together to address pressing community problems, it is easy to make assumptions about who is doing what and how decisions will be made. It is helpful to draft a memorandum of understanding (MOU) as the CBCAR project takes shape, so that the co-responsibilities are clearly delineated and understood. The essential components of a memorandum of understanding include: (1) a clear statement of project plans; (2) a detailed list of specific activities to be carried out by each partner organization; (3) a comprehensive statement of resources that each organization will contribute to the CBCAR project; (4) the responsibilities each organization will assume in administration of remuneration received from funding sources—specifically which organization will receive how much money for what services; (5) agreement on how the project will be presented to the public, including in what order organizations are listed and what funding sources must be acknowledged; and (6) the date when the MOU terminates, and thus must be reassessed and revised. **Box 4-2** provides the format for a sample MOU and **Box 4-3** includes sample activities to be included in an MOU. Having a signed comprehensive and detailed MOU will speak loudly to potential funders.

Box 4-2 Sample Memorandum of Understanding

Partner Organization A
Partner Organization B
(list all partner organizations participating in the CBCAR project)

MEMORANDUM OF UNDERSTANDING

I. Collaborative Partners

This memorandum of understanding is between <u>Name of Organization A</u> and <u>Name of Organization B</u>, as represented by <u>Name(s) of Individual(s) Representing Organization A, Title(s)</u> and <u>Name(s) of Individual(s) Representing Organization B, Title(s)</u>. By signing this document, <u>Name of Organization A</u> and <u>Name of Organization B</u> commit to details in this agreement for the time period specified.

II. Project Goals

As equal partners in <u>Name of Project</u>, we will work collaboratively to achieve the following goals (list project goals):

III. Project Activities

As collaborative partners in <u>Name of Project</u>, <u>Name of Organization A</u> and <u>Name of Organization B</u> will (list activities):

IV. Commitment of Resources

<u>Name of Organization A</u> commits the following resources to its collaborative partnership with <u>Name of Organization B</u> (list resources committed):

<u>Name of Organization B</u> commits the following resources to its collaborative partnership with <u>Name of Organization A</u> (list resources committed):

V. Compensation
Specify each organization's remuneration from funding source.

VI. Acknowledgements at Public Events and Publications
Formal Acknowledgements will be: Name of the Project, Name of Organization and Name of Organization (in collaboratively-determined order) and funded by (specify funding agencies or individuals)

VII. Term of Agreement
This memorandum of understanding is effective as of <u>Date</u> and ends on <u>Date</u>, at which point it will be revised as determined by the collaborative partnership. If at any time, additional sources of funding are procured, this memorandum of understanding will be revised to specify how funds will be allocated and administered.

_____   _____
Org. A Representative Name, Title   Org. B Representative Name, Title

_____   _____
Date   Date

Forming a Community Advisory Group and Research Partnership Group

Whether a CBCAR project is a partnership between two or more formal organizations, consists of a clinical practice group, or is a newly formed collaborative of individuals, it is helpful to have a community advisory group to oversee the direction of the CBCAR process and to serve as a liaison with the larger community of interest. To be a liaison with the larger community, the community advisory group needs representation from subgroups within the community. Optimally, the community advisory group has diverse yet equal voices so that the research project can be conceptualized, planned, and critiqued from multiple perspectives. It is of particular importance to have significant representation from the critical reference group, not

Box 4-3   Sample of Activities in a Memorandum
of Understanding

1. Plan of collaboration for the project in Year #1:
   - Network with community-based organizations.
   - Develop effective working relationships between partners.
   - Acknowledge and draw on one another's strengths to engage the community in answering questions of importance to immigrant women's and girls' health.
   - Study and analyze current literature on women's and girls' health experiences and concerns.
   - Study the community-based collaborative action research approach.
   - Dialogue with immigrant women and girls to develop a plan for how to best collect data on their perspectives about health concerns.
   - Formalize a plan for data collection and analysis to be conducted in Year #2.

2. Responsibilities of the academic partner in Year #1:
   - Administer the grant goals and budget.
   - Prepare for, participate in, and report on six scheduled NIH conference calls.
   - Prepare and submit all necessary grant reports to NIH.
   - Initiate, organize, and summarize the planning and working meetings between partnering organizations.
   - Supply all necessary materials for the meetings.
   - Coordinate activities to maintain the timeline.
   - Create a library of literature pertaining to community-based collaborative inquiry, women's and girls' health, and immigrant health disparities.
   - Maintain a working journal of all grant-related activities.
   - Prepare job descriptions for student assistants and pursue hiring process.
   - Prepare materials for approval from the Office for the Protection of Human Subjects.

3. Responsibilities of the refugee-assistance organization in Year #1:
   - Participate in planning meetings (approximately 6–8 meetings).
   - Approach community-based organizations who might be interested in participating.
   - Conduct inquiry and planning meetings with academic researchers and community-based organizations (approximately 3–5 meetings).
   - Share expertise on working with immigrant women and share insights from other projects conducted with immigrant women.
   - Participate in meetings with immigrant women and girls (approximately 3–5).
   - Offer guidance and participate in planning for Year #2.
4. Responsibilities of community-based partners in Year #1:
   - Participate in shared inquiry and planning meetings (approximately 6–8 meetings)
   - Share expertise gained from working with immigrant women and findings of other projects.
   - Study literature and offer additional resources and expanded perspectives on the literature.
   - Provide avenue for networking with African-born women and girls in the community.
   - Host meetings with African-born women and girls (approximately 3–5 meetings).
   - Offer guidance and participate in planning for Year #2.
5. Timeline (see Table 6-2 Task and Timeline Table for a detailed timeline)
6. Identify Year #1 remuneration for each partner.
7. Signatures of partnership members from each organization in the partnership

only on the advisory group, but also on the various work teams (data collection, data analysis, data presentation, and action planning). Depending upon the size of the CBCAR project, one group of people might carry out all of these tasks, or there could be various subgroups of the larger research partnership group, each assuming responsibility for a specific aspect of the CBCAR process. This does not mean that the same people have to work on all of the work teams. As indicated in **Figure 4-1,** *Fluid Collaborations in CBCAR,* the initial group of people who commence and conceptualize the CBCAR project in re-

Figure 4-1 Fluid Collaborations in CBCAR

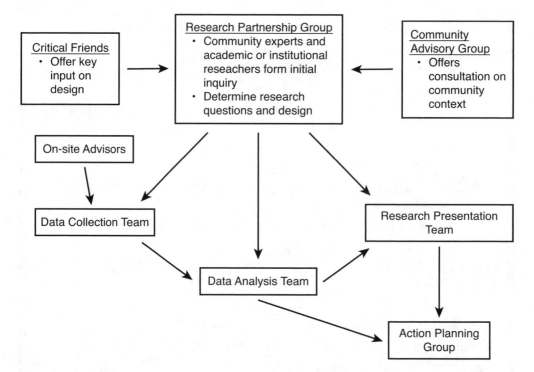

In some CBCAR projects, persons in the Research Partnership Group may also be on the Data Collection Team, Data Analysis Team, Research Presentation Team, and Action Planning Group (as indicated by the arrows). In other words, the entire group remains the same throughout the research process.

In other CBCAR projects, a core group may form out of the Research Partnership Group with different community members or institutional researchers flowing in and out of the project at different times and on different teams. With this model, some personnel changes will occur throughout the process. However, having a consistent core group of people is suggested.

sponse to community need is not necessarily the group that will eventually carry out all aspects of the research process.

For example, in the *Racism, Health, and Well-being* CBCAR project presented in Chapter 1, there were women on the women's advisory group who were essential to the project's conceptualization at the project's initiation, as well as in the discernment of action steps emerging from presentation of research findings; however, for a variety of reasons not all of the women on the women's advisory council were able to actively engage in the research process. Some of the women on the advisory council volunteered to be on the data collection team—a process for which they engaged in training related to the ethical conduct of research, methods of leading focus groups, and techniques for collecting data in one-on-one interviews. The data collection team was made up of members from the women's advisory council. The data analysis team included a new constellation of women from the advisory council and data collection team, along with university researchers. A few new community members with deep insight into the issues being studied were recruited for this effort. The data presentation team included women from the previously mentioned groups, along with women from the arts community who helped with transforming the data from numbers and words to a spoken-word narrative that would speak more loudly and holistically to the wider community. The data were woven together in a manner that engaged the wider community in dialogue about what the findings meant and what needed to be done. The dissemination team included people interested in organizing, filming, and writing to take the findings further. The entire women's advisory council—with all of the women involved in the project from start to finish—engaged in the action planning. Only a small group of women were involved in every step of the CBCAR process, an arrangement that worked well for that particular community. Each CBCAR partnership and project will be uniquely shaped, depending on the resources of the partners, the interests of each member, and the demands of the project.

In another project—on an inpatient renal unit of a hospital—a group of nurses came together at the inspiration of their nurse manager, who was at the time in a doctor of nursing practice (DNP) graduate program. She was learning to do systems improvement and wanted to use a CBCAR process for systems change. The idea came up in the break room one day when she was pondering ways to create systems change with three nurse colleagues. They wondered about a way to improve the patient experience and staff satisfaction without increasing the unit budget. Determined to engage in an action research project, they formed an advisory group that included six interested nurses, three nursing assistants (one of whom was also a nursing student), an MD hospitalist, two members of the housekeeping staff, the unit social worker, one of the nephrologists, the unit chaplain, two former patients, and one current patient and his caregiver. The four nurses who originally conceptualized the project began by organizing a dialogue centered on the patient experience and meaningful work. The nurse manager shared resources on CBCAR and conducting dialogues. Two of the nurses carefully prepared themselves to facilitate the dialogue.

The initial dialogue took place in a comfortable conference room at the hospital. A colorful woven cloth covered the sign-in table where participants found name tags with their first names. At the next table were flowers and an attractive array of nutritious food. To signify equality of participation, the chairs were arranged in open clam style (a circle with two opposing chairs removed, forming two equivalent arcs of chairs facing each other, which allows for passage in and out of the circle).

After a brief opening centering reflection, the facilitators explained the guidelines for dialogue—how it was different from a meeting full of discussion with a predetermined agenda and where some voices become directive and more dominant than others. They stressed that each person in the room holds a view of the whole and together, through dialogue, the group will reach greater understanding. Listening with one's ears, eyes, heart, and soul are essential. The facilitators encouraged participants to leave a space before talking and to focus on what they are feeling as people speak and what they perceive about their own opinions, assumptions, and judgments. The facilitators assured the group that the process of action research was based on 4 decades of scientifically tested theory demonstrating that when people who are closest to a situation gather in a spirit of dialogue to collectively analyze an issue from their varying perspectives, new insights arise that were previously unforeseen. Their focus this evening was to dialogue about what is meaningful in terms of patient and staff experiences.

The dialogue began slowly but soon delved deeply into what was meaningful to the group. At the end of 2 hours the group was energized to form an advisory group, for which they determined it was essential to involve more patient voices, a representative from the local kidney foundation, and a few more nurses who were identified as particularly insightful. The group also identified the need to invite someone from administration to be present so that the project outcomes would be more fully understood and felt by someone who could be a champion for necessary change at the administrative level. Since the patient experience was so central to this project, involvement of patients and patients' significant others was a major concern—they wanted to expand the patient voice right from the beginning, not when the current group was well into the project and would miss out on patients' direction of the research process—an idea strongly supported by the literature (Abma, Nierse, & Widdershoven, 2009; Prior, 2006; Smith, 1997; Stringer, 2007). A meeting for the project's advisory group was set. The purpose of that meeting would be to define the project focus and develop the research work teams.

The nurse manager who was doing this project for her DNP capstone project was tempted to take on the majority of the work herself, but, with the help of a wise advisor, she came to realize that her work involved creating community and being a catalyst—teaching her colleagues about the action research process and engaging as many people as possible in discerning how to proceed. Her role was that of teacher and facilitator; she needed to maintain a focus on dialogue, meaning, pattern recognition, and attending to emerging insights for action. She was alert to the fact that as different people's perspectives of truths and realities come together, a convergence of views constructs a new view of reality and presents new possibilities (Guba & Lincoln, 1989; Stringer, 2007). There is a joint construction of new meaning not visible without the collective dialogue. What the nurse manager learned in her DNP studies, she shared with others on the organizing team and listened to what they were learning. What she felt she needed to know to successfully engage in systems change, she explored in a manner that involved as many colleagues as possible. They began by looking at patient involvement in action research.

Focusing on the important role of patient participation in research that affects patients' lives, Abma et al. (2009) pointed out that through the choice of research design and data collection strategies, researchers preordain both the outcomes and the extent to which patients' voices are valued, collected, and presented in research reports. Different data collection methods open up varying amounts of space for participants to offer original ideas and new insights. When patients fill out surveys, they are answering questions predetermined by the researchers. Semistructured interviews leave a little more room for patient-directed input, and in-depth interviews and focus groups allow for more patient control of the direction of the conversation, yet the questions that are asked and the way they are analyzed, interpreted, and presented are controlled by the research team. The experience and concerns of patients are more adequately represented when patients are full research partners, not just participants. Abma et al. (2009) presented a laddered conceptualization of patient participation, from patients as the object of research, to patients as interviewer/moderator in the data collection process, to patients as full research partners, and finally, to patients as principal investigators. When patients participate in the research design and data collection process, they can lend insider insights as to what outcome indicators might need to be measured before and after interventions so that impact can be demonstrated. When partnering to design data collection protocols, patients can better gauge how much time and depth it is okay to ask of patients. Patients as partners "influence crucial decisions regarding research (aim, questions, design, data collection and analysis, dissemination, and implementation), not in the role as advisor to decision makers, but as co-decision makers in a research team" (2009, p. 403).When people from the target population are involved in every step of the research process—from the very beginning until the very end of the CBCAR cycle—the project is better informed, and the action steps more meaningfully address the problem.

Once project partners are certain that the community advisory group has representation from all necessary stakeholders, particularly from the populations most affected by the topic of interest, the first meeting is organized to identify the specific focus of the CBCAR project at hand. If this is a new advisory group that has been formed for a specific project, keep in mind that this may be the beginning cycle of many important projects. Once people learn how to change their environment through action research, they usually want to keep the process going. Building solid relationships at this point is central. In the action planning phase, new research questions are often generated. Who else should be involved is of constant concern. CBCAR teams constantly ask the question, *what voices are missing?* Margins are repeatedly stretched. Workload and team member well-being are held to heart at every step along the way.

Defining the Research Focus

After the advisory group has been organized so that the important voices within the community of concern are adequately represented, the next step is to bring the group together to clearly define the research focus and CBCAR project's organizational structure and process. Careful attention is again directed toward the meeting location, logistics, and process. In his book *Participatory Workshops*, Robert Chambers (2004) wrote a fine section on "messing up," in which he offered cautions by outlining what could go wrong, from the room being too hot or too cold, to a way too long introduction by a "PAIN (Pompous And Insensitive Notable)" who arrives late and sets the wrong mood (p. 62). Notably, Chambers recommended not being flustered or too preoccupied with the details before a meeting that you fail to adequately greet, acknowledge, and come to know participants as they arrive. CBCAR calls participants to be present to one another as well as to the process. It is not rushed or harried. It is built on strong relationships in which people are honored for who they are. To begin that process with groups where not everyone knows each other, Chambers (2004) proposed a technique for introductions in which those present form two lines facing one another. Advisory group members briefly greet the person they are facing, with each person repeating the other person's name. The group moves like a bicycle chain to the left; members move to the other line when they reach the end of the line they are in, greeting people until they have personally greeted and said the name of each person present. To do this exercise, there must be a space large enough to accommodate a line of half the people present. When choosing introductory exercises, select one where all participants are perceived as equally important (i.e., academic credentials or community member insider knowledge are not highlighted). The intention is to level the playing field and to equitably honor the importance of each person's voice.

There are several ways to engage the group in focusing the direction of their work; the method chosen will depend on the group's size and the complexity of the topic. The group could divide into small groups of around eight people to answer a question that would help focus the research. Sample questions might include:

> In your opinion, what is the major barrier to health for people in this community?
>
> What constitutes quality care for patients on this unit?
>
> What are the advantages and disadvantages of establishing a community birthing center?
>
> What is the major concern of women in this refugee camp?

The question should be broad enough to elicit a range of responses within each small group. Before breaking into groups, dialogue guidelines are reviewed to encourage equity of contribution and a spirited and meaningful process. Groups are asked to record their insights to report back to the large group within a specified time period.

Another technique is reflective interviewing (Sagor, 1992). Here, the group is divided into pairs for in-depth interviewing about the chosen topic. For example, a group of nurse midwives and interested women from the local community are engaging in an action research project to explore establishing a community birthing center. They have invited OB/GYN medical partners and representatives from the local hospital and health department to join the advisory group. All advisory group members have read the same articles and state regulations pertaining to community birthing centers. The group engages in dialogue to explore what the barriers and advantages are to community birthing centers. Members are reminded to let go of preconceived notions of what should happen and to honestly share with and to listen to others, attending to what they can learn from arising feelings, assumptions, opinions, and judgments. They are encouraged to trust the group process. The dyads are given 40–60 minutes to interview one another—20–30 minutes for one person to interview the other. A facilitator will tell them when the 20–30 minutes are up so that they can reverse roles. People must remember that this is not a discussion, but rather an interview, where "the person being interviewed has an opportunity to fully and deeply explore feelings and ideas" related to the issue (Sagor, 1997, p. 13). Sagor offers the following guidelines for interviewers:

1. Make the interview comfortable but challenging.
2. Keep it challenging but not threatening.
3. Try to elicit deep responses.
4. Try to elicit broad responses.
5. Keep the interview somewhat structured, but allow for flexibility and spontaneity.
6. Consider the rights and feelings of the respondent. (1997, p. 13)

The purpose of the interviews is to thoroughly explore what is known and what remains to be understood or discovered about a potential focus for the research. After the reflective interviews, the entire group gathers in a circle and each member shares for several minutes what they learned during their interview. If small group dialogues were used, the same large group sharing process would take place. Through this process, the most salient issues arise. At this point the advisory group can make a graphic representation of what is known about the topic of concern or problem at hand and what needs to be known. The facilitator double-checks that all important points are represented. From that representation, the group formulates clear problem statements and/or research questions. If the advisory group is also going to be the research partnership group (see Figure 4-1), then it is important to clearly define the specific research questions.

Otherwise the research methods group can shape the research questions from the problem statements.

The above processes are suggestions to massage the research topic so that the group can clearly identify what the problem is and what the research focus should be. Each CBCAR project develops its own unique process for problem identification and determination of the research focus. What is important is that it emerges from the entire group's efforts, that there is equity among voices (no one person or small group is directing the process), and that attention is paid to enhancing well-being for the target population in a meaningful way. Groups have often been surprised by the direction their CBCAR project takes, but it should not be surprising as this is a formative process with the meaning and direction evolving from the dialogue at each step. For example, the birthing center group may find that it is much more energized to begin with a breast-feeding promotion effort and move on to the birthing center as their second project. With time and experience using the CBCAR approach, team members learn to trust the process. **Box 4-4** provides questions to guide the organizing phase of the CBCAR partnership.

Essential Organizational Decisions

In addition to discerning the focus of the research, the research partnership group must decide how decisions will be made, how and where records of group process and decisions will be maintained, what principles will guide group work, and who will work on which CBCAR teams. To discern guidelines for group processes, it may be helpful to have the group spend some time thinking about groups they have worked with in the past and write down three to five factors that contributed to it being a positive experience and/or contributed to successful group work. They can then be asked to think of groups that did not work well and what three to five factors would have needed to be changed to make the group function more effectively (Becker, Israel, & Allen, 2005). Each CBCAR project will discern its own best method. It is also helpful to pull together the

---

Box 4-4   Questions for the CBCAR Organizing Phase

1. How will we make decisions? Consensus? Robert's Rules of Order? Majority vote?
2. Do we need a mission statement? What is our purpose?
3. Who is most affected by the topic at hand? Are they sufficiently represented in this group?
4. Will the community advisory group and the research work group be two separate entities?
5. Who will be the guardian of our agendas, meeting minutes, group processes, and data?
6. How will we maintain fidelity to our process?
7. How will the collaborative communicate and access information?
8. How often will the community advisory group meet? What is their role?
9. Who will be on the data collection, data analysis, data presentation, and action planning teams?
10. How will we decide when additional members are needed for a team?
11. Who are the critical friends we need on this project?
12. How will we protect the confidentiality and rights of vulnerable people while maximizing their voice? (Adhering to the *Belmont Report,* as described in Chapter 8)
13. What new knowledge and insights are emerging from our process?
14. How will we know we have done well when the project is completed?

---

principles that will guide the project (see **Box 4-5** for an example of questions based on one project's guiding principles and **Box 4-6** for an example of how these questions guide the evaluation of group processes).

As previously mentioned, each group will divide the tasks according to the complexity of the project and number of people involved. The group may be so enthused about the project

---

Box 4-5 CBCAR Work Team Questions

The following questions were posted at the bottom of every agenda for one CBCAR project. For that project, a team member painted one question in each of eight sea shells. At the beginning of each meeting, various members took shells to be guardians of the questions on the shells. Time was allotted at the end of each meeting to assess group process. A table tent or laminated card could serve the same purpose.

1. Are we staying focused on our purpose?
2. Is the workload equitably distributed?
3. Are we maintaining confidentiality?
4. Are we using principles of dialogue? Is there equity of voice in our process?
5. Is the voice of the people most affected being engaged yet not exploited?
6. How are we dealing with power imbalances in our process?
7. Are we archiving the process and content of our work?
8. Is our work meaningful?

---

that they decide they will all complete each step of the research process. Other groups may have many members with little spare time. These groups may end up recruiting additional community members to serve in various roles or they may write a grant to hire staff to conduct some of the work, while the group maintains control of the major decisions. CBCAR is a process that fluidly adapts to the local context.

■ Designing Research Questions

The process of formulating the research question(s) will be done by the research partnership group, or if the community advisory group has decided that they will serve the function of the research partnership group, they will formulate the question(s) after determining the focus of the research. Formulating

Box 4-6   Equity Process Evaluation in Action

For working team meetings, each agenda has eight questions at the bottom, with team members taking responsibility for being guardians of specific questions. During the data collection team organizing meeting of one CBCAR project, Ana volunteered to be the guardian of questions 4–6 listed in Box 4-5. Ana's questions were focused on equity of voice and participation, with special attention on equitable and just involvement of members of the critical reference group and members who come from the margins. The CBCAR project's aim was to identify and address barriers to retention and successful graduation for nursing students from ethnic minorities. Ana, who is a white learning lab assistant, knew that she might not notice the inequalities if she didn't systematically look for them because people from privileged populations (in this case white faculty and administrators) oftentimes fill the dialogic space without even noticing they are doing so, since it is the cultural norm they live in, and they are rarely, if ever, challenged. Ana unobtrusively placed a check mark by each person's name when they spoke and tried to estimate how many minutes or seconds they talked each time they spoke. She also attended to interruptions. The group consisted of three African-American nursing students, one Latina nursing student, one white nursing student, two African-American nursing faculty, two white nursing faculty, a white learning lab director, and one white and one African-American administrator. At the end of the meeting, when it was Ana's turn to offer her reflection on the process related to her questions, she couched her remarks in the fact that they are doing this study because of issues related to cultural racism, which is pervasive and difficult to measure; it is like the smog we breathe—we all take it in, usually without even noticing it. Ana then presented her findings in which she demonstrated that 75% of the dialogue was consumed by the two white faculty members and the two administrators. More disturbingly, all of the ethnic minority students were cut off by the faculty and administrators at least once when they attempted to speak. Ana's reflection of the group pattern generated some discomfort followed by very meaningful dialogue about leaving space, filling space, and honoring space; she was asked to take the same questions the next time, but when she saw someone's voice being silenced, to call a timeout. With time, the group became strong, cohesive, and equitable. New leadership strengths arose in each member.

a research question is a complex mental operation (Thorne, 2008). The question needs to be clearly defined and understood, which can be done by identifying its main concepts and determining how to measure, describe, or most fully understand each concept. Activities in the next chapter highlight the process of extracting concepts from the research questions and determining ways to collect data.

The research methods chosen need to be in alignment with the nature of the questions being asked. Research groups are often most interested in understanding the structures and processes that are behind the problem upon which the CBCAR project is focused. They are concerned with "the need to understand *how* things are happening, rather than merely *what* is happening, and to understand the ways that stakeholders—the different people concerned with the issue—perceive, interpret, and respond to events related to the issue investigated" (Stringer, 2007, p. 19). The group needs to develop a precise understanding of what they want to know in order to enhance well-being for the target population and effectively address the identified problem. They also must identify potential sources of information to answer the question(s).

For example, Pierre-Louis, Akoh, White, and Pharris (2010) reported on a CBCAR project that arose during action planning on the *Racism, Health, and Well-being* CBCAR project described in Chapter 1. This second-cycle CBCAR project was aimed at addressing the rising rate of diabetes for African-American women in the community. Faced with very high hemoglobin A1c levels in the clinic population, the physicians said, "These women are just noncompliant." The women on the advisory committee felt that there was more to the story. Clinic healthcare providers and members of the women's advisory group wanted to know what was behind this problem. The problem focus was the disproportionately high blood sugar levels for African-American women. After much dialogue, members of the research partnership group decided on two research questions:

1. What is the pattern of hemoglobin A1c levels for African-American women in the clinic?
2. What is the experience of African-American women with diabetes and high hemoglobin A1c levels?

The first question required collection of quantitative descriptive data and was fairly easy to answer since clinic data were computerized, and the variables of HgbA1c, ethnicity, and gender could be easily accessed and analyzed. The team had to decide if they were interested in entering any other variables into the data run, such as age, marital status, zip code, etc., to provide a more elaborate view of the pattern.

The second research question had three major concepts: experience, African-American women, and diabetes as measured by high HgbA1c. To recruit women with high HgbA1c levels, clinic data were used to generate a list of women. A protocol for inviting women into the study was developed, approved by the university IRB, and followed. To determine women's experiences involved a phenomenological process; the team decided to follow Margaret Newman's hermeneutic–dialectic process. The African-American community was tightly knit, which presented challenges for confidentiality in the process of data collection. It was therefore decided that the data collection team would be made up of African-American nursing students from the university who were not from the local community, and who were trained in the protection of human subjects. Again, to maintain confidentiality, the women who did the data collection also did data analysis, along with a faculty researcher skilled in CBCAR, and a nurse who was the director of community health initiatives and was knowledgeable about human subjects protection and the research process. This community nurse's insights during the preliminary data analysis were invaluable. All identifiers were stripped from the data. When it came time for data presentation, Mrs. Nothando Zulu from the Black Storytellers Alliance worked with Berline Pierre-Louis, who was funded as a student nurse community health intern and coordinator of the project, to weave the distinct stories into a dramatic spoken-word performance. To preserve confidentiality, each of seven voices written into the narrative included the experience of various women. Spoken word uses voice inflection and varying emotions to present a narrative. The narrative of research findings was performed by members of the Black Storytellers Alliance at a luncheon entitled, "Living the Sweet Life" which was held at a local church and advertised through community radio, the clinic, and word of mouth to invite African-American women with diabetes. After the performance, the women were invited to dialogue in small groups about what was presented during the spoken-word narrative and what needed to be added to better reflect their own experiences. Specifically, the women were asked to reflect on the following questions:

1. What is missing from the performance that is connected to your life? Share this with your sisters.
2. What feelings and insights arose as you watched the performance?
3. In what ways can the community help women with diabetes lead healthy lives?

The women's responses were recorded and analyzed to better understand the community pattern and to aid in action planning. Based on community feedback, the spoken-word narrative was made into a DVD to be used in community gatherings and healthcare provider training. The DVD, *Living the Sweet Life: Our Story, Our Voice, Our Wisdom. The Experience of African American Women Living with Diabetes,* ends with two questions on the screen: "What feelings and insights arose as you watched this performance?" and "What needs to happen so that women with diabetes can live happy, healthy lives?" Todd Marcus gave permission to include *ma'aelsalama* from his *In pursuit of the 9th man* album; this music creates a spirited environment in which small groups can ponder their responses to the two questions on the screen. The DVD is used to inspire action and transform practice. Women from the CBCAR partnership have made numerous presentations of this project, and the clinic has made significant changes in the way care is organized and delivered. Findings have been submitted for publication (Pierre-Louis, Akoh, White, & Pharris, 2010).

■ Choosing Research Methods

Following the principles of CBAR, each research partnership team carefully discerns who should be included in each step of their CBCAR process (e.g., represented on the data collection team, data analysis team, research presentation team). The work of the research partnership team is fluid and adheres to the guiding principles of CBCAR. The problem statement guides the research questions, which guide the selection of research methods.

Once the research question has been identified, academic researchers and community members must determine the research design by discerning appropriate data sources and methods of data collection for each question. Generally speaking, in CBCAR, attention is given to trying to keep people's experiences whole rather than collecting particulate data, while keeping in mind that findings may be richer if a variety of sources of data are used. Nonetheless, it is the clear definition of the research question that directs the research methods to be employed in the CBCAR project. The quality of the research depends on the match between the research question and the method. Because CBCAR projects respond to the questions generated by the community, the research partners who are responsible for determining the data collection and analysis techniques cannot anticipate in advance of the community advisory groups' formulation of the research questions which data collection and analysis methods they will be employing. The nature of the question drives the methods used in the research. Once the research questions are decided upon, the research partnership group carefully discerns which methods are best matched to the research question(s) that have been posed. It may be necessary to bring into the CBCAR process other researchers who are experts in the methods that are required to answer the questions posed. There should be a coherent thread and logical match between the research problem statement, question(s), methods, and the nature of the findings that are generated. To move from the research problem statement to the question may take investigation and study. For example, if the research problem is rising childhood obesity in the community, enough background needs to be collected to gain a full view and understanding of the community pattern. The group may decide on the following initial research questions to begin to explore structural factors related to obesity. Each question can be triangulated with a mixture of data sources and collection techniques:

- What has been the pattern of physical education in community schools over the past 5 years?
- What is the pattern of availability and cost of low-fat nutritious foods in relationship to high-fat processed foods in the community?
- What is the pattern of physical activity opportunities for youth in the community?
- What is the pattern of foods and snacks available in the schools over the past 5 years?

The group may also be interested in the experience of obese children in the neighborhood; generating the following initial questions:

- What is the experience of obese children in this community? (qualitative interviews)
- What does the average child eat during a typical day? (food diaries)
- How much time does the average child spend watching television or playing video games? (activity log)

The next step is to discern—given the project resources—what questions generate the deepest insight into the identified problem. In this situation, the group would have to decide what age range they are looking at—hopefully determined by demographic data of childhood obesity in their community. If they are collecting data from schools, they must decide which schools would provide the most relevant and representative data. These decisions take careful attention and time and should be recorded.

Coordinated, well-designed research projects can provide transformative insights into community patterns and result in significant policy changes. For example, the WE ACT partnership in New York City looked at community level exposure to diesel exhaust emissions and other related air pollution, which resulted in conversion of the city's bus fleet to clean diesel (Zimmerman, Tilly, Cohen, & Love, 2009). Studies such as this one might use traditional methods and research design, or they may use emergent designs. Decisions on which design to use involve discernment of the best scientific methods to answer the research question.

Traditional Design or Emergent Design?

Most community-based collaborative action researchers will use both qualitative and quantitative methods to answer the research questions posed; however, most CBCAR projects focus on the patterns of people's experiences within the community, and for this reason qualitative methods predominate. Because patterns are also discerned through the presentation of quantitative data, many CBCAR projects utilize a variety of methods of data collection. Quantitative data help us understand what is going on at the population level, and thus they supplement the qualitative data that inform the research endeavor. Sometimes the research method used to answer the questions posed comes from and follows traditional and familiar research methods such as grounded theory or ethnography. Most often in CBCAR, some degree of openness to emergent methods is necessary. Reason and Bradbury (2006) claimed that community action research is a "living, emergent process which cannot be pre-determined but changes and develops as those engaged deepen their understanding of the issues to be addressed and develop their capacity as co-inquirers both individually and collectively" (p. xxii). Similarly, addressing community action research in the face of power differentials, Prior (2007) presented an agenda of decolonizing research, which shifts the focus of the research from the aims of the researchers to the agenda of the people. The aim of decolonizing research is to evoke discourse, which Prior defined as "a process of developing meaning or 'truth' through a relationship of trust, reciprocity and co-operatively evolved methods of research that remain true to the context of the story being presented" (p. 165).

An emergent research design involves researchers listening to what the data is telling them and remaining open to modification in data collection or analytic strategies. It does not abandon scientific discipline, but rather pushes its boundaries to establish strategies that uncover more meaningful data. Hesse-Biber and Leavy (2008) stated, "Working with emergent methods is not about abandoning our disciplinary training but rather taking that training, adapting it, applying it, modifying it, and working beyond it as appropriate with respect to our research objectives" (p. 2). They go on to point out that emergent methods are "about methodological innovation for the purpose of enhancing knowledge building and advancing scholarly conversations" (Hesse-Biber & Leavy, 2008, p. 4). Chapters 5 and 6 delve deeply into issues related to data collection and analytic techniques that emerge from the identified research questions.

■ Partnering the Inquiry

After the research questions have been clearly defined, there are several major decisions that need to be considered prior to delving into the exciting work ahead of the group. Topics for an initial planning meeting include:

- Developing the structure, timeline, and communication strategies for the working teams
- Discerning the method for decision making
- Considering required resources needed
- Determining the process of facilitating meetings, setting agendas, and keeping records
- Deliberating on how to protect participants
- Strategizing for clear and honest communication about roles and expectations

This is also the time to dialogue about who would be best suited for which team—the data collection, data analysis, and data presentation teams.

Decision-making power and processes should be clearly deliberated and delineated before the research gets underway. It is important to talk about who decides what and when, for example: When should new partners be added? Who will invite them in? How will findings be disseminated? Who decides? Each working group in the CBCAR project must decide about the process for decision making. When important decisions are being made, will the group use consensus, majority vote, or another method of reaching decisions? How will differences be acknowledged, appreciated, and managed? Most CBCAR projects operate by consensus to maximize equitable participation.

Similarly, the distribution of resources for funded projects should be collaboratively determined; partners need to talk about what resources might be needed, who will receive which resources, how those decisions will be made, and which principles will guide these decisions. If a project is not funded, and it involves asking people without resources to travel or spend time away from young children, some fundraising may need to be done to assure equity of participation.

Another important aspect of group function is the use of agendas, taking minutes, and the facilitation of group meetings. Becker, Israel, and Allen (2005) stressed the importance of communication between meetings and the importance of deciding who calls the meetings, who facilitates, who takes minutes, and how minutes will be distributed. These decisions should be made from the point of view of the most potentially marginalized person in the group—consider how this person would best receive information and make sure that all information is accessible to this person to assure optimal participation. Some groups rotate meeting facilitation and recordkeeping, others designate a facilitator and record keeper.

At the point that the research questions have been determined, it is wise to consult the Office of Research Affairs or Institutional Review Board (IRB) for all involved agencies (university, institution, and community) to discuss their requirements for training project members who will be involved in research design and data collection and analysis, as well as to determine when their IRB meets to review project proposals. Data collection cannot commence without IRB approval of the project. Funders may also have specific requirements for training. It is essential that all research working group members clearly understand the ethical issues involved in working with human participants in research, as well as their responsibility for maintaining confidentiality and protecting research participants' rights. Some groups have found the IRB language and requirements to appear adversarial and legalistic, but can use dialogue about this as an opportunity for co-learning (Zimmerman et al., 2009). Groups can work with their IRB to design engaging and interactive training sessions that meet IRB requirements. Ideally, work group members would have several options for learning about ethical guidelines for research in an engaging manner best suited to their style of learning. The protection of participants is one of many topics of concern for the research partnership group. Being central to the research process and partnership, ethics is also emphasized in subsequent chapters.

Another issue of concern relates to the costs of involvement in the project. An ongoing, honest dialogue about these issues helps build trust and understanding. If people from a community agency are collaborating with university researchers, it is important for the university researchers to understand and acknowledge that the community partners' time on the project may be taken from the time community members would otherwise be spending fundraising and grant writing to sustain essential community programming and services. Individual community partners may also experience vulnerability. For example, in the case of involving people who are undocumented, involvement might mean deportation and abandonment of and separation from young children, who will be left without a parent. CBCAR members may experience strain. For example, if the collaborative consists of emergency department nurses trying to discern how to streamline their work to better serve patients, involvement may be very difficult for nurses with multiple family and community commitments. On the other hand, involvement in the project may give these very same nurses significant energy and enthusiasm, which often result from becoming an active participant in shaping one's own professional work environment and providing more meaningful patient care. This added energy and enthusiasm will be evident in all aspects of their lives. Similarly, there are costs and benefits to university researchers. In CBCAR, the community may determine it is best to publish the project results and findings in a community venue that does not count toward tenure and promotion within the university structure. On the other hand, working with community partners may offer academic researchers valuable lessons for classroom learning. Working alongside others to plan evidence-based action can also be very satisfying. It is beneficial to dialogue about costs and benefits to each partner at the time the collaboration has been established. These aspects of culture sharing deepen the bonds of understanding and trust.

Forming the Data Collection, Data Analysis, and Data Presentation Teams

One of the first tasks of the research working group is to determine who will be involved in which aspect of the project. When forming the data collection team, decisions are made about who would be best able to collect the data and how. Ideally, this team has a good mix of research and community experts. Community members have the best insight into who needs to be approached and how best to approach them. Rapport is more easily built within cultural groups. Research partners have knowledge of data collection strategies and processes that are consistent with the methods chosen for the project. Chapter 5 further examines the work of the data collection team. Open communication and clearly defined roles strengthen the working relationship.

The data analysis and presentation teams are also formed during this stage—usually with generous overlap from the data collection team and with the understanding that additional members may be recruited depending upon how the project unfolds. It is essential that academic researchers be on the data collection and analysis teams so that they can share their expertise, and that community members also be well represented as they will have a fuller view and deeper insight into context and what is in the data. The role of the data presentation team is to integrate and present the findings in a way that will engage the larger community in a dialogue about what the findings mean. Since this is often a creative process, additional artistic expertise that is not foreseeable at the time of team formation may be required. For example, if it is decided that the data are best presented in the form of a play to engage the wider community in action planning, it may be helpful to recruit a playwright to join the team. Chapter 6 further describes the work of data analysis and presentations teams.

Maintaining Strong Relationships

Strong, healthy relationships and processes are the fuel for smoothly running CBCAR projects that go the distance toward meaningful transformations. Seifer (2006) described the findings of 10 US-based organizations that collaborated to analyze the facilitators and barriers to success in prevention research within their own community partnership projects. Project staff stressed the importance of *time*, which they saw as playing an "important part in the quality of the partner relationships and the impact of the partnership's activities" (p. 992). Seifer (2006) found that community members often do not trust people from outside of the community in relation to how data will be used and where and to whom funds will be allocated. For this reason, when partnerships are being formed, it is important for each partner to know the history of other partners and to openly talk about who has been invited, why, and by whom. Seifer (2006) stressed the importance of "being open and honest, being able to listen well, and being able to directly address and speak frankly about contentious but important issues, such as power differentials, racism, and financial decisions" (p. 993).

It is important to remember that most everything takes longer than anticipated. This is especially true when working with university systems and timelines—students need advisor and committee approval, and then the university Institutional Review Board (IRB) schedule and process may involve delays that could be weeks or months—this can prevent academic partners from getting on the train that is moving full steam ahead toward community health and well-being. Worse yet, the delays and pressures to claim research findings can derail the entire process, causing an irreparable rift between academic researchers and community partners. This happened to a colleague who engaged in a CBCAR process, but had an advisor who was out of town and then not available for 3 months. She could not proceed without advisor and committee approval of the process. Meanwhile the community partners kept meeting, and since they could not proceed with the research project due to the student's delays, they kept adding more and more items to their survey. After a several-month delay by the university IRB, partners lost enthusiasm, and the tool became unwieldy, producing data that were difficult to analyze in a way that would produce a meaningful representation of what was occurring in the community. In the name of scientific rigor, university advisors, who did not know the community, were dictating how data needed to be analyzed and reported. The CBCAR project no longer involved the community as an equal partner. The student did not return to the community, and the research did not produce any change or benefit to the community. The end result was that community partners lost trust in the graduate student and the university. In order for graduate students to succeed in CBCAR endeavors, clear communication and commitment have to flow between the community, university students, advisors, committees, and IRBs. There is never too much up-front negotiation and clarification. Collaborative efforts have been supported by the National Institute for Health, which has taken an active role in advancing shared governance of research decisions and findings.

When university students who are working on graduate degrees are part of the CBCAR research team, they may find themselves caught between conflicting pulls. Graduate students are well advised to negotiate up-front with community collaborators, advisors, and committee members to be clear and realistic about: (1) expectations related to the project timeline (keeping in mind that most tasks take longer than planned), (2) funding streams, (3) data ownership, and (4) dissemination decisions and control. The theoretical underpinnings of CBCAR will guide students and their advisors in this process and provide firm ground on which to stand for working through university rules and policies.

The Influence of Funding Agencies

Seifer (2006) cautioned that funding agencies often do not "honor the time and money required to develop partnerships or to achieve tangible community benefits and outcomes" (p. 996). Many funders have established outcomes and processes they want organizations to meet and follow, which might put community-based collaboratives in the position of serving funders' needs over the community's immediate needs and long-term well-being. Additionally, when seeking funds, decisions about what organization is going to administer grant monies are extremely important. Issues to consider are organizational capacity, organizational overhead, equitable allocation of funds, and placing the greatest amount of control possible in the hands of the people most affected. Successful partnerships have shown that when larger funding streams are involved, all partners should be involved in decisions related to hiring staff for key positions, and attempts should be made to invest in the community through hiring community members and purchasing products from community businesses (Seifer, 2006). Chapter 9 provides further information on the funding process for CBCAR projects.

Attending to Self-Referentiality and Reflexivity

Everyone involved in the CBCAR effort has multiple identities and roles that impact their way of viewing the world. We are all "outsiders" and "insiders" in different arenas and aspects of each project we work on and every group we are a part of. Honest and reflective identification regarding one's positionality enhances the ability to be in authentic relationship with partners. Kristiansen and Bloch-Poulson (2004) cautioned against the power mechanism of *self-referentiality*, which involves the unconscious, nondialogic way of transforming the perspective of the other "into your own a priori categories and ways of relating"—a process that assumes that it is "only your reality that counts" (p. 372). We are reminded of a young student who came back to the US from a hitchhiking adventure through Europe. He recounted his concern when heading from France to Germany and the signs that kept pointing toward *Deutschland* rather than Germany. He was carefully following his map and assumed someone had made a mistake. Self-referentiality—the idea that the world works in the way that you know it—is a very common practice that takes conscious effort to notice and deconstruct. If we do not make the effort, we might not recognize our destination when we get there.

Being involved in CBCAR involves an intense and unrelenting practice of questioning one's own perspectives, assumptions, and ways of viewing and making sense of the world. In this way, the world can be seen through the perspective of multiple others' eyes, and thus more fully experienced and understood. To recognize our biases and blind spots takes a fair amount of critical reflection.

Self-reflexivity involves reflecting on and critiquing the influence of one's own gendered, class-based, and racialized position in order to fully and authentically engage in collective reflexive engagement (Chiu, 2006; Genet, 2009). Self-reflexivity is essential at the onset of a CBCAR project to make sure the research collaboration and design include all voices within the community, particularly those voices that have been silenced in the past and are most affected by the issue at hand. Self-reflexivity also informs the data collection and analysis processes and provokes researchers to make sense of data using varied lenses. For that reason, positionality and reflexivity are also examined in subsequent chapters.

Self-reflexivity occurs not only at the personal and interpersonal level, but also at the collective level, where CBCAR partners develop the skill of critiquing findings from a range of theoretical perspectives. For example, when looking at low health screening rates for ethnic minority women, Chiu (2006) and research partners used Black feminist theories to frame their critique of the narrative explanation that low screening rates were caused by women's cultural attachment and language deficits. The participatory action team reframed the issue of low health screening as a "symptom of the routinized professional practice perpetuated through colonial ideologies and racialized practice" that shifted "the responsibility for improving service accessibility for minority ethnic women back to the health professionals" (p. 196). Chiu (2006) referred to the work of sociologist Pierre Bourdieu to better understand the transformative process involved in seeing more clearly the structural forces behind health inequalities, stating, "Bourdieu suggests that cultural resources, practices and institutions function to maintain unequal social relations" (p. 196). CBCAR at its best exposes the cultural systems behind inequalities and aims to create a more just society. Reflexivity encourages all people engaged in conducting the research project to examine their perceptions and biases that could be blinding them to what the data are saying. Removing these blinders is an important aspect of looking behind the data to see a larger picture.

Honestly Unearthing and Addressing Power Differentials

Dialogue that identifies and deconstructs power differentials is an essential aspect of the CBCAR process. Becker et al. (2005) asserted that power and influence in groups come from "expertise, personal attraction, access to information, the ability to reward or punish, legitimate role-based authority, verbal skill, or even self-confidence" (p. 64). They suggested that small groups tend to balance power better than large groups. Kristiansen and Bloch-Paulsen (2004) drew on the work of Foucault to define power not as an individual possession, but rather as a discursive activity; power is produced and exercised through the discursive relationship between action researchers and participants. Seen this way, power can be identified and intentionally shared, once the processes of self-referentiality and self-reflexivity have been consciously attended to by individuals and the collective partnership.

Understanding the historical, political, and sociocultural underpinnings of positions of advantage and disadvantage is a necessary starting point so that the CBCAR process does not replicate societal forces of privilege and oppression, which are often not consciously acknowledged by those who benefit from them. Once the sources of power inequalities have been fully studied and stories adequately shared so that each member of the team is able to map the forces that shape the inequality or problem being addressed, a plan can be put into place to share sources of power. A horizontal rather than hierarchical relationship becomes part of the participatory work (Heron & Reason, 1997). In this way, empowerment becomes an equal process where everyone taps into the source of their own power and puts it on the table for others to examine and take on (Abma, Nierse, & Widdershoven, 2009). Partners from within the community can guide researchers to help them understand the culture within the community, how things work, and what might not work in this community even if it has been successful in other communities. Partners who are trained in the research process can help community members understand the mechanics of the research process and the potential pitfalls if research protocols are not followed. They can also explain the workings and history of the institutions they come from, making them more understandable and accessible to the community. Abma et al. (2009) asserted:

> The prime responsibility of the responsive researcher is not to delegate power to participants, but to enhance the quality of the dialogical process between stakeholders (both in terms of its meaningfulness and its relational quality). For a genuine dialogue to take place, the responsive researcher is sensitive to power imbalances and the subtle process of exclusion. (Mertens, 2002, p. 404)

In many communities margins exist that are known only to the people who are on the peripheral side of the margins. In the CBCAR project aimed at improving patient outcomes on a nursing unit, the people on the margin may be the housekeeping staff whose names and stories are not known by the nursing and medical staff, but who provide patients' frightened and tired partners a cup of coffee, a warm blanket, and a listening ear in the family lounge. In the CBCAR project aimed at reducing barriers to community health services, the people on the margin may be single mothers working two jobs to support their children. An effort needs to be made to erase the margins and address the barriers that prevent the involvement of people who are living beyond the margin, yet may have essential insight that could give rise to effective actions. Rabinovitch (2004) calls on action researchers to *[re]move* the margins, which involves getting beyond *us* and *them* thinking in order to move and remove the margins. When what had been *us* and *them* becomes *we*, we are more able to stretch the margins even further to welcome in even more diverse voices to the collaborative. Oftentimes, partners who thought that they were smack dab in the center, realize upon hearing the stories of the people "on the margins" that it was actually they themselves who had been on the margins when standing on a moral or relational plane. Once they make this realization, their world becomes larger and their life takes on new possibilities. It is within the honest, open, nonjudgmental dialogue—involving storytelling and story beholding between diverse stakeholders—that new possibilities become a reality.

The Role of Researchers

The role of the research partner in community-based action research is different from the role of a researcher in traditional or community-placed research. The research partner is someone who regardless of affiliation brings expertise to the collaborative to help design the research question(s), determine methods, guide data collection and analysis, and interpret results. The community partners are also engaged in these activities and have an insider's view that informs the collection and interpretation of data; they simply lack the technical skills of the researcher (Zimmerman et al., 2009). In action research, the researcher is socially available and walks humbly and attentively with a main focus on creating community and healthy relationships, actively learning all he or she possibly can about the community's history and the formal and informal groupings in the community (Stringer, 2007). CBCAR research partners see themselves as a catalyst serving a process that is by and of the community. Control of the research question and the final research results will not be theirs; but rather they will belong to the collaborative. Stringer (2007) encourages researchers to "aim to present themselves in ways likely to be perceived as skilled, supportive, resourceful, and approachable" (p.48). Ideally, they will teach well enough that their technical skills will be needed less and less as the CBCAR project matures through several cycles

Periodically Assessing Process, Workload, and Relationships

Successful CBCAR project teams schedule time to collectively assess their structure, culture, workload balance, resources, and relational strengths. It is also important to critically reflect on how the process is going for all partners—to evaluate whether there have been changes in process, power dynamics, and/or means of communication. Checking in on these issues can be the first item on the agenda of meetings, while attending to the balance between attention to group process and actually getting the necessary work done. Regularly scheduled critical reflection on group process helps CBCAR work teams function productively and stay true to the project's purpose; this is an essential aspect of process evaluation (see **Table 4-1**).

Creating a Process and Content Record that Is Accessible to All

The importance of keeping good records of CBCAR process and content cannot be stressed too often. These written records are often called audit trails, and they are presented in the literature as a way to advance the quality of the research study. Chapters 5 and 6 will also examine the use of audit trails, but they begin with detailing the collaborative process in the early stages of the project. Besides advancing scientific rigor, audit trails have other benefits. For example, when beginning a project, CBCAR team members often do not anticipate that further into the CBCAR process they might have differing recollections about earlier decisions that had been made. At the point of dissemination, the group may come to realize that it is actually their process itself that is the most important aspect of what needs to be disseminated. For this

Table 4-1 Aspects of CBCAR Evaluation

Type of evaluation	Who is responsible	Methods of collection	Time of collection
Group process	All work groups evaluate their process on a regular basis	Key process questions are placed on every agenda. Answers are analyzed to improve process. These determinations and decisions are recorded in the minutes. Particular attention is paid to critiquing whether the key stake-holders' voices are being adequately heard.	At the end of every significant work group meeting
Baseline and evolving pattern	The advisory group and/ or research partnership group or designees	Data are collected and presented to provide as complete a pattern as possible to view the phenomenon of interest and related variables. Pattern data are useful for clarifying the research focus and in funding proposals to demonstrate need.	Project initiation and as new patterns emerge; this pattern can be reassessed at the end of the project to identify transforma-tions in the pattern.
Project flow	Subgroup named by advisory group	Compare progress against timeline. Interview/group dynamics survey of members from each work group.	Set intervals during course of project
Emerging insights	Subgroup named by the advisory group	Interview work groups and conduct analysis of meeting records.	Set intervals during course of project
CBCAR process impact on team members	Subgroup named by the advisory group	Collect the stories of CBCAR team members.	End of project
Collective self-reflective critique	Advisory group and the entire project team	Group reflection on the question: How might life be better for the most vulnerable in the target population of this project because of our work?	End of project, before beginning another research cycle

reason, careful attention should be paid to creating a method to record group processes and decisions. A documents room where records of meeting decisions and descriptions of processes are safely stored becomes a very important CBCAR space; it will need at least one attentive guardian. This room may be a physical space, such as a secured filing cabinet, or it may be a website. Ideally all records are stored in at least two locations—hardcopy and electronically if possible—and are accessible to all project members, with the exception of data collected during the research process from participants. These confidential research data records are kept secured by the data collection team following Institutional Review Board guidelines for the protection of human participants. People who work in nursing academia or other institutions where periodic accreditation visits occur know how important good data recordkeeping is. If documents are in good shape and the system is organized, accreditation visitors can easily assess what has been happening over the years. CBCAR research projects are no different.

Another important aspect of the process recording or audit trail is that CBCAR teams might not realize how profound their work is until the end since a basic tenet of CBCAR is that essential actions emerge from the process. Addressing the importance of giving voice to the experience of participants, particularly presenting the voices of the oppressed, Chiu (2006) stated:

> [I]t is intellectually unsatisfying to hear these voices without knowing how they were generated and encouraged in dialogues, how they were previously disrupted and silenced, and how they reveal multiple identities and social locations thus leading to the unsettling of existing power relations. Voices that are just voices have no intrinsic claim to truth (Reason, 1994), neither do they have the practical value of informing others of how the central concerns for engagement, dialogue and pragmatic outcomes have been addressed. (p. 188)

Reflection on the CBCAR processes sheds light on how changes occurred. Documents of these reflections contain important CBCAR findings to be analyzed and disseminated.

■ Seeking and Engaging Critical Friends

The wider the perspective of the participants in the research process, the greater the view of the phenomenon of interest will be. For this reason, critical friends are actively sought out to critique the research design and process and to engage the academic researchers and community in dialogue about whose voice is being represented and how. The term "critical friend" was proposed by Sagor (1992) as someone who "has your interests at heart when she gives you constructive criticism" and is invited in to "guard against incomplete or short-sighted data collection" and surface additional questions for consideration (p. 46). Critical friends are sought who have expertise in the task at hand and who might challenge the theoretical underpinnings, research methods, and content perspectives on the phenomenon being studied. When the research team has heavy involvement from academia, critical friends from the community will be essential. Similarly, when the researchers are all primarily situated within the community, critical friends with methodological and theoretical expertise will be essential to the process. A critical friend is not a consultant. Sagor (1992) shared the following set of guidelines that Project LEARN developed for their cadre of critical friends:

1. The critical friend will be chosen based on the needs and desires of the project participants.
2. The critical friend will not have any stake in the problem being addressed or in the outcome of the project unless such ownership is granted by the participants.
3. The critical friend is a positive friend whose primary agenda is to assist in moving the project toward success.
4. The critical friend may have a personal agenda complementary to the project agenda. The critical friend will share with the participants their motives or intents at the time of the first interaction.
5. The critical friend is a visitor and participates only at the continued invitation of the project participants.
6. The critical friend will respond and act honestly at every juncture.

7. It is the obligation of the critical friend to declare any conflict of interest or conflict of values with the project focus or methods.

8. The critical friend will assume that the project's interactions, work, and findings are confidential unless the project directs otherwise.

9. The participants are expected to assist the critical friend by fully informing them of all agendas prior to each consultation. (Sagor, 1992, p. 47)

As critical friends become engaged and invested in the process, they often become good friends who lose their critical stance and join the CBCAR team. At this point there must be an intentional effort to widen the circle and invite a new and more critical set of critical friends.

■ Evaluating the CBCAR Process: Capturing Patterns Now and Then

In CBCAR, the team attends to how the work and process will be evaluated prior to the time that they begin collecting data, but the evaluation methods are not fixed at the initiation of the project. Just as knowledge and methods emerge during the CBCAR process, so too, evaluation insight and process become constructed and reconstructed as the project marches along. Data from reflective meetings lend insights to project evaluation (Chui, 2006). To not think about evaluation at the beginning of a CBCAR project would be like deciding to cut your own hair without first getting a mirror; the outcome might leave something to be desired. Periodic evaluation also helps the group assure that they are maintaining a focus on and listening to the voices of people within the critical reference group. Participatory processes call for participatory methods of evaluation. Schultz, Israel, and Lantz (2003) drew on the work of Knight to define participatory evaluation as a systematic inquiry that involves "collaborative self-critical communities" assessing "their process and progress toward intermediary and outcome objectives" (p. 252). Other evaluation theorists propose emergent designs in which it is impossible to identify the exact goals of the evaluation or the specific design prior to initiating the project (Baur, Abma, & Widdershoven, 2010). So too, in CBCAR, due to its theoretical understanding of change as not being predictable and its expectation of emergent realities, objectives are not written in a prescriptive sense, and attention is focused on the quality of the process and emergent outcomes from a perspective of justice and community well-being, particularly for the most vulnerable. For a hospital collaborative team, the focus may be on quality care and organizational performance. Evaluation sheds light on how the project is operating, whether timelines are being met, how the process is working, what intermediary outcomes are being achieved, and whether new directions and outcomes are emerging from the CBCAR process (see Table 4-1).

For many projects, engaging community members in the CBCAR process of discerning pattern and meaning is in and of itself transformative. Systems changes take place well before the team gets to the action planning. An example is a health department and rural community clinic partnership focused on increasing health screening in a migrant community, which is largely Spanish-speaking. The research partnership group had decided to collect patient satisfaction data and health screening records prior to the initiation of the project; however, there were other outcomes that arose from the process. The CBCAR community advisory group had several very strong, charismatic migrant workers who at the second meeting shared dramatic stories about their experiences with the clinic, as well as the experience of their neighbors. The advisory group members from the community health clinic were so moved by the stories they heard, that they initiated substantial changes within a week of the meeting. The team also learned that there were no curtains in the pelvic rooms, and male interpreters simply turned their back on the patient—not a comfortable situation for female patients, who told their friends, who subsequently avoided having pelvic exams. Needless to say, within 1 week there were curtains in the pelvic rooms and an additional female interpreter was added to the staff. By the end of the project, several CBCAR team members who worked at the clinic were enrolled in Spanish language classes, and a trip was being planned to the town where most of the migrant workers came from. None of these actions were part of the original plan; they simply emerged from the process.

CBCAR team members will experience growth in many aspects of their lives. They will certainly have developed many very meaningful relationships that have made them better persons and more responsible citizens of society. Their relational expertise and critical analysis skills will have grown exponentially. Many community members go on to university to study new areas of interest; research partners find their work more fulfilling and meaningful. At the end of the project a complete CBCAR project evaluation will collect people's stories—particularly people whose voices have traditionally been marginalized—to grasp the full flavor of what has happened, not simply the consensus of experience (Widdershoven, 2001). Simple, open-ended questions will elicit deep responses—questions like: "Tell me the story of your participation in this project." and/or: "Tell me about what was most meaningful in your work on this project."

If there is any inkling that in spite of the group's best efforts and attention to equity of voice, the most marginalized stakeholders in the project do not feel they have been equal partners in the project, the group may want to invite in a critical friend or two to engage in a process designed to gain insight into these dynamics.

■ Summary—Convergence of Relationships, Methods, and Work Plan

We begin the CBCAR process by developing strong, respectful, caring relationships that extend beyond our immediate social and work groups. People come together to address a particular issue of concern and to understand it more deeply. They discern how to relate to one another and learn how to dialogue. They talk about what they would like to do and how they might evaluate whether they have done good work at the end of their project. They learn about the CBCAR approach, how to formulate a research question, how to choose research methods and carry them out, and how to ask and answer hard questions—often mainly focused on themselves. They learn about joy and meaning in life. They notice patterns. They find new ways of being in the world and new ways to be part of positive change. As action research theorist Ernie Stringer (2007) stated:

> Action research seeks to develop and maintain social and personal interactions that are nonexploitative and enhance the social and emotional lives of all people who participate. It is organized and conducted in ways that are conducive to the formation of community—the "common unity" of all participants—and that strengthen the democratic, equitable, liberating, and life-enhancing qualities of social life." (pp. 27–28)

The underpinnings of CBCAR suggest that change is unpredictable and that the world is a unitary whole, and when we are guided by principles of social justice and human rights to participate in uncovering, analyzing, and addressing patterns of health and well-being, our participation in the world brings about meaningful change and human flourishing for all.

The first and most important step in the CBCAR process is preparing the soil before planting the tree. It may involve some research and dedicated study of how big of a hole to dig, what kind of mulch is needed, how much water should be added, whether a fertilizer is necessary, and how to prepare the roots for their new environment. This careful tending will bear great fruit in the years to come.

■ References

Abma, T. A., Nierse, C. J., & Widdershoven, G. A. M. (2009). Patients as partners in responsive research: Methodological notions for collaborations in mixed research teams. *Qualitative Health Research, 19*(3), 401–415.

Baur, V. E., Abma, T. A., & Widdershoven, G. A. M. (2010). Participation of marginalized groups in evaluation: Mission impossible? *Evaluation and Program Planning, 33,* 238–245.

Becker, A. B., Israel, B. A., & Allen, A. J. (2005). Strategies and techniques for effective group process in CBPR partnerships. In B.A. Israel, E. Eng, A. J. Schultz, & E. A. Parker (Eds.), *Methods in community-based participatory research for health* (pp. 52–72). San Francisco, CA: Jossey-Bass.

Bohm, D. (1992). On dialogue. *Noetic Sciences Review, 23,* 16–18.

Bohm, D., & Nichol, L. (Ed.). (1996). *On dialogue.* London, UK: Routledge.

Bohm, D., Factor, D., & Garrett, P. (1991). *Dialogue—A proposal.* Retrieved from http://www.david-bohm.net/dialogue/dialogue_proposal.html

Chambers, R. (2004). *Participatory workshops: A sourcebook of 21 sets of ideas & activities.* London, UK: Earthscan.

Chiu, L. F. (2006). Critical reflection: More than nuts and bolts. *Action Research, 4*(2), 183–203.

Genat, B. (2009). Building emergent situated knowledges in participatory action research. *Action Research, 7,* 101–115.

Guba, E. G., & Lincoln, Y. S. (1989). *Fourth generation evaluation.* Newbury Park, CA: Sage.

Heron, J., & Reason, P. (1997). A participatory inquiry paradigm. *Qualitative Inquiry, 3*(3), 274–294.

Hesse-Biber, S. N., & Leavy, P. (2008). Pushing on the methodological boundaries: The growing need for emergent methods within and across the discipline. In S. N. Hesse-Biber & P. Leavy (Eds.), *Handbook of emergent methods.* New York, NY: Guildford Press.

Kristiansen, M., & Bloch-Poulsen, J. (2004). Self-referentiality as a power mechanism. *Action Research, 2*(4), 371–388.

Mertens, D. M. (2009). *Transformative research and evaluation.* New York, NY: The Guildford Press.

Nichol, L. (1996). Foreword. In D. Bohm (author) & L. Nichol (Ed.), *On dialogue.* London, UK: Routledge.

Phillips, M. E. (2004). Action research and development coalitions in health care. *Action Research, 2*(4), 349–370.

Pierre-Louis, B., Akoh, V., White, P., & Pharris, M. D. (2010). The pattern of African American women with diabetes. *Nursing Science Quarterly,* at press.

Prior, D. (2007). Decolonising research: A shift toward reconciliation. *Nursing Inquiry, 14*(2), 162–168.

Rabinovitch, J. (2004). *Transforming community practice: [Re]moving the margins.* Retrieved from http://comm-org.wisc.edu/papers2005/rabinovitch

Reason, P. (1994). Three approaches to participatory inquiry. In N. K. Denzin, & Y. S. Lincoln (Eds.), *Handbook of qualitative research* (p. 324–338). London, UK: Sage.

Reason, P., & Bradbury, H. (2006). Preface. In P. Reason, & H. Bradbury (Eds.). *The handbook of action research*. London, UK: Sage.

Sagor, R. (1992). *How to conduct collaborative action research*. Alexandria, Virginia: Association for Supervision and Curriculum Development.

Schaffer, M. A. (2009). A virtue ethics guide to best practices for community-based participatory research. *Progress in Community Health Partnerships, 3*(1), 83–90.

Scharmer, C.O. (2009). *Theory u: Leading from the future as it emerges*. San Francisco, CA: Berrett-Koehler.

Schultz, A. J., Israel, B. A., & Lantz, P. (2003). Instrument for evaluating dimensions of group dynamics within community-based participatory research collaborative. *Evaluation and Program Planning, 26*, 249–262.

Seifer, S. D. (2006). Building and sustaining community-institutional partnerships for prevention research: Findings from a national collaborative. *Journal of Urban Health: Bulletin of the New York Academy of Medicine, 83*(6), 989–1003.

Smith, S. (1997). Deepening participatory action-research. In S. Smith, D. G. Willms, & N. A. Johnson (Eds.), *Nurtured by knowledge: Learning to do participatory action-research* (pp. 173–263). New York, NY: The Apex Press.

Stringer, E. (2007). *Action research*. Los Angeles, CA: Sage.

Thorne, S. (2008). *Interpretive description*. Walnut Creek, CA: Left Coast Press.

Widdershoven, G. A. M. (2001). Dialogue in evaluation: A hermeneutic perspective. *Evaluation, 7*(2), 253–263.

Wright, M. T., Roche, B., Von Unger, H., Block, M., & Gardner, B. (2010). A call for an international collaboration on participatory research for health. *Health Promotion International, 25*(1), 115–122.

Zimmerman, S., Tilly, J., Cohen, L., & Love, K. (2009). *A manual for community-based participatory research: Using research to improve practice and inform policy in assisted living*. Retrieved from http://www.shepscenter.unc.edu/research_programs/aging/publications/CEAL-UNC%20Manual%20for%20Community-Based%20Participatory%20Research-1.pdf

Creating the Real-Life Narratives: Engaging in Data Collection

*T*rees have many elements, intersections, and angles. When examining a tree, we often focus on its appearance—noting and frequently appreciating how large the tree stands, how wide the branches stretch, how cool the leaves shade. However, as scientists, we query beyond appearances and systematically scrutinize behind, underneath, around, and inside. The tacit elements of the tree only speak if deliberately explored. Studying inside the tree's existence means examining its unique features: how the tree has grown, developed, and adapted; its resilience and frailties; and its immediate and far-reaching environmental interactions. Each tree offers a story of living contextual realities, and as scientists, we formulate relevant questions and use various tools to elicit information and subsequently learn various facets of the tree's existence and environment.

The systematic process of collecting data by reaching deeply for authentic individual, collective, and contextual understandings of human realities is the subject of this chapter. Data collection about people's realities generally involves qualitative data collection strategies such as interviews and focus group sessions. Listening to narrations of participants' experiences, CBCAR investigators explore perspectives, contexts, conditions, and social interactions. For example, participants may be asked in a variety of ways to describe how they perceive or find meaning in the research phenomenon. Subsequently, data are collected that provide insight into the meaning of the phenomenon being researched and dynamics underlying community or system patterns. Dialogue ensues, narratives are constructed, and patterns emerge. Data collection continues until patterns are understood.

Other sources of data, such as demographic and/or survey data may assist the research team in seeing the emerging patterns. For example, statistical data that describe particular characteristics and community context may supplement our understanding of participants' situations. Social epidemiologic research can measure and assess the effects of contextual variables, such as average neighborhood income or green space access on population health risks (Torres-Harding, Herrell, & Howard, 2004). Quantitative data often provide valuable background and contextual information regarding understandings of people's health and well-being. Similarly, statistical data on organizational performance, such as medication error variables or hospital-acquired infection rates provide fuller understandings of system operations. However, since CBCAR's primary data source pertains to people and their narrations of contextual reality, this chapter focuses on qualitative data collection principles and processes. After describing principles, we offer a flexible data collection pathway. We then consider issues associated with data collection site entry. Perspectives on collaboratively developing and implementing a data collection plan are offered. We integrate pertinent ethical principles and provide suggestions for advancing data quality. Finally, we describe data collection strategies and offer examples of tools for collecting people's narrations.

■ Principles of CBCAR Data Collection

Similar to other primarily qualitative research designs, data collection within a CBCAR framework draws on many strategies such as in-depth interviews, participant observation, and focus groups. If a traditional research design is being used, then specific data collection tools can be developed within a particular design, such as an ethnographic interview guide. If an emergent design is being used, then focus groups that explore perspectives about the research topic are particularly helpful early in the CBCAR process (Genat, 2009; Morgan, Fellows, & Guevara, 2008). Subsequent data collection strategies and tools emerge from data collected in those early focus groups. Additionally, data gathering tools that are associated with participatory data collection such as mapping, diagramming, and ranking contribute valuable information about participants' perspectives and offer ideas for action planning (Barnidge, Baker, Motton, Rose, & Fitzgerald, 2010; Chambers, 1997; Ellsberg & Heise, 2005; Kumar, 2002; Pretty, Guijt, Thompson, & Scoones, 2002; Sethi & Belliard, 2009). Therefore, CBCAR teams must be knowledgeable about the options and deliberately select from a variety of data collection strategies and tools. Whether using data collection strategies associated with traditional research designs or developing strategies and tools relevant to participatory and emergent designs, certain data collection principles are especially pertinent to CBCAR (see **Box 5-1**).

Data Collection as Relevant, Practical, Rigorous, and Action-Oriented Inquiry

Investigating practical and pressing issues relevant to the daily lives of people in communities and organizations, CBCAR researchers should scientifically collect data that is oriented toward deeper understandings of problem situations and their potential solutions. Research teams investigate, analyze, and carefully select data collection strategies that not only relate to the research question and design, but also provide insight on community context and relevant actions. First, from the research question, research partners extract key concepts that are subsequently explored during data collection. If, for example, a CBCAR team's research question is, "What are the factors that contribute to ethical dilemmas in critical care nursing?" the key concepts are "ethical dilemmas" and "contributing factors."

Box 5-1 Principles of Data Collection

Data collection is:

- Relevant, practical, rigorous, and action oriented
- Circular, progressive, and iterative learning
- Paradoxical positioning
- Collaboratively planned and implemented
- Ethical and authentic human interaction
- Contextual diagramming
- Pluralistic and triangular
- Joint meaning construction within research conversations

When considering their own projects and contexts, research teams may expand or revise these principles while remaining grounded in CBCAR's foundational elements.

Second, context is considered. In the previous example, the context would be critical care settings in acute care facilities. From context, research teams extract pertinent data sources such as stakeholders who have a shared interest in the research phenomenon, people who are particularly affected by the phenomenon, or demographic information that offers valuable insight into the setting's characteristics. Finally, CBCAR teams select data collection strategies that yield practical information and also create action opportunities for changing people's beliefs and behaviors and systems' policies and practices. Research partners should consider key concepts and context when selecting or developing data collection strategies and tools.

Data Collection as Circular, Progressive, and Iterative Learning

Data collection is portrayed as an ongoing learning cycle in CBCAR projects. Chambers (1997) described data collection in participatory action research as "Conscious exploration, flexible use of methods, opportunism, improvisation, iteration, and cross-checking" (p. 157). According to Senge and Scharmer (2006), data collection is an active learning process that balances attentive inquiry with reflective stillness. Key components of progressive learning during data collection include heightened awareness and the ability to "presence"—to be still and become aware of inner reflections in the presence of data. Recording and sharing inner reflections often shape emergent learning and guide further data collection (Stringer, 2007).

Additionally, as learning ensues during data collection, CBCAR teams refer back to the research question to assess whether pertinent insights are developing and move forward to data analysis to query whether further data collection is required. For example, if using a grounded theory design within the CBCAR approach, research partners usually initiate data analysis after conducting the first few interviews, and subsequently, use theoretic sampling to seek participants with special knowledge of the ideas emerging from initial data analysis (Charmaz, 2008). In ethnographic CBCAR projects, data analysis often occurs concurrently with data collection—with ongoing analysis often guiding the collection of subsequent data (Roper & Shapira, 2000). This iterative movement between research question, design, data collection, and analysis contributes to the circular and ongoing learning that occurs during data collection (Creswell, 1998; Pawar, 2004; Suarez-Balcazar et al., 2006).

Data Collection as Paradoxical Positioning

As deliberative, scientific work within a particular research setting, CBCAR data collection poses important paradoxes. For example, research teams cannot distance themselves from the research setting and yet, to collect data, they need to establish some distance from the social experiences being studied. Shkedi (2005) asserted that during data collection research partners should seek a balance between "involvement and immersion on the one hand and distance and critical thinking on the other" (p. 47). The former is necessary for negotiating access, establishing rapport, being sensitive to community or organizational concerns, and understanding participants' perspectives. However, this involvement requires careful reflection, to stand apart from what is being learned in order to understand the multiple angles and interpretations that are inherent in the information (see **Box 5-2**). Additionally, data collectors must earn the trust of participants and be genuinely present to their difficulties while remaining politically and personally neutral to the data that are being collected in the research setting (Stringer, 2007). Finally, as data are collected and knowledge is accrued, the tendency for researchers to view themselves as experts increases. While CBCAR partners gain valuable information and expanding expertise during data collection, they should paradoxically view themselves as humble learners and informed novices who sit beside the real experts, i.e., the research participants whose daily lives occur in the situations and settings being studied (Thorne, 2008). The various tensions inherent in these paradoxical positions are an inescapable component of data collection in CBCAR projects.

Data Collection as Collaboratively Planned and Implemented

Collaborative planning for data collection benefits from community members' knowledge of community context and academic researchers' knowledge of various sampling strategies and data collecting techniques. The cognitive mingling that results from dialogue between community members and academic researchers yields valuable guidance in designing a research-specific and community-appropriate data collection plan. Furthermore, when community members partner with academic researchers to collect data, the capacity for developing deeper understandings about the research phenomenon and its context blossoms both ways. This bi-directional learning relationship is particularly significant for emergent research designs where data collection is partially dependent on what is being learned within the research process and not just as a result of the research process.

Box 5-2 Paradoxical Positioning During Data Collection

Using a variety of strategies and tools, data collectors engage with people to elicit information regarding the research topic. This requires data collectors to adopt paradoxical stances of unity and separation, detachment, and engagement with data sources and resulting data (Patton, 2002). Referring to simultaneous activities of developing data insights and evaluating their meanings and impacts, these paradoxes can be difficult to maneuver during data collection. Similarly, Haraway (1988) described "passionate detachment" (p. 585) as developing close relationships with participants, and subsequently, detaching oneself from those relationships enough to critically examine their influence on data, data meanings, and self as data collector—becoming a part of participants' worlds while remaining apart from the data.

Occasional opportunities for data collection team members to debrief can be helpful (Naples, 2003). Additionally, attending to these paradoxes in field notes or reflective notebooks capitalizes on the data collector's potential to expand data meanings and develop significant insights (Patton, 2002).

Data Collection as Ethical and Authentic Human Interaction

Data in CBCAR projects are usually gathered during interactions with people in their community or work settings. Additionally, observations of people as they interact with their environments might be included. Describing work with an Aboriginal community, Genat (2009) described data collection as a "space of interaction [among research partners] where emergent meaning [is] examined, contested, debated, reviewed, recorded, and constructed" (p. 107). Ideally, interactions are characterized by mutual respect, shared interests, open communication, joint meaning construction, and authenticity. Lincoln and Guba (1985) claimed that researchers are the research instrument in qualitative data collection. As such, they should be responsive, sensitive, adaptable, inquisitive, and able to clarify, link, and summarize data within various interactive data collection strategies.

Ethical interactions during data collection require attention to the principles of respect for persons, beneficence, justice, and respect for communities (Kitchener & Kitchener, 2009; Lincoln, 2009; Mack, Woodsong, MacQueen, Guest, & Namey, 2005; Smith, 2000). Full disclosure during informed consent, noncoercive tactics when recruiting participants and gathering data, keen sensitivity to any potential harm to participants or communities, attention to confidentiality, and emphasis on the voluntary nature of participation are vital researcher responsibilities during data collection and throughout the research process.

Data Collection as Contextual Diagramming

As CBCAR researchers enter research settings and, through data collection, into participants' lives, they should view narrated perspectives and experiences within a larger context. Creating visual diagrams of systems and structures that influence participants' experiences is a valuable part of data collection. Genat (2009) asserted that "the research question is at the hub of a social arena, a system of social worlds of various stakeholders each who have some interest in the research question" (p. 109). Contextual diagramming avoids isolating human experiences into parts and instead encourages CBCAR researchers to search for patterns and interactions that depict the whole.

Data Collection as Pluralistic and Triangular

Multiple data collection strategies are usually necessary to examine the complex human, health, and social questions that pertain to CBCAR projects (Stringer, 2007; Suarez-Balcazar et al., 2006). Triangulation refers to using multiple data collection strategies within the same research project to expand, clarify, compare, and cross-check meaning (Thurmond, 2001; Pawar, 2004). In some CBCAR projects, triangulation may mean multiple data collection strategies within a single qualitative-constructivist paradigm. In other projects, triangulation, sometimes called a pluralistic (Pawar, 2004) or mixed-methods (Mertens, 2005) approach, indicates multiple data collection strategies across qualitative and quantitative methods. The pluralistic approach embraces both objective and subjective aspects of reality—reaching across traditions to discover multiple meanings in people's realities. Claiming that quantitative and qualitative data collection strategies complement each other, Suarez-Balcazar et al. (2006) stated, "As community researchers, we are not only interested in numerical data descriptions of participants and context, but also rich stories and voices that help explain or illustrate those numbers" (p. 109). The ultimate aim of triangulation and pluralism is to produce trustworthy and credible evidence; however, using multiple data collection strategies does not ensure credibility. A rigorous study requires several built-in mechanisms to enhance trustworthiness.

Data Collection as Joint Meaning Construction Within Research Conversations

Gathering qualitative data in interviews, focus groups, and other data collection strategies is more than seeking and recording descriptions of experiences. Research teams simply cannot claim to understand people just by what is seen or heard (Shkedi, 2005). Instead, scientists actively and patiently pursue understanding through the art of questioning for meaning (Holstein & Gubrium, 1995). Gadamer (1960/1995) asserted that the skill of inquiry requires gentle persistence in questioning and preserving an orientation towards openness. Although data collection may start with a question/answer format, CBCAR inquirers should transition rather quickly into creating a "context for conversation" where questions open the quest for meaning (Herda, 1999, p. 113).

Advising researchers to specifically aim for joint construction of meaning within data gathering sessions, Mishler (1986) suggested that inquirers avoid assuming to understand and instead pursue questions that elicit participants' tacit understandings of their experiences. Polanyi (1962) distinguished between explicit and tacit knowledge. Representing customary explanations and scientific descriptions, explicit knowledge is readily expressed information. However, as unarticulated understandings and assumed truths, tacit knowledge is much more difficult for research teams to access, and yet also more important since tacit understandings often form the basis for human perceptions and actions. CBCAR researchers may initiate research conversations by seeking explicit knowledge about the research phenomenon but should move beyond the explicit and seek tacit understandings—or the meanings that participants attach to their experiences. The essential element for CBCAR inquirers during data collection is to avoid assuming they know and instead use "indwelling" with participants, i.e., staying within the experience while focusing away from explicit knowledge of the experience and instead attending to the experience's tacit meanings (Polanyi, 1962). This is not an easy task and requires being open to learning, creating shared understandings, and reaching a fusion of horizons between text (written or spoken) and inquirer (Gadamer, 1960/1995).

Summary of Data Collection Principles

The principles of CBCAR data collection should be reviewed and discussed by collaborating research teams prior to designing data collection strategies and tools. Adjustments and expansions to these principles may be necessary as research teams consider their own projects and contexts. Our only caution is that if principles are added or revised, those changes are rooted in theories and concepts that are compatible with the foundational principles of CBCAR process—that is, action science, unitary–transformative participatory paradigm, and social justice.

■ Overview of the Data Collection Process

The process of creating real-life narratives nestles inside the entire CBCAR process, and therefore, is inherently related to all other CBCAR steps. Extracting the data collection phase from the larger CBCAR process, we illustrate the progressive steps and circular motion of planning and creating the research text (see **Figure 5-1**). Most often, CBCAR projects occur within organizations or communities. Social scientists, anthropologists, and other scholars frequently label the settings where data are collected as field sites and data collection as fieldwork (Denzin & Lincoln, 2000; Patton, 2002; Thorne, 2008). However, this nomenclature can create false images of geographic distance, colonizing ideologies, foreign realms, and power hierarchies. We believe that

Figure 5-1 Data Collection Pathway with Site Entry Points

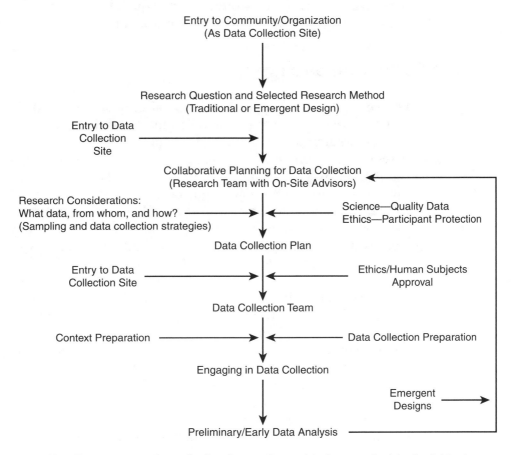

Note: Team can enter data collection site at various points; however, the later the field entry point, the less site-specific the project might become (can still be collaborative in planning).

CBCAR projects can occur in any setting. For example, some CBCAR projects might develop within collaborative groups who seek to study themselves and the processes they use in everyday practices. Entry into the research setting in that situation pertains more to a certain mindset or mental space rather than an actual physical place. So for clarity and inclusivity, in this chapter we use the terms *data collection sites* to indicate the settings in which the research occurs; *research participants* to identify people who supply information on the research topic; and *data collection strategies and tools* to indicate the means by which data are accrued. Data collection as emergent, iterative, and circular indicates that the research team is constantly questioning whether additional participants, settings, or strategies are required for deeper and more authentic understandings of the research topic.

■ Data Collection Site Entry

During CBCAR projects, researchers collect data in community and organizational settings that are politically, socially, economically, and culturally dynamic and complex. The research team bases site selection on the research question and generally selects specific sites when designing the study. Data collection sites can range from patient care units to major medical centers, from local neighborhoods to expansive metropolitan areas, and from small nonprofit agencies to multi-organizational alliances. In any given CBCAR project, more than one data collection site may be required. For example, in research situations when findings might reflect poorly on the setting, Thorne (2008) suggested that researchers use multiple settings and avoid naming specific institutions unless expressly approved. She stated, "It can help to remember that [the] ultimate goal is to engage systems in making constructive change, not alienate them from the findings [the research team] produces" (p. 122). Using multiple data collection sites also provides opportunities for pluralities and comparisons. Keep in mind that adding sites requires further approval by the original institutional ethics committee (such as an IRB) and usually an ethics representative or committee in each new setting.

As illustrated in Figure 5-1, if entry into a data collection site is required, that entry can occur at various points in the data collection planning process. When members of the research partnership are part of the setting that will be studied in CBCAR projects, site entry generally occurs at the outset of CBCAR projects. For example, a nurse practitioner who is employed by a hospital may partner with nurses in several patient care units to study the institutional factors that contribute to elevated rehospitalization rates for elderly, congestive heart failure patients. Since site-insiders conduct the study, site entry has already occurred. In contrast, the research partnership may choose to examine the full spectrum of care and include home healthcare factors that also contribute to rehospitalization rates. Adding a home care agency site—which may be an unfamiliar setting for the research team—would result in site entry further into the collaborative planning process. In emergent designs, as other settings are added, site entry continues to occur along the research process as needed.

In situations involving geographic distance, research experts, community partners, and on-site staff may collaborate electronically and plan the entire data collection process while academic research partners are outside the data collection site. Therefore, some members of the research team may not actually enter the setting until late in the process. The key component in any CBCAR project is collaborative planning among all research partners. Ideally, site entry occurs early in the collaborative process; however, each research project has its own particular pathway, and therefore, site entry could occur at different points for different projects.

Site Entry Guidelines

Whether early or later in the data collection pathway, site entry is an important aspect of CBCAR projects and requires careful planning. Certain guidelines may be helpful (see **Box 5-3**). First, scientific data collection in any setting requires careful preparation. Although human beings are natural observers of their environment, disciplined and scientific observing is not natural. Before entering research settings to collect data, research team members should deliberately and carefully prepare for the

---

Box 5-3 Site Entry Guidelines

- Prepare to enter the setting as scientific rather than casual observers.
- Start learning about context before entering the field and continue learning while in the field.
- Establish credibility without becoming the expert.
- Keep a descriptive and insightful notebook about information being learned, questions and opportunities to pursue, and critical reflections that arise.
- Plan site entry carefully and determine who should be early contacts in the setting:
  - Community residents
  - Community groups
  - Community leaders—informal and formal
  - Stakeholders
  - Gatekeepers
  - Site advisors
  - Project advisory group
  - Critical friends
- Seek wise site advisors who can help navigate the setting and, if appropriate, invite them into the research partnership and/or process.
- Prepare a clear, crisp purpose statement that also implies opportunities for collaboration.

---

transition of simply being a casual, everyday observer to becoming a scientist who has the following characteristics:

- Systematic and focused attentiveness
- Perceptive and discerning ears
- Observant and inquiring eyes
- Respectful and nonjudgmental attitude

- ■ Disciplined and descriptive writing and recording skills
- ■ Critical and reflective pauses

Patton (2002) claimed that preparing to become a skilled data collector is as rigorous as training to become a proficient statistician. All members of the data collection team should deliberately prepare themselves mentally, physically, intellectually, and psychologically for the intense concentration required during scientific data collection. In addition, actively practicing data gathering techniques and pilot testing data collection tools are helpful ways to prepare for data collection (Herda, 1999; Patton, 2002).

Second, being informed about research settings eases site entry. Representing 11 community-based organizations that participated in CBCAR projects, Van der Eb et al. (2005) claimed that community members appreciate researchers who spend time learning about local cultures, customary activities, historical events, and social and political realities. Occasionally, community representatives "test" researchers' knowledge and genuine interest in their communities or organizations by asking researchers specific questions pertaining to the site. This "testing" might represent on-site members' attempts to assess the research team's readiness to collect data in the community or organization. Additionally, site representatives could be identifying researchers' positions on a specific topic or analyzing the amount of orientation work that will be required to prepare the data collection team. Therefore, advanced preparation about the setting is important.

Third, research team members should record the information that they glean prior to entering the setting and keep recording information that is gathered at the site. These descriptive notes about the setting are a valuable resource for contacts and context. However, information about the setting, whether written or spoken, is usually shared from a particular viewpoint, so becoming aware of and reflective about how early information could potentially influence data collection is important. Early information gathering is meant to benefit and inform—not bias—researchers. Therefore, a reflective notebook (often called field notes) that not only records descriptive information, but also critical reflections on the potential for bias, is particularly helpful in CBCAR projects. Several reflective questions can be considered in researchers' notebooks and later considered in dialogue with one another during team meetings, including:

- What are we learning?
- Who are we learning it from?
- Are there other viewpoints about this?
- How does this influence us as researchers?
- What else do we need to learn about this and who might we learn that from?
- What does this tell us about the setting and the circumstances?
- How does this information affect our data collection plan?

These questions assist research teams to chronicle early information in a beneficial rather than biased manner and provide opportunities for critical examination of ourselves as researchers. We should consistently consider how our backgrounds and predispositions can constrain what is observed and understood—not only during the planning process but also during data collection (Patton, 2002).

Fourth, prior to site entry for data collection, the research team should consult with site advisors such as a Community Advisory Group (Chapter 4). These site advisors provide valuable assistance in establishing contacts and informing research teams about important gatekeepers and stakeholders. Additionally, site advisors may subsequently help research teams plan data collection and gain required community and ethics approval for the research. Patton (2002) labeled this type of site entry, "the known sponsor approach" (p. 312) and indicated that using the "legitimacy and credibility" (p. 313) of a person or group to establish the research team's credibility is often the best approach. However, caution is warranted. Ulin, Robinson, and Tolley (2005) cautioned on-site researchers to avoid seeking assistance from controversial persons in the community or seeking people in positions of authority and power to collaboratively govern data collection. Although these persons may provide valuable information for the research study and could be included as key informants, they should be avoided as decision makers and major research partners in data collection since other potential participants might view people in authority as coercive or intimidating.

Moreover, while Community Advisory Groups and other site advisors often facilitate entry and provide valuable guidance on contacts, these people or groups can also serve as gatekeepers and prevent access to certain important sources of information. For example, when meeting with the all-male section chiefs in the refugee camp to discuss the possibility of planning and conducting a participatory action research study on women's health, we were advised not to speak directly to refugee women because "they are too shy" to talk about their health concerns. Instead we were advised to interview healthcare providers and male section chiefs. The female language interpreter listened carefully but negotiated firmly by asserting that refugee women were the best source of information about their own health concerns and that an action-oriented study without women's perspectives would be incomplete. Even though the interpreter was not a field insider, she shared an East African heritage with the section chiefs that provided a strong base for negotiating at least a planning meeting with refugee women. In the end, we did have the opportunity to plan the study with female community health workers. However, we were also required to include male section chiefs as key informants, which actually provided valuable information for project planning and follow-up research. The primary point is that site advisors and gatekeepers can provide valuable guidance, but their suggestions should be considered carefully. Research experts and team members should critically analyze which data collection strategies and sources are most appropriate for the research question. Respectfully negotiating access to certain populations within the research setting may be necessary. Seeking guidance from site advisors who are knowledgeable and generally well known and respected by their peers is important (Ulin et al., 2005). Developing respectful relationships requires careful attention and adequate time in CBCAR projects.

Fifth, research team members should carefully consider how to introduce the project to gatekeepers, stakeholders, and community or organization members. Research partners should develop a clear and consistent purpose statement along with a concise explanation that not only structures the project and informs the listener but also invites collaboration. This is a delicate balance. If, on the one hand, the CBCAR project explanation is too detailed, the research plan sounds predetermined and does not invite on-site collaboration. On the other hand, if community members have had prior experience with traditional research in their communities, they may be expecting to hear about an established project with a set process. Therefore, in their initial presentation, the CBCAR team needs to provide enough structure to satisfy their listeners' expectations—and yet offer a framework that encourages meaningful input from community members. This type of entry statement represents a negotiated, reciprocal model of entry (Patton, 2002) which invites conversation about the project. According to Creswell (1998), the information that most site gatekeepers and stakeholders seek from project introduction includes succinct answers to the following questions:

■ What is the reason for the project?
■ Why was the site selected?
■ What will be done at the site during the study (time and resources required by participants and amount of time to be spent at the site by the researcher)?
■ Will the research team's presence be disruptive to the research setting?
■ How will results be reported and to whom? Who decides this?
■ What will the gatekeepers/community gain from the study?

Additionally, CBCAR explanations should include avenues for collaboration, an invitation for active participation by people in the research setting, and an emphasis on practical utility for research results.

Research teams should also consider the style in which they present a CBCAR project. A conversational tone, relaxed approach, friendly and professional manner, and genuine interest in collaborating with community organization members are just as important as the purpose statement—and yet, often not considered as carefully. Acknowledging the importance of the organization or community to the CBCAR project and opening a space for listeners to shape the research plan are significant aspects of project introduction.

Research partners who are informed yet neutral and respond genuinely in these early, on-site interactions often set an effective, collaborative tone that eases subsequent research steps. Additionally, during this early phase, establishing the research team's credibility is important. However, researchers should avoid establishing themselves as the experts (Thorne, 2008; Ulin et al., 2005). In CBCAR and other qualitative research methods, true experts are the people inside the research question and setting—not the research team.

■ Collaborative Planning for Data Collection

The original research partnership may have proposed a data collection plan when designing the research project. In some CBCAR situations, the original research partnership implements the data collection plan. In other situations, team composition shifts during the data collection phase. Figure 4-1 in Chapter 4 on page 110 illustrates how team formation may change during the CBCAR process. Keep in mind, CBCAR projects benefit from both stability and flexibility. If a new group forms for data collection, stability is provided by including some members of the original research team. Flexibility is demonstrated when research site representatives or community residents are invited to become part of the data collection team. New ideas and important voices are gained when adding members to the data collection team.

Degrees of collaboration vary along a continuum in CBCAR projects (Patton, 2002). Therefore, research teams need to deliberate on types and styles of collaboration. Three concepts, positionality, reciprocity, and role clarity have particular relevance when considering collaboration during the data collection phase.

Positionality

Ideally, data collection teams should invite a representative from each research site to be part of the data collection effort (Ulin et al, 2005). Described by Naples (2003) as the "study of one's own social group or society" (p. 46), insider research has some advantages. For example, insider research could potentially lead to expanded understandings about deeply embedded beliefs and practices than if the research was conducted by people outside of the setting. Insiders can also provide access to hidden voices in the community, i.e., those persons whose voices are not usually included or queried. An additional benefit is that inside researchers have knowledge about context, required contacts, and approval routes. However, disadvantages of insider research also exist. For example, role confusion can occur if insiders have difficulty stepping out of their daily roles and into the researcher role. Moreover, inside researchers are more likely to be uncritical of their assumptions about data and miss opportunities to explore meaning during data collection (Thorne, 2008). Furthermore, study participants may not be as honest when offering information to inside researchers (Ulin et al., 2005). Naples (2003) questioned whether inside researchers share dual and sometimes conflicting accountability to the research project and the research setting.

Full collaboration with site representatives is not always possible given practical issues such as time commitments, resource constraints, and ethical considerations such as confidentiality. In some CBCAR projects, data collection by site outsiders can be beneficial. For example, Zimmerman, Tilly, Cohen, and Love (2009) described a multisite, collaborative research study to explore medication administration in assisted living centers. The study protocol required outside data collectors to observe staff members administer medication to assisted-care residents. According to the authors, if staff members were part of the data collection planning team, biased data could have resulted. So, to increase validity of findings, outside researchers collected data in each site.

However, potential disadvantages of outside researchers also exist. For example, some sites could be reluctant to collaborate with the research team (Naples, 2003; Smith, 2001; Wallerstein, Duran, Minkler, & Foley, 2005). Resistance to outside researchers in some communities may be based on historical trauma such as colonization and slavery (Minkler, 2004). Also, more time is frequently required to develop relationships within the setting. Without inside knowledge of community or organizational culture, outside researchers might make more mistakes and could be seen as "intruders" to the setting (Thorne, 2008, p. 119).

Some researchers have contested the inside/outside debate. **Box 5-4** offers further considerations about insider–outsider positions and perspectives during data collection. Whether data collectors are site-insiders or site-outsiders, position should be carefully considered.

Box 5-4   Contesting Insider/Outsider Perspectives

Some feminist researchers (Bays, 1998; Naples, 2003; Wasserfall, 1997; Williams, 1996) have contested the inside/outside debate and claim that people's identification with multiple groups within dynamic settings where roles and relationships are constantly shifting precludes simple categorization of insider/outsider positions. Naples (2003) stated, "Outsiderness and insiderness are not fixed or static positions. Rather, they are ever-shifting and permeable social locations that are differentially experienced and expressed by community members" (p. 49). These researchers conclude that the key is for research teams to consistently reflect on power implications of who they are and how they are construed in the setting and by whom in relation to what they are doing and how these factors might influence the data they are collecting. These critical reflections can be included in each researcher's field notes or reflective notebook.

Reciprocity

As noted in Chapter 4, partnerships are a two-way learning relationship. Inviting suggestions for data collection from site advisors helps to establish reciprocity. For example, if local staff members suggest altering data collection strategies or tools, the research team should carefully consider the scientific and ethical implications of the suggested change. Being flexible enough in planning to consider shifting directions or altering data collection strategies is important. However, research partners should also maintain fidelity to their ethical and scientific responsibilities. Foster and Stanek (2007) described the importance of community perspective in their community-based participatory research on HIV. Because of a growing HIV infection rate, university researchers sought to partner with community members to use qualitative methods and explore the community's understanding of HIV infection. However, as community members and university researchers worked on the research question and subsequent data collection, differences became apparent. Rather than focusing on HIV infection, community members preferred a broader research agenda that explored gender and lived experiences. For example, women who lived in the community expressed more concern about intimate partner violence than expanding HIV rates. Acknowledging the process for working through difference to co-create knowledge is not smooth; academic researchers concluded that "strategies for mobilizing the community around HIV infection . . . need[ed] to be redesigned to assume a more holistic approach to risk reduction that include[d] structural interventions based on the everyday experience of community members" (p. 48). Researchers also reflected on how their cultural assumptions influenced their research focus and that "to stay at the table" with community members meant that academic researchers needed to listen as community members provided valuable contextual understandings that made data collection and action planning more relevant to the community setting (p. 48).

As part of reciprocity, the data collection team should carefully and continually cultivate positive and collaborative working relationships with site advisors, decision makers, workers, and groups whose interests are at stake in the research project (Herda,

1999). Researchers often underestimate the time required to develop trust and maintain effective working relationships within data collection settings. If site-insiders are part of the research partnership, less time is generally required than in circumstances where trust with community residents or organizational staff must evolve from point of entry. All interactions should be guided by respect, equity, community, and reciprocity. Thorne (2008) described various disruptions that research teams introduce when entering sites to collect data. Workflow and responsibilities, time requirements, and normal relationships may be altered, and these interruptions are not always welcomed by local staff and community members. In fact, Thorne claimed that some people in these settings find researchers "a bit of a nuisance" (p. 119). When researchers respectfully acknowledge these disruptions, significant progress in establishing good working relationships with people whose work has been altered is made.

Emphasizing the importance of collaborative working relationships and demonstrating an emergent data collection approach, Salina et al. (2006) described their organization-based project, Women's Health, Empowerment, and STD/HIV Prevention Project, with the legal staff that provide services to female detainees. The research partnership, which included academic researchers and Department of Women's Justice Services staff, collected data in questionnaires and focus groups. The original questionnaire was devised by researchers, reviewed by staff members, legal counsel, and formerly incarcerated women, and subsequently revised. The authors claimed that the process of seeking feedback and revising their data collection instrument "yielded a questionnaire that was inclusive of all stakeholders' perspectives" (p. 170). For example, in an effort to develop additional health-related programs, justice department staff members suggested questions related to health concerns other than STD/HIV. Additionally, female detainees in early focus group sessions indicated that HIV education was not as important to them as information about housing, health care, and substance abuse treatment options. Consequently, during HIV-related program offerings, participants were asked to voice their own concerns and needs regarding a health-positive life. Originally focused on STD/HIV prevention, the program's initiatives were broadened to respond to participants' expressed needs. By listening to research participants, who in this case were women detainees, describe concerns that differed from the research purpose, the research partners added questions in the focus groups. Being responsive to community needs while preserving the scientific and ethical integrity of any research project is important (Thorne, 2008).

Role Clarity

Clear role descriptions for the multiple collaborators on the research and data collection teams and the on-site staff contacts and advisors should be developed. Role clarity is especially important in CBCAR projects because roles often shift during the collaboration (Suarez-Balcazar et al., 2006). For example, from one step of the CBCAR process to another, researchers might shift between learner, facilitator, and advocate roles. Additionally, decision-making roles should be distinguished from advisor and implementer roles. For example, local residents may be involved in data collection but not necessarily included in deciding what data to collect and how to collect it. In large, formal projects, creating written role or job descriptions is part of the planning process. Data collection can proceed in a more systematic, efficient, and effective manner when role clarity is established. Patton (2002) claimed that "clarity about roles and divisions of labor can make or break collaborative, participatory forms of inquiry" (p. 321). While collaborators may share similar visions and values, how these values are actually implemented may differ. Developing clear role descriptions prevents confusion, redundancy, and gaps during data collection. Because CBCAR projects are dynamic and emergent, these role descriptions should be periodically reviewed for necessary changes and revised accordingly.

■ Strategic Planning for Data Collection

Research science and ethics are important considerations when planning data collection. Everyone on the team should be knowledgeable about the project and how data collection relates to all other steps of the research project. Additionally, since people are the primary data source in CBCAR projects, protection of human subjects should be the core of all data collection plans. Consulting with and seeking approval from an ethics committee or representative is essential before any contact with potential participants can occur. Additionally, all data collection team members may be required to complete ethics training and certification prior to project approval. We urge data collection teams to study ethical action in data collection and carefully research all institutional and federal guidelines for the ethical conduct of research before planning data collection. Centralizing and converging research science and ethics in all data collections discussions and plans is of paramount importance. Many excellent references are available for planning ethical research (Mertens & Ginsberg, 2009). The United States Department of Health and Human Services, Office for Human Research Protections publishes the federal policies that guide the ethical conduct of research along with many ethics resources (http://www.hhs.gov/ohrp). Chapter 8 also emphasizes the ethical principles that are essential in planning and implementing CBCAR projects.

In addition to research science and ethics, practical issues pertaining to each CBCAR project and setting should be considered when making decisions about data collection. Representing the voices of community-based organizations and community members, Van der Eb et al. (2006) claimed that "Assistance of academia in solving community problems is welcome when researchers are committed to valuing the individual's real-world experience and to being sensitive to cultural and personal differences" (p. 221). Researching real-world experiences within a cultural context requires grounding data collection in natural settings and pragmatic, everyday human experiences. Therefore, as research teams collaboratively plan data collection, practical elements such as access, resources, time, personnel, and logistics are important to consider.

Figure 5-2 illustrates four questions that data collection teams should ask as they collaboratively plan data collection. Specifically, considering what data to collect, from whom, how to collect the data, and subsequently, circling back to the research question to evaluate whether the decisions on what, who, and how make sense.

Figure 5-2 Data Collection Decisions

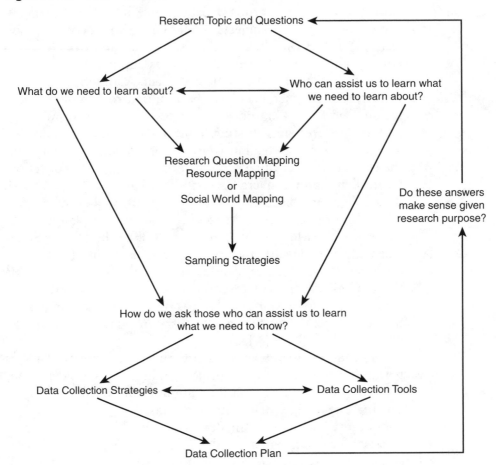

Developing the Data Collection Topics

Reviewing the research question facilitates the process of determining what data to collect and how to do it. Specifically, the data collection team should examine the research question(s) and ask:

■ What do we need to learn to answer the research question(s)?

■ Who can assist us in learning what we need to learn?

- How do we ask those who can assist us in learning what we need to know?
- Do our answers to the above questions make sense for the research question(s)?

Three mapping exercises may benefit data collection team members as they consider these questions. First, in contrast to quantitative researchers who critically study relevant literature, create a framework of pertinent variables to be examined, and subsequently test their framework by using research instruments to collect data, qualitative researchers review relevant literature to become informed about the topics inside the research question. However, being informed does not mean knowing relevant variables and hypothesizing their relationships. Instead, by studying the phenomenon of interest, carefully designing data collection strategies, and being open to new dimensions and meanings that participants bring to the research question, qualitative researchers encourage participants to identify and define the variables within the experiences being studied. If, for example, a research team of intensive care nurses believed that current nurse–physician communication patterns interfere with quality of care, but the nurses are uncertain about the communication dynamics that operate, a CBCAR project seeking deeper understandings about communication patterns and its variables could be planned. After collaboratively writing the research questions, the data collection team carefully dissects each question to identify pertinent content areas (what needs to be learned) and significant data sources (who can tell us). Without attempting to link these concepts, team members then use the map to facilitate choosing data collection strategies and sources (see **Figure 5-3**).

An alternative mapping exercise that also facilitates data collection planning is the resource map (see **Figure 5-4**). Conceived from an ecological perspective, the resource map identifies what really matters in this research: who "resides" in the research questions; who illuminates the way toward deeper insights about the research questions; what voices are currently missing; who has a stake in the outcome; what information is required for situational and contextual understandings; and what information is required for deeper experiential understandings.

Figure 5-3 Research Question Mapping

A group of ICU nurses express concern that communication between nurses and physicians sometimes diminishes quality of patient and family care. Therefore, nurses seek assistance to design a CBCAR project to explore communication patterns. They write and map the following research questions:

- Question #1: What communication patterns between nurses and physicians currently exist in the Intensive Care Unit (ICU) at this medical center?
- Question #2: What are the characteristics of good communication between nurses and physicians in ICU?
- Question #3: What factors facilitate effective communication between nurses and physicians in ICU?
- Question #4: What factors pose barriers to effective communication between nurses and physicians in ICU?

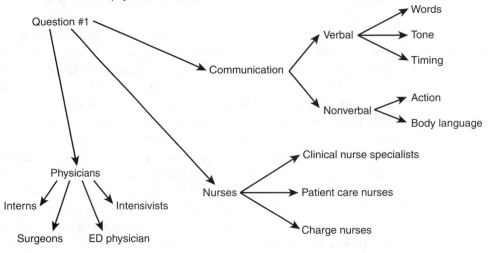

Try mapping questions #2, #3, and #4

Resource mapping is guided by the question, "What persons, groups, organizations, systems, and other resources (such as the literature) provide insight on the research topic?"

A final strategy for crafting a data collection plan is mapping social worlds. Clarke (2005) described social world mapping as a data analysis technique. However, the social worlds concept also facilitates analysis of a research question. In this exercise, team members consider the relevant actors in the research question and their social worlds. In other words, what actors and social interactions pertain to the research question?

Figure 5-4   Resource Map for Research Topic

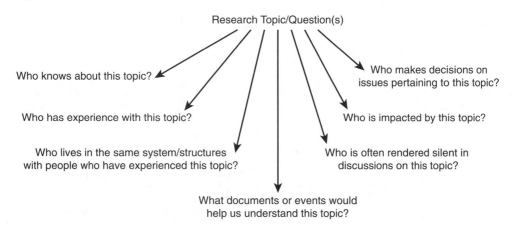

For example, if they are studying nurse–physician communication patterns, the team might map the actors' social worlds, i.e., who the nurse and physician interact with during a typical day and/or quickly evolving emergency events. Examining what is known about the social worlds of both actors as they operate with other actors within larger systems and structures will yield insight about who to include in data collection and what to pursue. A word of caution about social world mapping, however, is required. The social world maps that are drawn prior to data collection are vastly different from the social world maps that are created during the data analysis that is described in Chapter 6. The data collection social world map is pragmatic and based on team members' everyday observations. Designed to provide guidance about data collection, these maps are not scientific or evidence-based; they are simply a tool for devising a data collection plan. In stark contrast, the social arena maps that are drawn during data analysis are based on careful examination of the research data; they are scientific and evidence-based. Distinguishing between the data collection map and the analytic social world map is important. **Figure 5-5** illustrates a data collection social world map that is useful for considering data sources. As data collection ensues, the map is periodically reviewed and revised to determine whether additional data sources are required.

Figure 5-5   Social World Map for Data Collection

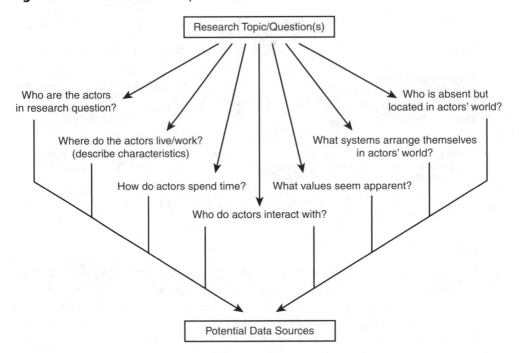

All three mapping activities guide collaborative analysis of the research questions so researchers can formulate a data collection plan. As research topics and populations within the research question emerge, researchers turn their attention to sampling strategies.

Selecting Research Participants

Decisions about who to invite as participants into the CBCAR project are primarily dependent on the research questions, population characteristics, community context, and available resources. The previous mapping exercises facilitate team discussion about these complex considerations. Analyzing information in these maps generally provides a potential pool of participants who would most likely have experience or insights about the research topic and context. Knowledge of various sampling strategies is also important. One of the most commonly-used strategies, purposeful sampling, identifies potential participants according to preselected criteria. These criteria should emerge from one of the mapping exercises. If, for example, researchers are examining the effectiveness of a hospital-based bereavement program, then criteria for participant selection will become more evident as researchers map the question.

Patton (2002) described several types of purposeful sampling strategies such as maximum variation, homogenous, intensity, and theory-based sampling. Additionally, an emergent sampling strategy might be considered. In this approach, new sampling criteria emerge once initial data collection has started (Thorne, 2008). For example, early data analysis might reveal new avenues to explore and possibly new participants to pursue. An emergent sampling strategy could be built into the study design.

Purposeful sampling options should be considered in light of the information research partners agree they want to gather. Keep in mind that sampling strategies may change during different phases of the CBCAR project. For example, Kieffer et al. (2005) described a three-phase project that used different populations and sampling strategies in each phase. Seeking critical friends who are ethics experts on sampling might be appropriate. Once a sampling strategy is determined, community partners and critical friends can provide valuable contact information. Who contacts potential participants and how they are recruited depends on participants' vulnerabilities to potential harm or exploitation (as established by federal guidelines on ethical research). Dialogue between ethics and community experts may shed light on additional vulnerabilities. Additionally, recruitment efforts are generally more effective if community members rather than academic make the initial contact (Baker & Motton, 2005).

Ideally in CBCAR projects, all pertinent actors and stakeholders are included in data collection; however, this inclusive approach can be difficult to navigate (Zimmerman et al., 2009). Political entanglements can occur. For instance, when researching women who have been battered, Kendrick (1998) noted how pressures from law and social welfare professionals, government officials, and funding agencies prevented women who have been battered and other community residents from being a strong voice in research on program and policy decisions. Limited access to potential participants, privacy concerns, resource constraints, and timeline requirements are practical research issues that must be considered when designing a sampling strategy. If major restrictions in sampling impair research integrity, then a new research approach, design, or set of data collection strategies should be considered.

Compensating Participants

A decision about reimbursing participants for their time and possible expenses such as travel and child care should be made while planning data collection. Policies about compensation differ in communities and organizations, so team members should seek advice from people inside the research setting. Providing monetary compensation or another resource that directly benefits participants often improves recruitment efforts (Krieger, Allen, Roberts, Ross, & Takaro, 2005). However, appropriate type and amount of benefit should be carefully considered and contextually grounded. Coercion might result if reimbursement is inappropriate. All compensation for participants must ultimately be approved by relevant ethics committees.

Developing Data Collection Strategies

Frequently seen as advocacy research, CBCAR projects seek information that is useful to policy makers, local leaders, and community members in creating change to improve community circumstances or organizational performance (Van der Eb et al., 2006). As such, data collection strategies should yield practical and useful data from relevant sources in order to develop action plans for transforming problems into solutions. Dissecting this statement, the data collection team should build at least three elements into their strategic plan. First, collecting information on people's experiences and perspectives is important. Second, context matters. Data collection in

CBCAR projects should include information about the community or organization in which people's experiences occur. Third, people's ideas about solutions and transformative action to improve community circumstances or organizational climate and performance should be included. Grounding action planning in a wide variety of participants' experiences is key to CBCAR and often distinguishes this approach from other qualitative methods. As data collection teams plan their strategies, they should select the techniques that are most likely to yield these three elements about the research question. A variety of data collection strategies exist and are described later in this chapter.

Developing Data Collection Tools

Since information gathered and action planned in CBCAR projects depends on what and how questions are asked, data collection tools such as interview guides or standardized questions should be collaboratively developed and carefully constructed by all research partners (Baker & Motton, 2005; Minkler & Wallerstein, 2003). This generally requires an iterative process that includes the following elements:

- Creating and sequencing pertinent questions and/or participant activities
- Reviewing content and sequence for coherence with the research question and setting
- Revising until content and sequence are appropriate to the research question and community context

Because appropriate language use during data collection leads to better data (Christopher, Burhansstipanov, & McCormick, 2005; Herda, 1999; Smith 2001), at least some tool developers should know the "community language" (Van der Eb et al., 2006, p. 223). Keep in mind, community language might refer to formal languages such as Swahili and Spanish or informal linguistics such as healthcare or organization-specific terminology.

The final version of the data collection tool should "make sense to and be useful for all partners" (Baker & Motton, 2005, p. 309). The data collection team can then assess tool effectiveness by role playing and pilot testing questions and activities.

Bias often accompanies instrument development (Mertens, 2005). So when evaluating their data collection tools, researchers should keep in mind that people have a right to be different from one another and assess the openness of their research instruments and protocols. For example, after developing data collection tools and protocols, the data collection team should consider critical questions such as the following:

- Are the data collection strategies and tools appropriate for the people and context?
- Does the instrument contain biased language? Consider potential biases in gender, race, ethnicity, age, class, or varied abilities.
- Has the instrument been reviewed by a heterogonous group of people?
- Were multicultural issues considered throughout the data collection plan?
- Have data collectors been adequately prepared in working across cultures?
- Is it possible to collect data with at least two team members (preferably from different races, ethnicities, ages, genders, classes, abilities)?
- Have data collecting team members reflected on the potential for bias in their notes taken immediately after each data collection session?

We suggest that critical friends, site advisors, and community insiders review all data collection strategies and materials before these materials are finalized and sent to an ethics committee for consideration and approval. Data collection tools should be culturally sensitive and language appropriate and should focus on learning about context and people's perspectives, experiences, and ideas for change.

Box 5-5 Collaborative and Strategic Planning for Data Collection

- Include plenty of time for establishing relationships and building trust.
- Establish reciprocity by being responsive to community needs while still maintaining scientific and ethical integrity of the project.
- Seek ethics consultation and approval from IRB for the original research plan and any subsequent alterations in data collection tools and protocols or sampling strategies.
- Collaboratively develop and describe roles clearly with research team, data collection team, and site advisors; communicate frequently and clearly.
- Match data collection strategies and tools to research questions and design.
- Select participants who are most likely to provide insight on the research question.
- If community members or organization staff assist with data collection, plan to prepare them well, support them consistently, and compensate them adequately.
- Consider practicality in the context of ethical responsibilities.

Many decisions must be made as teams collaboratively and strategically plan appropriate data collection topics, sources, and techniques for their CBCAR projects. **Box 5-5** summarizes some important points to consider.

■ Advancing Scientific Rigor During Data Collection

Cohesiveness of the CBCAR project is always a central factor when planning data collection. Pawar (2004) suggested that researchers incorporate reflective pauses throughout the research planning process to consider cohesiveness. We suggest that the data collection team periodically incorporate reflective moments about data collection appropriateness by standing back and querying along the following lines:

- What is the purpose of our research?
- Does our chosen question and design relate to the purpose?
- Do the realities we plan to seek provide insight into the research question? Are we missing anything?
- Do our selected data collection strategies attain those realities? Are there alternative strategies to consider?

By periodically reviewing cohesiveness of the research project, researchers might discover gaps that suggest further data collection. The emergent quality of data collection should be carefully considered through the lens of research cohesiveness so researchers avoid pursuing data collection paths that do not pertain closely to the research question and design.

After implementing a participatory action research project with street youth to evaluate the effectiveness of an urban drop-in center, Whitmore and McKee (2006) recommended three ways to improve data collection, and hence, data quality. First, for better participant engagement during data collection, they suggested combining conventional data collection methods with Participatory Learning and Action (PLA) tools such as mapping and ranking. Various PLA strategies are described later in this chapter. Second, data collection tools should fit the capacity of data collectors. This pertains not only to tool development but also to effective team member preparation. Third, examine data collection strategies and tools for possibility of bias. Pilot test selected strategies and critically evaluate data quality during early phases of data collection. When collaboratively developing data collection strategies and tools, technical quality of data collection is important to consider.

Careful recordkeeping during all meetings also enhances scientific quality of data collection. Consider audio-recording and transcribing the transactions that occur. A transparent audit trail that chronicles all steps and decisions in the collaborative data planning and collection process provides traceable procedural evidence. This is especially important with CBCAR projects, which tend to last longer and involve more people

---

Box 5-6 Enhancing Trustworthiness During Data Collection

- Prolonged engagement with people and groups in the research setting
- Triangulation by multiple sources, methods, and data collectors
- Team communication and coaching—periodic meetings with data collectors to support consistent application of research ethics and protocols
- Careful recordkeeping on data collection process in an audit trail
- Reflexive journaling where data collectors reflect on themselves and potential for bias in data collection
- Participant checking—asking participants to explain meaning within data collection sessions

---

than other research projects. An audit trail enhances the dependability of research evidence (Mertens, 2005). Additionally, all data collectors should record technical and reflective comments after their contact with participants. As mentioned previously, these field notes provide valuable information on context and an opportunity to assess researcher bias. Field notes contribute toward confirmability of research findings (Mertens, 2005). To enhance data trustworthiness, CBCAR should consider multiple ways to advance scientific rigor during data collection (see **Box 5-6**).

■ Preparing Data Collectors

Part of preparing for data collection is considering who should collect the data. Prior to making that decision, community and research partners should consider:

- Tasks and actions that are required to collect the data (such as interviewing or facilitating focus groups)
- Skills that are necessary in accomplishing the tasks
- Who is best prepared to reliably complete the required tasks

As stated previously, in ideal CBCAR situations, project partners collect data (Zimmerman et al., 2009). However, in some CBCAR situations, practical needs of the project might necessitate hiring community members or other persons outside the data collection team to be data collectors. Employing community or organizational staff members as data collectors can be beneficial to the community by providing employment and skill development (Krieger et al., 2005). For example, the Congolese community health workers who participated in the research project on women's health concerns requested a Certificate of Learning that documented their attendance at workshops that prepared them to plan and conduct the research. According to the community health workers, these certificates were valuable evidence of qualifications as they pursued future job opportunities. In addition to benefitting the community, hiring community members can also benefit the CBCAR project. For instance, Van der Eb et al. (2006) claimed that community members' skill development during CBCAR projects contributes effectively to program sustainability. Community members often provide valuable feedback regarding respectful and effective data collection approaches. They also guide appropriate wording for project introduction and data collection tools that increases accuracy of the data (Christopher et al., 2005; Suarez-Balcazar et al., 2006).

Regardless of who collects CBCAR data, they should be carefully prepared. Instruction should occur prior to data collection and include periodic review and coaching throughout the data collection process. Careful and structured preparation is particularly significant if numerous data collectors are hired. Instructional support for data collectors enhances consistency and data quality. When preparing nonresearch persons to collect data, researchers should emphasize ethics and science and carefully consider cultural context. For example, as mentioned in Chapter 2, before collaborating to explore refugee women's health concerns, the data collection team had to identify the skills needed to collect data in an ethical, scientific, and culturally appropriate manner. A 5-day, interactive, learning and planning workshop resulted. As we engaged with one another during this workshop, cultural differences that impacted the data collection plan occasionally surfaced. **Box 5-7** provides a few examples and how we addressed these tensions.

During our data collection workshop, focus group practice and debriefing sessions were very valuable. **Box 5-8** provides adult learning principles that guided our work. Free-flowing ideas shared in open dialogue resulted in a collaboratively developed list of focus group guidelines and

---

Box 5-7 Tension Between Ethics, Science, and Context

In the Congolese culture, once private information is shared in a public space, the information is considered public and can be freely shared with neighbors and larger community. However, according to ethical guidelines for the protection of human subjects, information shared during focus groups should be kept confidential. Even though we clearly stated that we could not guarantee confidentiality of information shared during focus groups, we still needed to emphasize the importance of privacy. We also had to consider ways to seek general rather than personal information from focus group participants. The Congolese culture has an oral tradition of sharing information through personal story so we had to construct focus group questions very carefully to avoid personal storytelling. Because of our ethical responsibilities, privacy and confidentiality were discussed extensively during the workshop sessions—not in a didactic and directive way, but rather in open dialogue about the mutual cultural value of respect for persons. We engaged in role play to imagine how private information shared with the larger community could harm women. We also tried different ways to politely interrupt personal stories. The experiential learning in these role play situations was important for all of us.

Asking for informed and ongoing consent was also foreign to CHWs and focus group participants. The Congolese culture is based on a strong sense of community responsibility; the individual right to choose whether to participate and what information to share (i.e., the ongoing nature of consent) was novel. Therefore, in addition to acquiring informed consent prior to each focus group session, CHWs periodically inserted deliberately stated reminders of the voluntary nature of participation during the sessions. Afterwards, several focus group facilitators remarked that participants appreciated messages about their right to choose whether to participate and what to say.

(continues)

Box 5-7 Tension Between Ethics, Science, and Context
(continued)

Another ethical consideration pertained to people's expectations of the research. Seeking people's input during data gathering sessions potentially raises the expectation that discernable and quick action will follow. Part of our ethical responsibility was to emphasize that no personal or community benefit could be expected and that focus group sessions were strictly for information gathering with no promise of subsequent action. However, Hyvärinen (2008) claimed that human expectations are deeply embedded in almost every human interaction. When people exchange ideas with one another, they develop expectations. Therefore, we had to emphasize in the introduction and throughout the focus group session that participants would not directly benefit. Follow-up action could not be promised.

Box 5-8 Principles of Adult Learning

Adult learning:
1. Takes place within a democratic framework
2. Respects cultural context
3. Is based on what learners are concerned about
4. Poses questions and problems
5. Acknowledges unequal power relations in society (seeks to develop voice)
6. Encourages everyone to learn and everyone to teach
7. Includes people's emotions, actions, intellects, reflections, creativity, and curiosity
8. Uses varied activities/incorporates best practices in adult learning theory
9. Involves high levels of participation in all phases (planning, implementation, and evaluation)
10. Begins with people's own experiences, proceeds to analysis, moves to collective learning and action, and finally reflection and evaluation of the learning process

interview questions. The workshop's participatory learning activities along with our eagerness to learn from one another were key elements in reciprocal trust and skill development. Scientifically sound, ethically based, and culturally sensitive data collection resulted.

Data collection by community members requires careful preparation and ongoing coaching and supervision (Krieger et al., 2005). Reinforcing data collection protocols and ethics guidelines is particularly important. Being readily available as consultants to the data collection team also facilitates data gathering. Periodic site visits to observe data collection, offer feedback, and answer questions can be particularly helpful (Krieger et al., 2005).

■ Data Collection Strategies

This section describes various data collection strategies that are appropriate for CBCAR projects. These include conducting interviews, facilitating focus group discussions, observing behaviors in natural settings, and engaging in participatory and dialectic techniques such as card sorting and process mapping. Each of these strategies is explained briefly with some examples provided. For more in-depth and specific guidance on implementation, readers are urged to read the vast array of CBCAR exemplars that currently exist in the nursing and social science literature.

Conducting Interviews

One of the most common forms of qualitative data collection is the guided interview (Ellsberg & Heise, 2005). Researchers pose questions pertaining to the research topic and participants describe their knowledge, perspectives, experiences, beliefs, observations, and feelings about the topic in their own words. As the researcher and the participant interact within the interview, relationships are explored and meanings are uncovered. To gain a wide perspective on the research topic, researchers usually conduct multiple interviews. In-depth interviewing is appropriate for most research topics and especially useful for sensitive, controversial, or personal topics. With one-on-one interviews, researchers adopt measures to protect data privacy and can assure confidentiality. Researchers cannot make the same assurance of confidentiality when collecting data in focus group discussions or using participatory strategies. Researchers also use in-depth interviewing in combination with other data collection strategies. For example, key informant interviews (which are discussed later in this section) provide valuable insights on community context that effectively supplement information from focus groups.

Individual interviews are often characterized by the degree of structure that data collectors impose (Robson, 2002; Ulin et al., 2005). In structured interviews, researchers create an interview guide that is carefully worded and sequenced. Data collectors simply ask questions exactly as worded and record participants' responses. The interview guide is consistently applied in each interview. As a result, not much interviewing skill is required. In contrast, semistructured interviews are more flexible and spontaneous. Data collectors still use interview guides that focus the conversation. However, when applying the interview guide, researchers interact with participants and use follow-up questions that seek detail, clarification, and meaning. Data from semistructured interviews typically result in more expansive data than data collected in structured interviews. Finally, in unstructured interviews, the interviewer poses the research topic without a prescriptive interview guide and engages with the participant to explore the topic's many dimensions. Researchers allow conversation to develop within the interview. As a result, respondents have more control over topic flow and content. In contrast to structured interviews, both unstructured and semistructured interviews require highly skilled researchers who can create a comfortable atmosphere, listen attentively, and question astutely (Ulin et al., 2005).

As a process, interviews have identifiable and progressive steps. Combining suggestions from several sources, (Robson, 2002; Rubin & Rubin, 1995; Ulin et al., 2005), we offer a process that CBCAR interviewers might find helpful (see **Box 5-9**). The first stage of an interview is an information exchange in which attention is immediately focused on participants' rights and researchers' ethical obligations as outlined in in-

---

Box 5-9   Interview Phases

- Informational exchange
  - Informed consent with research purpose explained
  - Orientation to the interview
- Conversational, descriptive, straightforward questions
  - Warm-up for interviewer and participant
- Experiential and explanatory questions
  - Early main body of interview—focused primarily on descriptions
- Perspective and meaning-seeking questions
  - Main body of interview—focused on beliefs and meaning construction
- Closure
  - Toning down and fading
  - Ask participant to identify most important topic
  - Ask if participant has anything more to say or any questions

---

formed consent. Voluntary participation, the ongoing nature of consent, and confidentiality should be emphasized. Also during this stage, researchers orient participants to the interview task by distinguishing interviews from ordinary conversations, clarifying the researcher's role as learner (as opposed to expert or advisor), and setting the time frame. As a result, participants know what to expect during the interview. They should also be encouraged to ask questions.

In the second phase of the interview, researchers ask relatively easy questions in an informal manner. For example, a researcher might review the participant's work responsibilities or living arrangements. Once both persons become comfortable in conversation, the researcher transitions into the main body of the interview. Researchers usually start this stage of the interview by asking experiential and explanatory questions before seeking participants' personal perspectives and beliefs. Participants usually describe experiences more easily than beliefs and meanings. So this sequencing follows an arrangement of increasing complexity. Once experiences and perspectives are described, the researcher might start the quest for meaning. However, because interviews are iterative, the researcher and participant are constantly moving between experiences, perspectives, and meaning. All three parts of the main body—experiences, perspectives, and meaning—should be covered within the interview time frame so pacing becomes significant.

Finally, the researcher transitions toward summarizing and closure. Researchers might conclude the interview with one or two fairly straightforward questions. Considering interview phases is an important part of planning effective data collection. Once the interview process is planned, researchers consider the specific interview questions.

Questions are designed to engage participants and researcher in an open and honest conversation where researchers primarily query, prompt, and listen while participants inform, describe, and clarify. Together, they explore meaning. Asking the right questions is critically important for providing a context for knowledge and understanding. Two particular types of questions are most commonly used during interviews (Patton, 2002; Ulin et al., 2005). First, researchers write main topic questions that pursue information about the research topic and community or organizational context. Main topic questions formulate the interview guide for structured and semistructured interviews. Second, for unstructured and semistructured interviews, researchers should develop a repertoire of productive follow-up questions that they are comfortable asking during an interview. These questions encourage further description, explanation, or clarification regarding the information provided by participants in response to the main topic questions that are asked by the researcher. Since follow-up questions pertain to the conversation in the moment, they cannot be specifically written ahead of time. However, follow-up questions are important to consider and practice when planning interviews so researchers are more ready to use them during interviews.

Together, main topic and follow-up questions guide interviewers during most interviews. However, because of the particular type of information researchers seek in CBCAR interviews, we have added two other important types of questions to consider. First, since participants and researchers co-construct meaning in interview sessions, questions that specifically seek meaning should be added to the repertoire of follow-up questions. Second, reflective questions that encourage participants to reflect back on earlier comments and consider how different situational elements might relate can provide additional insights. **Box 5-10** distinguishes between

---

Box 5-10   Types of Interview Questions

1. Main topic questions
   - Related to concepts and subtopics in research question
   - Open-ended, yet specific and clear
   - Sequenced in a logical, thoughtful, deliberate manner (e.g., easy to complex or broad to specific)
2. Follow-up questions (sometimes called probes or prompts)
   - Seek further explanation about topic or experience mentioned by participants
   - Seek clarity and depth
   - Seek detailed description with who, what, when, where, how?
3. Meaning-seeking questions
   - Co-construct meaning with participant
   - Avoid assumptions
   - Seek definition and examples of abstractions
   - Sample question—When you say "peaceful death" what do you mean by that? Can you provide an example that illustrates the meaning of a "peaceful death?"
4. Reflecting back and relating questions
   - Seek connections in concepts and ideas
   - Seek explanations
   - Sample question—Earlier you described risk factors for adolescent depression and now you are describing early indicators. How do you think those two ideas are related?

types of interview questions and provides sample questions for CBCAR researchers to ponder when planning data collection in interviews.

Once complete, the interview guide is usually reviewed and revised by critical friends and setting insiders. Additionally, data collectors should practice applying the guide in mock interviews with one another. These practice sessions offer valuable opportunities for reviewing and revising the interview guide (Eng et al., 2005). Feedback on follow-up questions that interviewers use during these mock interviews is also valuable. All questions should be open-ended, neutral, clear, simply stated, and singular. Distinguishing between questions that commonly occur in informal conversations but are not productive during interviews is important. See **Box 5-11** for examples of unproductive questions that should be avoided during research interviews (Mack et al., 2005; Patton, 2002; Stringer, 2007).

Besides developing an interview process and constructing a sound interview guide, data collectors should consider other aspects that pertain to planning and conducting effective interviews. First, being familiar with the research topic and community or organizational context is important. However, "bracketing" or setting aside that knowledge during the interview is also important (Stringer, 2007). Data collectors should approach each participant's interview as eager learners ready to absorb important new information on the research topic. Second, arranging to meet participants for the interview in a convenient, private, and quiet place is usually suggested. Besides allowing for fewer interruptions and better audio recording, a quiet space is usually more conducive to private, in-depth conversations than busy locations. However, safety and convenience are also considered when deciding on an appropriate location. Third, practicing with the recording equipment ahead of time and bringing backup equipment, such as recorders and batteries, to the interview is advised. Allow plenty of time for arranging and testing the equipment prior to the interview. Fourth, prior to the interview, the researcher should review whether all ethics guidelines have been carefully followed. Also, interviewers should center themselves before meeting the participant. Data collection requires intense concentration so researchers should deliberately prepare themselves to transcend daily busyness and

> ## Box 5-11　Types of Questions to Avoid During an Interview
>
> - Dichotomous questions—can be answered with one-word or brief responses
>   - Did you enjoy your experience?
>   - Were you lonely?
>   - Do women avoid that or do they address it?
> - Leading questions—wording potentially influences participant's response
>   - Were you trying to avoid infection?
>   - Don't you think people are afraid of being stigmatized?
> - Long questions—respondent will only respond to the parts that are remembered
>   - In previous interviews, people have commented on their frustrations with the logistics of transferring or discharging patients from the Emergency Department. In addition, we have noted in the research literature that other researchers have identified common barriers to the smooth flow of ED patients through the hospital system. Things like required documentation and communication barriers were identified. What has been your experience with that?
> - Multiple questions
>   - What happened? How did you feel about it? When did it occur?
> - Double-barreled questions
>   - Can you tell me how that felt compared to when you were growing up?
> - Questions with jargon or unfamiliar words
>   - What did the foley feel like?
>   - What did you do for gainful employment?

mentally enter a quiet, attentive, and focused space. During the interview, researchers should build rapport, listen attentively, enter and remain in the participant's descriptions, adapt their interview style to fit the participant's personality, and be flexible in applying the interview guide (Mack et al.,

2005). Also, researchers should refrain from inserting their own perspectives, correcting or arguing with participants' statements, judging behaviors or beliefs, and counseling participants. Fifth, occasional note-taking during the interview might be helpful for follow-up questioning. Finally, documenting observations, impressions, and lessons immediately after each interview is very valuable. These written notes often supplement interview transcripts in important ways. Also, in emergent designs, these notes may suggest new avenues to consider.

Key informant interviews, a particular type of interview, can be particularly helpful in CBCAR projects (Eng et al., 2005; Israel, Schultz, Parker, & Becker, 1998). Key informants are particular people who have specialized knowledge and experiences. Offering researchers access to information that might not otherwise be available to the research team, key informants usually speak on behalf of others when being interviewed (Gilchrist & Williams, 1999; Ulin et al., 2005). For example, we collected data from healthcare professionals and women advocates who worked inside the refugee camp when researching women's health concerns. These key informants had practical and first-hand knowledge regarding women's daily struggles and health concerns and spoke eloquently on their behalf. Key informants generally provide information on organizational or community history and culture, social arrangements and relationships, and perceived system barriers and facilitators (Eng et al., 2005). This information can be especially valuable when designing intervention research with communities and organizations. A sample interview guide is provided in **Box 5-12**. While researchers usually gain valuable insights from key informants, they should also recognize that key informant information can be limited, selective, and biased (Patton, 2002). Therefore, interviewing a number of key informants who represent several aspects of the community or organization is beneficial to CBCAR projects.

Interviews can potentially provide highly illuminating, in-depth information about the research topic, population, and context. However, quality of interview data is dependent on researchers' planning and interviewing skills (Patton, 2002). Therefore, researchers should carefully prepare for interviews, observe ethical responsibilities throughout the data

Box 5-12   Sample Key Informant Interview Guide

Opening Question
- What is your current job title?
- How long have you worked in that capacity?
- How long have you worked in (name of organization/school, etc.)?

Introduction Question
- What is your overall assessment of the health of African immigrant women and girls as you interact with them in this organization?

Key Questions
- How does your organization support African immigrant females' health and well-being?
- What are the strengths to those systems and structures?
- What are the actual and potential barriers to those systems and structures?
- How are the barriers being addressed/how would you like to see the barriers addressed?
- What would you like to see in the future for programs that seek to improve the health and well-being of African immigrant women and girls?

Ending Questions
- Of all the things we talked about today, what aspects seem most important to you?
- Of all the things we talked about today, what aspects seem most urgent to you?

collection process, follow interview protocols carefully, and develop and practice their interview skills prior to conducting interviews. Researchers should also evaluate their interview skills and monitor for bias in following leads, forming questions, and interpreting responses. Advantages of interviews include that they are designed to be flexible, iterative, emergent, and opportunistic. However, limitations include the potential for biased interpretations within the interview. In CBCAR projects, interviews are usually triangulated with other data collection strategies such as surveys, participant observation, focus groups, or participatory techniques. As previously mentioned, triangulation generally enhances data quality and trustworthiness.

Facilitating Focus Groups

Focus groups have been successfully implemented in a variety of healthcare settings and cultural contexts (Davidson, et al., 2003; Hennink, 2008; Kieffer et al., 2005; Koniak-Griffith, Nyamathi, Tallen, González-Figueroa, & Dominick, 2007; Morgan et al., 2008; Nyamathi, Thomas, Greengold, & Swaminathan, 2009; van Eyk & Baum, 2003). Moreover, an increased acceptance of using focus groups to collect data in health and human science research is evident (Hennink, 2008; Morgan, 2002; Morgan, et al., 2008). Vissandjée, Abdool, and Dupéré (2002) claimed that focus groups are especially appropriate for cultures with a strong oral tradition. Barbour and Kitzinger (1999) edited a book describing 21 participatory action research projects that utilized focus groups as a data collection strategy. The editors encouraged researchers to incorporate focus groups when planning action research projects.

Focus group data collection generally involves gathering a group of people and creating a comfortable environment that is conducive to open, honest dialogue on carefully planned questions. Being collectivistic rather than individualistic, focus groups capture the rich multivocality of participants' attitudes, experiences, and beliefs (Madriz, 2000). Researchers specifically design focus groups to be interactive, a place where diverse ideas spiral toward new insights that the group then collectively explores. Skilled facilitators encourage participants to share their views with one another, and skilled note-takers record their observations of human interactions that occur within the social context of the focus group. Most focus group sessions are audiotaped, although they can also be videotaped for subsequent transcription and observation.

Focus group dialogue is particularly useful for exploratory research on topics that are generally understudied. Focus group data collection is particularly suitable for exploring sociocultural or organizational norms, beliefs, and practices. Additionally, data from focus groups are often helpful in revealing community or organizational concerns and priorities. Some researchers collect focus group data in formative studies prior to developing research instruments, community health interventions, or social programs. In these situations, focus group findings provide information to prepare large-scale CBCAR projects. Focus group data can also be helpful in interpreting results of quantitative studies (Pawar, 2004). For example, if a large-scale research study reveals health outcome disparities between ethnic groups, ethnic-specific focus groups could lend insight on why differential outcomes occur. Chiu (2003) proposed a three-stage process for using focus groups during action research projects. The author asserted that focus groups generate experiential knowledge for problem identification. Then focus groups can create practical knowledge for constructing an intervention program, and finally, focus groups can engage in critical reflection for evaluating program effectiveness. The author concluded that collecting data in focus groups is very versatile and contributes valuable knowledge for action research projects.

Researchers should decide whether to have homogenous or heterogeneous focus groups in their study. Pawar (2004) suggested avoiding extreme homogeneity or heterogeneity when planning focus group composition. A more comfortable atmosphere for group dialogue is generally created by a homogenous group of participants. Participants might be similar in terms of age, gender, social class, health condition, professional preparation, or ethnic group. Experienced focus group facilitators generally recommend at least two groups that are characterized in a certain way (Ellsberg & Heise, 2005). In contrast, heterogeneous groups usually offer more diversity and, if facilitated well, richness that emerges from different perspectives. Hierarchical relationships within groups, however, should be avoided. Subtle power differences can silence some participants. In our human rights research, we formed groups based on gender and age. We arranged two women-only groups, two men-only groups, and two mixed-gender groups. Additionally, one of the mixed-gender groups was designated for participants ages 19–25.

Group size varies with the topic and social context. Generally 5 to 10 respondents per session are recommended (Ellsberg & Heise, 2005; Krueger & Casey, 2000; Mack et al., 2005). This number balances diversity with sufficient time for everyone to share their views. Focus group questions that pursue in-depth explanations are best answered in smaller groups of 4 to 6 respondents (Krueger & Casey, 2000). Furthermore, if people feel passionate about a particular research topic or have intense experiences to share about the topic, smaller-sized sessions are advised. A larger group size (8–10 participants) can be useful if focus groups seek breadth on a topic or aim to pilot test programs. Considering appropriate group size should be part of focus group planning.

Participant recruitment is sometimes challenging. Planners should prepare a succinct purpose statement, create an ethically appropriate and personalized invitation, and consider participant incentives. Some researchers also suggest scheduling focus group sessions to coincide with regular gatherings, such as staff meetings or trainings. This strategy might be more successful than asking participants to schedule a separate time to meet.

Researchers generally collect two kinds of data in focus groups. First, researchers seek participants' perceptions on social norms, customs, and practices relevant to the research topic. This is accomplished by exploring general, community-wide experiences rather than specific, personal narratives (Ellsberg & Heise, 2005; Krueger & Casey, 2000). So, focus group questions should not seek details of participants' lives or experiences. Individual, in-depth interviewing would be more appropriate for gathering personal accounts. Sensitive topics should also be avoided in focus group sessions. Instead the subject should pertain to social norms and practices—drawing on participants' general rather than specific life experiences.

Second, researchers seek information on social interactions relevant to the research topic (Hollander, 2004). Who speaks, in what sequence, and how they speak with one another to discuss their shared context are important observations. **Box 5-13** distinguishes between content and interaction data in a human

Box 5-13 Two Types of Information from Focus Groups on Human Rights

Sample human rights *content* findings:

- Men claimed that everyone had the same rights and especially emphasized the right to materials for daily survival such as agricultural tools and seeds.

- Women in the women-only groups noted their daily responsibilities and the numerous struggles associated with meeting their daily obligations; women could not identify any claims or rights for themselves.

- In mixed-gender focus groups, women talked about the difficulties in feeding their families; women described what families and family members had a right to (such as food and water) but not what women in particular had a right to.

Without soliciting personal narratives, we learned valuable information on cultural and community context.

Sample human rights *interaction* findings:

- Most women in women-only focus groups spoke freely and listened carefully to one another. However, they generally did not establish conversations within focus groups; in this case, women tended to provide responses but did not comment to one another on each other's situations or women's issues in general.

- During mixed-gender groups, men spoke freely to one another; when asked to provide perspectives, women were primarily silent.

- In mixed-gender groups, women consistently avoided commenting on men's observations or descriptions.

- Older men spoke freely and more frequently than younger male participants; younger participants listened carefully to older participants.

- Younger women spoke more often than older women; many older women were silent even when asked specifically for comments.

rights research project (Pavlish & Ho, 2009). Occasionally in CBCAR projects, group process and interactions might be the primary focus of data collection. In other projects, data is gathered about both content and group interactions.

To capture the complexity of group dialogue and dynamics, every focus group session should have at least two experienced focus group moderators. One person usually facilitates group dialogue, and the other person takes notes. The facilitator's overall responsibility is to encourage focus group members to interactively address a specific set of issues. Specifically, other roles include:

- Introducing informed consent; describing confidentiality but acknowledging limits on assurance of confidentiality in focus groups
- Fostering an informal and comfortable environment where all focus group members are offered an opportunity to participate
- Managing group dynamics for balance and cohesion
- Extracting information on the topic while being open to new, emerging issues
- Eliciting depth, clarity, and diversity in the dialogue
- Acknowledging participants as the topic experts
- Listening with focused attention and without a need to explain or defend
- Encouraging group members to dialogue with one another rather than with facilitator
- Avoiding controlling the dialogue as long as it revolves around the topic area

For group dialogue, facilitators might consider establishing some ground rules, such as speaking one at a time and not interrupting one another. These ground rules should encourage conversation that is respectful and orderly without sacrificing spontaneity and provide equal opportunity for everyone to participate.

The note-taker generally assists the facilitator as needed with promoting smooth flow to group dialogue. Specifically, the note-taker's responsibilities include observing group dynamics, careful recordkeeping of dialogue content and participant interactions, operating audio or video recording equipment, and handling session interruptions such as latecomers or inadvertent distractions. Furthermore, toward the end of the session, the facilitator often asks if the note-taker has any follow-up or clarification questions. Sometimes note-takers provide a brief, 2-minute summary for participants at the conclusion. Immediately after the session has concluded, the note-taker provides valuable input during a debriefing session with the facilitator.

The benefits of two people moderating each focus group session include an expanded capacity to absorb information so more data accumulates. Moreover, data trustworthiness generally improves because two people listened to the dialogue and observed group interactions (Krueger & Casey, 2000).

A dialogue guide is often used to systematically and consistently collect data across focus groups (Greenbaum, 2000). For example, when researching human rights, we developed a dialogue guide that encouraged reflective responses on the topic. Starting with concept definition to elicit participants' ideas about human rights, moving toward concrete experiences to clarify meaning, and finally, proceeding toward key questions to procure reflections about the topic, we consistently applied the dialogue guide in all focus groups so we could compare responses across focus groups (see **Box 5-14**). This type of question sequencing is often referred to as the "funnel" approach (Morgan et al., 2008, p. 192). Using the funnel approach, facilitators generally ask broad questions in the initial phase and proceed to narrow the focus toward the research topic. In contrast, an emergent focus group session might employ the "hourglass" approach, which starts with broad, open-ended questioning, proceeds to narrow the topic to researchers' interest, but concludes by broadening the questions so participants can raise new concerns or provide more detail about concerns that were previously expressed. Additionally, the last portion of the hourglass format might provide new avenues to pursue in subsequent focus groups (Morgan et al., 2008). Another strategy to allow for emergent topics when using focus groups is to hold repeated or reconvened focus groups. This strategy allows for more in-depth exploration of social interaction and deeper discussion on the research topic. Participants might even be

---

Box 5-14   Sample Semistructured Dialogue Guide for Focus Groups

Introduction Question(s)
- What do the words "human rights" mean to you?

Transition Question(s)
- What rights/entitlements are important to you as a human being, as a man/woman in this community?
- What are some situations in this community that involve human rights? Avoid names, identifiers.
- What in the community serves as a resource or barrier for those situations?

Key Question(s)
- What are the human relations issues in this community and how do they link to human rights?
- If we wanted to explore more deeply the human relations issues and human rights in this community, how would you suggest we proceed?

Conclusion Question(s)
- Of all the things we talked about today, what aspects seem most important to you?

(Adapted from Krueger & Casey, 2000)

---

asked to complete an assignment, such as keeping a diary, between focus group sessions to deepen topic exploration (Morgan et al., 2008). Additionally, many participatory strategies, such as context mapping or trend analysis, can be incorporated into focus group dialogue.

The advantages of collecting data in focus groups include democratic, spiraling dialogue as group members share ideas that elevate discussion beyond single responses and vacillates between what is currently happening and what is possible (Heron & Reason, 2006). Group dialogue generally creates more diversity and breadth in topic exploration and provides an opportunity to co-construct meaning. This usually leads to more elaborate accounts of social norms and practices and plans for social action. Another advantage is the opportunity to examine communication patterns and social interactions within a specified social context (Hollander, 2004). The focus group strategy also tends to generate good quality information relatively quickly at a reasonable cost. Additionally, the strategy works well with emergent designs and provides sound information as the basis for planning larger studies. Finally, this strategy gains important access to participants' own meanings and cultural language.

The limitations of data collection in focus groups include the possibility of restricted disclosure and losing sensitive data (Hollander, 2004; Mack et al., 2005), the artificial effort to elicit data (Morgan, 2002), and the possibility of peer influence on participants' responses (Hollander, 2004). Additionally, focus group dialogue may be difficult to manage. For example, some participants dominate the discussion; some respondents veer off track; and sometimes recording becomes difficult because people talk all at once. Depending on the research question and design, researchers may consider triangulation by using focus groups with other data collection strategies.

Collecting data in focus groups is an effective and appropriate strategy for many CBCAR projects. Careful planning and moderator preparation are essential to focus group effectiveness. We advise data collectors to practice their moderating skills in several mock focus group sessions before initiating actual data collection. Additionally, seeking counsel from critical friends and testing the dialogue guide are important to focus group planning and moderator preparation. Focus group data accumulates rapidly, so monitoring the amount and quality of focus group data is also important to the data collection process.

Engaging in Observation

Scientific observation as a data collection strategy involves researchers watching people in their natural settings, participating to varying degrees in the setting's daily activities, and writing detailed notes about what is seen and experienced. Observation provides valuable information on physical, sociocultural, and economic contexts. Using geographic maps, genograms, social maps, organizational charts, and other visual diagrams will amplify observations on the research setting. Additionally, observation yields valuable data on people's behaviors, relationships, activities, norms, and events.

Observation is rarely used as a sole data collection strategy (Robson, 2002). Instead, observation complements other data collection strategies in CBCAR projects. For example, extensive observation can be a way to triangulate data collection and provide a more thorough data set. Participant observation can also be useful in determining who to recruit for subsequent phases of a project and how to recruit them. Moreover, if used before interviews, observation data can facilitate development of an interview guide or alert data collectors to concepts or situations that require clarification during an interview (Mack et al., 2005). Observation can also be an inherent part of other qualitative data collections strategies. For example, when writing descriptive notes about interviews or focus groups, researchers often record their observations about setting and participant behavior.

During observations for CBCAR projects, specific dimensions of social experiences are noted, including space, chronology, actors, actions, group activities, events, objects, goals, and feelings (Patton, 2002; Robson, 2002). Additionally, observing appearance, verbal interactions, human movement from one space to another, and characteristics of people who receive attention and those who do not often provides interesting and pertinent data (Mack et al., 2005). Researchers may also find noteworthy what was expected in their observations but not actually evident in the setting.

Observation as a data collection strategy is often characterized according to the observation structure. For example, observations in some projects might be open and unstructured, and the data collector systematically records as much descriptive information as possible while immersed in the setting. This type of observation is more typical of studies seeking qualitative data. In other projects, researchers use structured observations to identify specific actions. Observers in this situation might use a checklist to record the number of times they see a specified action or event. Researchers might collect quantitative and qualitative data in structured observations. For example, while immersed in a nursing care unit, data collectors might use an observation checklist to record the number of times and how well nurses follow an established medication administration protocol.

In addition to structure, observations may be characterized according to the observers' roles. For example, data collectors may actively participate in the setting's normal activities as observations are being made. This is often referred to as participant observation, and researchers observe and record details of their participation with others in the natural flow of the setting's events and activities. In contrast, data collectors might not participate in any of the activities that are being observed. This is usually referred to as nonparticipant observation or passive participation (Mertens, 2005). In this situation, observers quietly watch people in their natural settings while participating minimally, if at all, in the setting's activities. Determining how much the observer participates depends on the type of information being pursued. For example, if researchers are examining nurse–physician communication, they may obtain better data as a participant observer since communication may flow more naturally without silent observers standing by.

Careful and descriptive note-taking accompanies every observation session. Notes for structured observations are usually prescriptive and specific. In contrast, notes for unstructured observations are generally open and wide-ranging. These notes are still detail-oriented but not necessarily focused on looking for specific actions or events. When writing, data collectors should focus on describing and not evaluating what they observe (Pawar, 2004). In some cases, notes may be taken during the observation session with reflections noted after the observation period concludes. In other cases, observers participate in the activities and record their descriptive notes and reflections immediately after leaving the setting. For data quality, each observation period should be thoroughly described before attempting to participate in subsequent observation sessions (Robson, 2002). Additionally, at the conclusion of each session, observers should note particular questions to pursue and pertinent suggestions for improving future observation.

Carefully described observations contribute effectively to a clear and rich picture of the research setting. When triangulated with interviews and focus groups, observations provide even deeper understandings of emerging patterns. However, observations also have limitations. Observers' values, beliefs, and life experiences often influence what is selected for observation. These selectivity biases in both attention and memory potentially limit data gathered. Additionally, observers' expectations potentially affect their descriptions of observed behaviors. However, if multiple observers who are diverse in age, gender, and ethnic characteristics are collecting data in the same setting, they can compare their observations and notes. This cross-checking can diminish the potential for observer bias. Additionally, multiple observation opportunities over longer time periods can result in more trustworthy observations.

The complexities of human experiences are more fully realized when observation is added as a data collection strategy to any CBCAR project. However, scientific observation requires extensive practice in both keen watching and detailed, descriptive writing. One way to practice is to become a stranger in a familiar place. Observers might select a setting they know well and while there, focus all their attention on collecting data through the five senses. After writing extensively and descriptively about the data absorbed by the senses, observers can then return their attention to observing the setting and analyze whether their descriptions clearly illustrate the experience of being immersed in the setting. Also consider what observations seem particularly important or helpful. Practicing observation with another person also facilitates skill development. Comparing notes afterwards can provide valuable information on the potential for selectivity biases. Developing both observational and writing skills contributes to the quality of CBCAR data, which, in turn, influences the nature and quality of research findings.

Using Participatory Data Collection Strategies

When numerous development projects that neglected to understand local perspectives and contexts failed, participatory strategies were developed and became popular as effective ways to access local knowledge. Often labeled participatory rural appraisal (PRA) or participatory learning and action (PLA), these strategies are distinguished from other data collection techniques by participants creating shared visual representations and analyses that depict some aspect of their realities. These visual illustrations are elicited through the use of data collection tools such as card sorting and ranking, spatial mapping, and process sequencing. Chambers (1997) claimed these strategies represent "handing over the stick" of problem identification and meaning making to people who are most affected, and therefore, most knowledgeable (p.117). Advantages of participatory data collection include representation of multiple perspectives, depiction of data relationships, specific attention to context, and focus on change. Potential disadvantages might include limited transferability and trustworthiness of findings. However, these possible disadvantages can be minimized by providing accurate and thorough descriptions of context; triangulating methods, sources, and investigators; and careful recordkeeping in data collection audit trails (Kumar, 2002; Pretty et al., 2002). Several participatory strategies exist; only four are explained in this chapter. Several references provide additional strategies and specific examples (Ayala, Maty, Cravey, & Webb, 2005; Barnidge et al., 2010; Chambers, 1997; Ellsberg & Heise, 2005; Kumar, 2002; Pretty et al., 2002; Sethi & Belliard, 2009; Whitmore & McKee, 2006).

Free-listing and card-sorting is a participatory strategy aimed at gaining breadth in topics about which the team has little previous knowledge (Ellsberg & Heise, 2005; Ulin et al, 2005). For this strategy, data collectors ask each participant to list all instances of a particular phenomenon—or a group can create a list together. For example, if researching violence against women in a community where limited information about violence exists, then participants might be asked to individually or collectively list all the ways in which violence against women and girls occurs in their community. After each instance of violence is transferred to its own card, participants (individually or as a group) are asked to sort the cards into whatever categories make the most sense to them. Participants then label their piles or categories. After the listing, sorting, and labeling activities have been completed, researchers ask participants to explain the items that they identified, the categories into which they sorted the items, and the labels that they used to describe the various categories. The examples and explanations that participants provide are usually rich with meaning on how they perceive and structure the phenomenon of interest and fit it into their own lives. Researchers should provide clear instructions for the activity and effectively elicit participants' descriptions and facilitate group discussion.

The initial free-list/card-sort activity can be followed by additional participatory strategies. For example, data collectors can use a second free-list/card-sort activity that explores participants' perspectives on categorizing causes of violence. Comparisons between participants or groups of participants might also provide valuable insights about the research topic. For example, data collectors might first use the strategy with young, middle-aged, and older women and then use the same strategy with young, middle-aged, and older men. These age and gender comparisons might reveal whether perspectives on violence against women differ among different age and gender groups. Another variation is for researchers to create their own categories such as sexual trafficking or intimate partner violence and ask participants to assign particular examples of violence that they identified in the free-list exercise to the researcher-created categories. During discussion, data collectors explore participants' reasoning behind their assignments of particular instances to specific categories. All versions of free-listing/card-sorting are important ways to access tacit knowledge, i.e., perceptions and behaviors that might not otherwise be apparent. This strategy can also be an effective means for uncovering local linguistics and "indigenous expressions" regarding a particular topic (Ulin et al., 2005, p. 97).

Ranking is a strategy in which participants identify what is most urgent, prevalent, important, or severe. Ranking information often yields useful insights on local priorities. Researchers facilitate group dialogue to determine criteria people apply to determine urgency, prevalence, or severity. Additionally, cross-group comparisons may be valuable since different groups might use different criteria to rank situations and set priorities. Since ranking often assigns numbers to items, certain statistical models can also be applied to the results of ranking exercises (Kumar, 2002). Ranking well-being, which is a specific type of ranking activity, has been applied in various health and development projects as a method for examining people's perspectives on socioeconomic disparities and identifying vulnerable populations in communities (Chambers, 1997; Kumar, 2002; Pretty et al., 2002).

Pair-wise ranking is another data gathering strategy in which participants collectively determine the most significant issue or greatest preference in a given circumstance (Kumar, 2002). The strategy also yields information on participants' decision-making processes and criteria for arriving at primary preferences. The activity starts with group members composing a list of responses to questions such as, "What health problems do women experience in this community?" or "What actions prevent violence against women in this community?" Subsequently, researchers create a grid that lists responses on both the horizontal rows and the vertical columns (see **Table 5-1**). Comparing the first item on the row with the item in each column (except the first column), researchers systematically ask participants questions such as:

■ Between respiratory and sexually transmitted infections, which is more important?

■ Between respiratory and sexually transmitted infections, which is more severe?

Participants in discussion with one another consider their responses but must arrive at one answer to record in the cell. Researchers should listen for differences in ranking criteria as participants discuss the comparisons and their reasons for ranking one condition higher than the other. The group must reach consensus on one answer and note pairs that are particularly difficult to rank. Continue comparing the row issues with column issues until all comparisons have been made and responses recorded. Researchers then count how many times each item was preferred. The higher the item frequency, the higher the priority or preference score. Explore the results with participants— noting particularly what criteria were applied to priority setting, what trends or changing patterns are occurring, and whether ranking reflects the community reality. Pair-wise ranking is also an effective strategy for community members to prioritize particular actions. For example, participants list various actions to prevent violence against women, create a matrix, and then

Table 5-1 Pair-Wise Ranking on Women's Health Concerns

	Respiratory infections	Sexually transmitted infections	Lack of money to buy medications	Intimate partner violence	Sexual violence
Respiratory infections	X	STIs	Lack of money	Violence	Violence
Sexually transmitted infections	X	X	Lack of money	Violence	Violence
Lack of money to buy medications	X	X	X	Lack of money	Violence
Intimate partner violence	X	X	X	X	Sexual violence
Sexual violence	X	X	X	X	X
Totals	0	1	2	2	4

X = redundant matrix box

perform pair-wise ranking to determine priorities for preventive programs.

Process mapping is another participatory data collection technique. In this strategy, participants outline their perceptions of steps in an identified process. For example, women in a rural Southern Sudan community described the process of reporting incidents of violence. Each step was written on a card and then arranged sequentially by participants to represent the process. Variations were immediately evident to all participants, and these differences provided excellent dialogue about process gatekeepers and system barriers that women encounter after a violent event (see **Box 5-15**).

A final participatory data collection example is the causal flow diagram (Ellsberg & Heise, 2005; Kumar, 2002). In this activity, a problem or concern has already been identified by community or organization members. For example, a nursing leadership group might decide to research the high hospital-acquired infection rates at their institution. One of the data collection strategies could include gathering key players' perspectives on the root causes and multisystem impacts of high infection rates. After identifying all pertinent actors and stakeholders, the research group conducts several focus group discussions with a mix of actors and stakeholders. During each focus group, facilitators draw a circle in the middle of a large flipchart and place the hospital-acquired infection rate in the circle. Asking focus group members to identify root causes of the situation, facilitators visually create on the left side of the flipchart multiple circles. Each circle flows into the large center circle and represents an identified cause (see **Figure 5-6**). Focus group members are also asked to identify causes of each cause, so the branching of circles can become quite extensive. Once participants are satisfied that the diagram depicts all root causes, facilitators then ask about the effects of high infection rates. New circles placed on the right side of the flipchart depict each identified effect. Once this discussion is exhausted, attention is turned to the entire flow diagram. Facilitators ask open-ended questions about each cause and each effect. Group dialogue ensues and often leads to deeper understandings about cause–cause, cause–effect, and effect–effect links in problem

Box 5-15 Process Mapping: Gatekeepers and Barriers Women Encounter When Seeking Help After a Violent Event

Process Gatekeepers

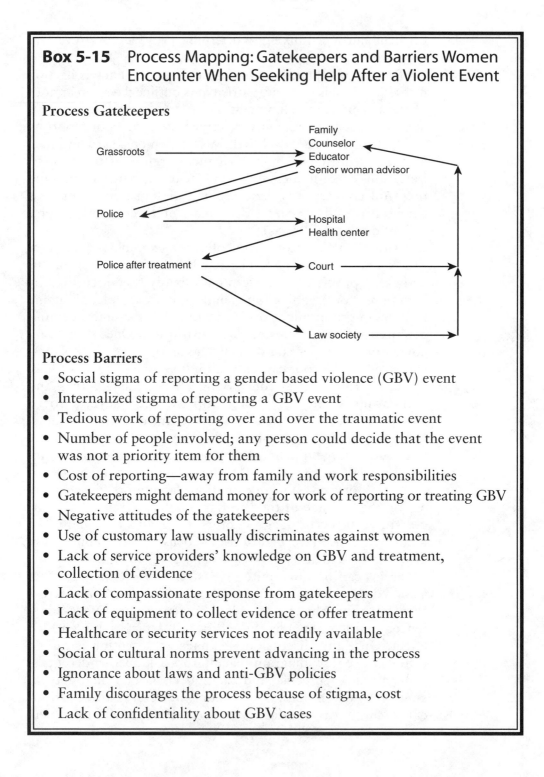

Process Barriers
- Social stigma of reporting a gender based violence (GBV) event
- Internalized stigma of reporting a GBV event
- Tedious work of reporting over and over the traumatic event
- Number of people involved; any person could decide that the event was not a priority item for them
- Cost of reporting—away from family and work responsibilities
- Gatekeepers might demand money for work of reporting or treating GBV
- Negative attitudes of the gatekeepers
- Use of customary law usually discriminates against women
- Lack of service providers' knowledge on GBV and treatment, collection of evidence
- Lack of compassionate response from gatekeepers
- Lack of equipment to collect evidence or offer treatment
- Healthcare or security services not readily available
- Social or cultural norms prevent advancing in the process
- Ignorance about laws and anti-GBV policies
- Family discourages the process because of stigma, cost
- Lack of confidentiality about GBV cases

Figure 5-6 Causal Flow Map

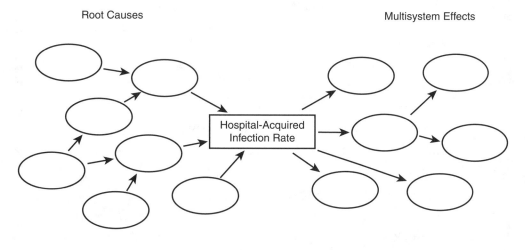

analysis. This data collection strategy is particularly helpful for system-wide analysis and action planning.

In summary, participatory strategies tend to engage participants very actively in the identification and analysis of problem situations. Each strategy embraces multiple perspectives and contextual understandings. The interactive nature of these data gathering techniques can be quite lively. Participatory strategies are particularly relevant to CBCAR projects since they delve into analyzing pragmatic, everyday concerns and often access tacit knowledge that can be useful for action planning. Additionally, wider analysis often results from participatory data collection that leads to more effective action planning (Kumar, 2002). Several participatory data collection strategies exist and are easily tailored to fit CBCAR projects (see **Box 5-16**).

■ **Summary—Circling Between Data Collection and Analysis**

The tree has a tale to tell. Our task as data collectors is to uncover the story. We persistently and patiently pursue the elements, and gradually, step by step, patterns unfold. Early patterns often present new avenues to pursue, which then reveal

Box 5-16 Participatory Data Collection Strategies

- Body mapping
- Community mapping
- Venn diagram
- Photovoice/photo elicitation strategies
- Timeline/seasonal diagramming/trend analysis
- Transect walk
- Participatory video
- Services and opportunities map
- Dream map
- Network diagram
- Spider diagram

new lines and new designs that require exploring. The quest for deeper understanding continues. Data collection is indeed a fascinating aspect of research that cannot be separated from the stages that precede or follow. Emerging from research questions that seek insight and from the research partnership that pursues change, the data collection plan is carefully and collaboratively crafted. Ethics, science, and context create the maps that guide collaborative planning. Researchers then enter new relationships in various settings and employ multiple strategies with research participants to embark on shared exploration and construction of meaning. Transcending simple data accumulation, joint construction of meaning implies stepping into data analysis and, as meaning unfolds, allowing for the possibility that data collection plans may shift. The circling between data collection and analysis requires researchers to be alert to the dynamic possibilities that unfold in the living, emergent process that typifies CBCAR projects. So even though chapter headings separate data collection from data analysis in this book, readers will find themselves circling between the two chapters as their own projects find life and gradually emerge.

■ References

Ayala, G., Maty, S., Cravey, A., & Webb, L. (2005). Mapping social and environmental influences on health: A community perspective. In B. Israel, E. Eng, A. Schultz, & E. Parker (Eds.), *Methods in community-based participatory research for health* (pp. 188–209). San Francisco, CA: Wiley.

Baker, E., & Motton, F. (2005). Creating understanding and action through group dialogue. In B. Israel, E. Eng, A. Schultz, & E. Parker (Eds.), *Methods in community-based participatory research for health* (pp. 307–325). San Francisco, CA: Wiley.

Barbour, R., & Kitzinger, J. (1999). The challenge and promise of focus groups. In R. Barbour & J. Kitzinger (Eds.), *Developing focus groups research: Politics, theory and practice* (pp. 1–20). Thousand Oaks, CA: Sage.

Barnidge, E., Bake, E., Motton, F., Rose, F., & Fitzgerald, T. (2010). Participatory method to identify root determinants of health: The heart of the matter. *Progress in Community Health Partnerships: Research, Education, and Action, 4,* 55–63.

Bays, S. (1998). Work, politics, and coalition building: Hmong women's activism in a central California town. In N. Naples (Ed.), *Community activism and feminist politics: Organizing across race, class, and gender* (pp. 301–324). New York, NY: Routledge.

Chambers, R. (1997). *Whose reality counts?: Putting the first last.* London, UK: ITDG.

Charmaz, K. (2008). Grounded theory as an emergent method. In S. Hesse-Biber & P. Leavy (Eds.), *Handbook of emergent methods* (pp. 155–170). New York, NY: Guilford.

Chiu, L. (2003). Transformational potential of focus group practice in participatory action research. *Action Research, 1,* 165–183.

Christopher, S., Burhansstipanov, L., & McCormick, A. (2005). Using a CBPR approach to develop an interviewer training manual with members of the Apsáalooke Nation. In B. Israel, E. Eng, A. Schultz, & E. Parker (Eds.), *Methods in community-based participatory research for health* (pp. 128–145). San Francisco, CA: Wiley.

Clarke, A. (2005). *Situational analysis: Grounded theory after the post-modern turn.* Thousand Oaks, CA: Sage.

Creswell, J. (1998). *Qualitative inquiry and research design: Choosing among five traditions.* Thousand Oaks, CA: Sage.

Davidson, P., Introna, K., Daly, J., Paull, G., Jarvis, R., Angus, J., & Dracup, K. (2003). Cardiorespiratory nurses' perceptions of palliative care in nonmalignant disease: Data for the development of clinical practice. *American Journal of Critical Care, 12*, 47–54.

Denzin, N., & Lincoln, Y. (2000). Introduction: The discipline and practice of qualitative research. In N. Denzin & Y. Lincoln (Eds.), *Handbook of qualitative research* (pp. 1–28). Thousand Oaks, CA: Sage.

Ellsberg, M., & Heise, L. (2005). *Researching violence against women: A practical guide for researchers and activists.* Geneva, Switzerland: World Health Organization.

Eng, E., Moore, K. S., Rhodes, S., Griffith, D., Allison, L., Shirah, K., & Mebane, E. (2005). Insiders and outsiders assess who is "community." In B. Israel, E. Eng, A. Schultz, & E. Parker (Eds.), *Methods in community-based participatory research for health* (pp. 77–100). San Francisco, CA: Wiley.

Foster, J., & Stanek, K. (2007). Cross-cultural considerations in the conduct of community-based participatory research. *Family and Community Health, 30*, 42–49.

Gadamer, H. G. (1995). *Truth and method.* (J. Weinsheimer & D. Marshall, Trans.). New York, NY: Continuum Publishing (Original work published 1960).

Genat, B. (2009). Building emergent situated knowledges in participatory action research. *Action Research, 7*, 101–115.

Gilchrist, V, & Williams, R. (1999). Key informant interviews. In B. Crabtree & W. Miller (Eds.), *Doing qualitative research* (pp. 71–88). Thousand Oaks, CA: Sage.

Greenbaum, T. (2000). *Moderating focus groups: A practical guide for group facilitation.* Thousand Oaks, CA: Sage.

Haraway, D. (1988). Situated knowledges: The science question in feminism and the privilege of partial perspective. *Feminist Studies, 14*, 575–599.

Hennink, M. (2008). Emergent issues in international focus group discussions. In S. Hesse-Biber & P. Leavy (Eds.), *Handbook of emergent methods* (pp. 207–220). New York, NY: Guilford.

Herda, E. (1999). *Research conversations and narrative: A critical hermeneutic orientation in participatory inquiry.* Westport, CT: Praeger.

Heron, J., & Reason, P. (2006). The practice of co-operative inquiry: Research "with" rather than "on" people. In P. Reason & H. Bradbury (Eds.), *Handbook of action research* (pp. 144–154). Thousand Oaks, CA: Sage.

Hollander, J. (2004). The social contexts of focus groups. *Journal of Contemporary Ethnography, 33*, 602–637.

Holstein, J., & Gubrium, J. (1995). *The active interview.* Thousand Oaks, CA: Sage.

Hyvärinen, M. (2008). Analyzing narratives and story-telling. In P. Alasuutari, L. Bickman, & J. Brannen (Eds.), *The Sage handbook of social research methods* (pp. 447–460). Los Angeles, CA: Sage.

Israel, B., Schultz, A., Parker, E., & Becker, A. (1998). Review of community-based research: Assessing partnership approaches to improve public health. *Annual Review of Public Health, 19,* 173–202.

Kendrick, K. (1998). Producing the battered woman: Shelter politics and the power of the feminist voice. In N. Naples (Ed.), *Community activism and feminist politics: Organizing across race, class, and gender* (pp. 151–173). New York, NY: Routledge.

Kieffer, E., Salabarría-Peña, Y., Odorns-Young, A., Willis, S., Baber, K., & Guzman, R. (2005). The application of focus group methodologies to community-based participatory research. In B. Israel, E. Eng, A. Schultz, & E. Parker (Eds.), *Methods in community-based participatory research for health* (pp. 146–166). San Francisco, CA: Wiley.

Kitchener, K., & Kitchener, R. (2009). Social science and research ethics: Historical and ethical issues. In D. Mertens & P. Ginsberg (Eds.), *The handbook of social research ethics* (pp. 5–22). Los Angeles, CA: Sage.

Koniak-Griffith, D., Nyamathi, A., Tallen, L., González-Figueroa, E., & Dominick, E. (2007). Breaking the silence: What homeless 18–24 year olds say about HIV vaccine trials. *Journal of Health Care for the Poor and Underserved, 18,* 687–698.

Krieger, J., Allen, C., Roberts, J. Ross, L., & Takaro, T. (2005). What's with the wheezing? Methods used by the Seattle-King County Health Homes Project to assess exposure to indoor asthma triggers. In B. Israel, E. Eng, A. Schultz, & E. Parker (Eds.), *Methods in community-based participatory research for health* (pp. 230–250). San Francisco, CA: Wiley.

Krueger, R., & Casey, M. (2000). *Focus groups: A practical guide for applied research.* Thousand Oaks, CA: Sage.

Kumar, S. (2002). *Methods for community participation.* London, UK: ITDG.

Lincoln, Y. (2009). Ethical practices in qualitative research. In D. Mertens & P. Ginsberg (Eds.), *The handbook of social research ethics* (pp. 150–169). Los Angeles, CA: Sage.

Lincoln, Y., & Guba, E. (1985). *Naturalistic inquiry.* Thousand Oaks, CA: Sage.

Mack, N., Woodsong, C., MacQueen, K., Guest, G., & Namey, E. (2005). *Qualitative research methods: A data collector's field guide.* Research Triangle Park, NC: Family Health International.

Madriz E. (2000). Focus groups in feminist research. In N. Denzin & Y. Lincoln (Eds.), *Handbook of qualitative research* (pp. 835–850). Thousand Oaks, CA: Sage.

Mertens, D. (2005). *Research and evaluation in education and psychology: Integrating diversity with quantitative, qualitative, and mixed methods.* Thousand Oaks, CA: Sage.

Mertens, D., & Ginsberg, P. (Eds.) (2009). *The handbook of social research ethics.* Los Angeles, CA: Sage.

Minkler, M. (2004). Ethical challenges for the "outside" researcher in community-based participatory research. *Health Education & Behavior, 31,* 684–697.

Minkler, M., & Wallerstein, N. (Eds.). (2003). *Community-based participatory research for health.* San Francisco, CA: Jossey-Bass.

Mishler, E. (1986). *Research interviewing: Context and narrative.* Cambridge, MA: Harvard University.

Morgan, D. (2002). Focus group interviewing. In J. Gubrium & J. Holstein (Eds.). *Handbook of interview research: Context and method* (pp. 141–160). Thousand Oaks, CA: Sage.

Morgan, D., Fellows, C., & Guevara, H. (2008). Emergent approaches to focus group research. In S. Hesse-Biber & P. Leavy (Eds.), *Handbook of emergent methods* (pp. 189–205). New York, NY: Guilford.

Naples, N. (2003). *Feminism and method: Ethnography, discourse analysis, and activist research.* New York, NY: Routledge.

Nyamathi, A., Thomas, B., Greengold, B., & Swaminathan, S. (2009). Perceptions and health care needs of HIV positive mothers in India. *Progress in Community Health Partnerships: Research, Education and Action, 3,* 99–108.

Patton, M. (2002). *Qualitative research and evaluation methods.* Thousand Oaks, CA: Sage.

Pavlish, C., & Ho, A. (2009). Displaced persons' perceptions of human rights in Southern Sudan. *International Nursing Review, 56,* 416–425.

Pawar, M. (2004). A pluralistic approach to data collecting methods. In M. Pawar (Ed.), *Data collecting methods and experiences: A guide for social researchers.* New Delhi, India: New Dawn Press.

Polanyi, M. (1962). *Personal knowledge: Towards a post-critical philosophy.* Chicago, IL: University of Chicago Press.

Pretty, J., Guijt, I., Thompson, J., & Scoones, I. (2002). *Participatory learning and action.* London, UK: International Institute for Environment and Development.

Robson, C. (2002). *Real world research: A resource for social scientists and practitioner-researchers.* Malden, MA: Blackwell.

Roper, J., & Shapira, J. (2000). *Ethnography in nursing research.* Thousand Oaks, CA: Sage.

Rubin, H., & Rubin, I. (1995). *Qualitative interviewing: The art of hearing data.* Thousand Oaks, CA: Sage.

Salina, D., Hill, J., Solarz, A., Lesondak, L., Razzano, L., & Dixon, D. (2006). Feminist perspectives: Empowerment behind bars. In L. Jason, C. Keys, Y. Suarez-Balcazar, R. Taylor, & M. Davis (Eds.), *Participatory community research: Theories and methods in action* (pp. 159–176). Washington, DC: American Psychological Association.

Senge, P., & Scharmer, C. (2006). Community action research: Learning as a community of practitioners, consultants and researchers. In P. Reason & H. Bradbury (Eds.), *Handbook of action research* (pp. 195–206). Thousand Oaks, CA: Sage.

Sethi, S., & Belliard, J. (2009). Participatory health assessment in Haiti: Practical tools for community empowerment. *Progress in Community Health Partnerships: Research, Education, and Action, 3,* 257–264.

Shkedi, A. (2005). *Multiple case narrative: A qualitative approach to studying multiple populations.* Philadelphia, PA: John Benjamins.

Smith, L. T. (2001). *Decolonizing methodologies: Research and indigenous peoples.* New York, NY: Zed.

Smith, M. B. (2000). Moral foundations of research with human participants. In B. Sales & S. Folkman (Eds.), *Ethics in research with human participants* (pp. 3–10). Washington, DC: American Psychological Association.

Stringer, E. (2007). *Action research.* Los Angeles, CA: Sage.

Suarez-Balcazar, Y., Davis, M., Ferrari, J., Nyden, P., Olson, B., Alvarez, J., & Toro, P. (2006). University-community partnerships: A framework and an exemplar. In L. Jason, C. Keys, Y. Suarez-Balcazar, R. Taylor, & M. Davis (Eds.), *Participatory community research: Theories and methods in action* (pp. 105–120). Washington, DC: American Psychological Association.

Thorne, S. (2008). *Interpretive description.* Walnut Creek, CA: Left Coast Press.

Thurmond, V. (2001). The point of triangulation. *Journal of Nursing Scholarship, 33,* 253–258.

Torres-Harding, S., Herrell, R., & Howard, C. (2004). Epidemiological research: Science and community participation. In L. Jason, C. Keys, Y. Suarez-Balcazar, R. Taylor, & M. Davis (Eds.), *Participatory community research: Theories and methods in action* (pp. 53–69). Washington, DC: American Psychological Association.

Ulin, P., Robinson, E., & Tolley, E. (2005). *Qualitative methods in public health: A field guide for applied research*. San Francisco, CA: Jossey-Bass.

van Eyk, H., & Baum, F. (2003). Evaluating health system change: Using focus groups and a developing discussion paper to compile the "voices from the field." *Qualitative Health Research, 13,* 281–286.

Van der Eb, C., Peddle, N., Buntin, M., Isenberg, D., Duncan, L., Everett, S., & Molloy, P. (2006). Community concerns about participatory research. In L. Jason, C. Keys, Y. Suarez-Balcazar, R. Taylor, & M. Davis (Eds.), *Participatory community research: Theories and methods in action* (pp. 221–226). Washington, DC: American Psychological Association.

Vissandjée, B., Abdool, S., & Dupéré, S. (2002). Focus groups in rural Gujarat, India: A modified approach. *Qualitative Health Research, 12,* 826–843.

Wallerstein, N., Duran, B., Minkler, M., & Foley, K. (2005). Developing and maintaining partnerships with communities. In B. Israel, E. Eng, A. Schultz, & E. Parker (Eds.), *Methods in community-based participatory research for health* (pp. 31–51). San Francisco, CA: Wiley.

Wasserfall, R. (1997). Reflexivity, feminism, and difference. In R. Hertz (Ed.), *Reflexivity and voice* (pp. 150–168). Newbury Park, CA: Sage.

Whitmore, E., & McKee, C. (2006). Six street youth who could . . . In P. Reason & H. Bradbury (Eds.), *Handbook of action research* (pp. 297–303). Thousand Oaks, CA: Sage.

Williams, B. (1996). Skinfolk, not kinfolk: Comparative reflections on the identity of participant-observation in two field situations. In D. Wolf (Ed.), *Feminist dilemmas in fieldwork* (pp. 72–95). Boulder, CO: Westview.

Zimmerman, S., Tilly, J., Cohen, L., & Love, K. (2009). *A manual for community-based participatory research: Using research to improve practice and inform policy in assisted living*. Retrieved from http://www.shepscenter.unc.edu/research_programs/aging/publications/CEAL-UNC%20Manual%20for%20Community-Based%20Participatory%20Research-1.pdf

Analyzing Data and Reflecting Patterns

*J*ust as roots provide trees with sturdy foundations, tree trunks function to sustain life. On first glance, a trunk appears simply as a lofty structure that connects roots to branches. However, coaxing organic materials into its structure and dispersing nutrients throughout the system, the trunk actually reveals complex patterns. If, for example, we burrow deeply into the trunk's structure, we find channels for material transport, membranes for nutrient absorption, and matrices for tensile strength. The trunk reflects a dynamic, living system that reveals meaning about the tree's existence—not only about longevity, but also about environmental stressors and the tree's adaptive capacities. Similarly, research data, sometimes appearing simple on its surface, have many complex patterns living beneath. The process of carving into data to understand its complexities is the subject of this chapter. Although we mention the benefits of quantitative analysis, we focus primarily on the principles of qualitative data analysis. Subsequently, we present ideas on forming a collaborative data analysis team before describing options for constructing an analytic pathway. We also offer suggestions on creating an iterative and flexible yet rigorous qualitative data analysis process accompanied by specific examples of collaborative analytic techniques. Finally, we describe options for representing and re-presenting research findings to a larger community.

■ Principles of Data Analysis

More than word and number crunching, data analysis represents a rigorous yet fluid set of cognitive processes that requires extensive time and energy. In community-based collaborative action research (CBCAR) studies, researchers seek to uncover patterns of the whole in human experiences. Whether analyzing qualitative or quantitative data, some general data analysis principles include the following:

- Data analysis is determined by the research design and theoretical framework as well as emerging questions and gaps in understanding patterns of the whole.
- Researchers should know a variety of data analysis techniques and understand which techniques will best answer the research questions posed.
- As the analysis proceeds, researchers should recognize how weaknesses in the data or data analysis influence the conclusions that can be drawn.

Even though community-based collaborative action researchers might use both qualitative and quantitative data analysis procedures, we believe that CBCAR is primarily concerned with narrations of human experiences as lived within a sociopolitical world, and therefore, qualitative data analysis is the cornerstone of this work. The conventions of quantitative analyses can be used to fill knowledge gaps and expand the picture that is emerging from analyzing people's narratives. Quantitative data analysis may also be important for developing more thorough understandings about specific population characteristics and community or organizational context. For example, community-based research regarding prolonged labor patterns and poor infant health outcomes could explore women's perspectives about personal and structural factors that influence their decisions about seeking health care. However, quantitative data on infant mortality patterns and pregnancy outcome variables could also contribute important information to our understanding of the problem.

Table 6-1 briefly summarizes various quantitative data analysis techniques that CBCAR researchers might find useful. Numerous texts and resources on quantitative data analysis are available for readers to consult (Grove & Burns, 2008; Mertens, 2005; Munro, 2004; Polit & Beck, 2008; Robson, 2002). In addition, we encourage readers to consult with statistical analysts and software experts in determining the best approach for analyzing numerical data.

The remaining information in this chapter focuses on strategies for collaborating on qualitative data analysis. Lawler (2002) claimed, "If we want to find out how people make identities, make sense of the world and of their place within it—if we want to find out how they interpret the world and themselves—we will have to attend to the stories they tell" (p. 255). Attending to and finding meaning in people's narrations and experiences is the work of qualitative data analysis. According to Denzin (1989), the goal of qualitative analytic techniques is deep and "authentic understandings" of key troubling aspects within ordinary people's lived experiences (p. 33). Using various analytic techniques, researchers abstract meaning from people's experiences to produce *verisimilitude*, or in other words, explanations that resemble people's realities. These rich and thick descriptions (Geertz, 1973) provide nourishment for developing action plans that improve systems of care and people's health and well-being.

■ Principles of Qualitative Data Analysis

Data analysis within a CBCAR process incorporates many of the data analysis principles found in other qualitative research methodologies. However, a few specific principles also pertain (see **Box 6-1**). Whether incorporating analytic techniques associated with specific research methods such as phenomenology,

Table 6-1 Quantitative Data Analysis

Type of analysis	Sample analytic strategies	Sample questions
Descriptive analysis (univariate analysis)	Central tendency of a distribution • Mean • Median • Mode	What is the typical value of a variable? For example: • What is the prevalence of reported incidents of violence against women?
Descriptive analysis (univariate analysis)	Spread of distribution (measures of variability) • Range • Inter-quartile range • Variance • Standard deviation • Standard error	What is distribution of a specific variable? • What is the age distribution of women who report violence?
Inferential analysis (bivariate analysis)	Relationships between two variables • Scatterplots • Cross tabulation • Chi-square • Correlation coefficients	To what extent are two variables associated? • Is women's risk of intimate partner violence associated with reported history of child abuse?
Inferential statistics (multivariate analysis)	Relationship between three or more variables • Multiple regression • Factor analysis • Structural equation modeling	To what extent are three or more variables associated? • To what extent are poverty, age, education level, and rural/urban residence associated with women's reports of partner violence?
Inferential statistics	Differences between groups • Chi-square as "goodness of fit" • Analysis of variance • 2-group t test	How similar are effects or processes of two or more programs? How similar are characteristic(s) of two or more groups? • How do self-efficacy and empowerment measures of women in Program A compare to those of women who are receiving standard treatment?

Box 6-1   Principles of Data Analysis

Data analysis is:

- A rigorous and fluid cognitive process
- Intentional, strategic, methodical yet emergent
- Iterative
- Co-constructed
- Dialectic with divergent voices converging
- Inductive, reflexive, and transparent
- Interpreted yet grounded in data descriptions
- Approached with confident humility

---

grounded theory, or ethnography, or using emergent analytic techniques within the CBCAR approach, these principles should guide data analysis teams throughout the collaborative data analysis process.

Data Analysis as a Rigorous and Fluid Cognitive Process

Maintaining scientific rigor while thinking holistically and fluidly through data analysis is complex work. Hasty assumptions about meaning, selective focus on easily-available understandings, overinscription of researchers' own voices, excessive confidence in findings, and the tendency to ignore conflicting information are hazards inherent in qualitative data analysis (Patton, 2002; Robson, 2002). To avoid these pitfalls, researchers using qualitative analysis must adhere to rigorous evaluation criteria and also develop awareness about their own processes of thinking through their data. In addition, while working together on data analysis reaps multiple benefits, collaboration also expands the amount of time required to review and reflect on data meanings.

Data Analysis as Intentional, Strategic, Methodical yet Emergent

Data analysis teams should approach data analysis with the research purpose, utility, and rigor in mind. In addition, deliberate, ongoing, and open dialogue with the data and analytic process creates an opportunity for data analysis to be systematic, transparent, and always emerging. In other words, during analysis of people's lived realities and dynamic search for patterns of the whole, new questions emerge that open possibilities for unanticipated lines of inquiry within the CBCAR framework. Data analysis techniques are linked to method (for example, open coding and analytic memoing to grounded theory) but can also be emergent as data are analyzed and reveal new analytic pathways (Charmaz, 2008; Hesse-Biber & Leavy, 2008).

Data Analysis as an Iterative Process

Even though the data analysis team systematically plans the data analysis process and identifies progressive steps toward uncovering research results, those steps are not necessarily accomplished in a set order (Coenen & Khonraad, 2003; Stringer, 2007; Thorne, 2008). Movement between steps is partially dependent on researchers remaining open to the data messages. Therefore, rather than establishing a firm pathway toward findings, researchers must remain flexible and willing to reexamine data as new patterns arise, surprising combinations evolve, or relationships emerge.

Data Analysis as a Co-Constructed Process

Shared data analysis such that multiple voices are invited into the data analysis process yields valuable rewards in thickening and contextualizing the data. However, multiplicity can also tangle the process. The key is for team members to trust one another and create safe spaces for open and nondefensive dialogue. Listening without an agenda and speaking without the need to be right provide rich opportunities to co-construct meaning in research data. All data analysis team members whether from the community or academic setting are considered researchers and have an equal voice in constructing findings from the analysis.

Data Analysis as a Dialectic Process with Divergent Voices Converging

When analysis teams share diverse perspectives about data meanings, new complexities and possibilities emerge in the dialogue that ensues. Contradictions become visible, and the entire group grapples with channeling multiple voices toward common pathways that become even more expansive because of divergences mixing and merging. Polyvocality abandons "right" and "wrong" perspectives on data and instead presents opportunities for newer and deeper understandings of the whole.

Data Analysis as Inductive, Reflexive, and Transparent

Because the phenomenon of interest resides in participants' narrations, researchers generally approach qualitative data openly, without a priori theory or concepts. In other words, researchers work with openness and curiosity to pull meaning from participants' descriptions. In addition, all members of the data analysis team need to think carefully about where they stand in relation to the question(s) being asked and the experience(s) being studied (Morse & Field, 1995; Thorne, 2008). Gadamer's (1960/1995) philosophy of science encourages researchers to be completely open to an understanding of the research text by being aware of personal history and its possible influence on textual readings and by preventing theoretical pre-understandings from controlling learning from the text. The key is visibility in how inductive decisions are made during data analysis.

Data Analysis as Interpreted yet Grounded in Data Descriptions

Because qualitative data resides in meaning extracted from words, and words potentially have multiple meanings, researchers who work with qualitative data recognize that their portrayal of phenomena in the social world is interpreted rather than an exact replica of that world (Charmaz, 2006; Denzin & Lincoln, 2000; Lincoln, 1998; Reissman, 1993; Thorne, 2008). However, part of researchers' responsibilities in maintaining a rigorous data analysis process is that data interpretations are traceable to data descriptions as provided by research participants. Without that link, interpretations can dissolve into abstract speculation and vague theorizing.

Data Analysis as Approached with Confident Humility

Shared data analysis requires sound research and context knowledge, analytic skills, synthesizing capacities, and clear communication. Research team members have to be confident in themselves and each other as well as confident that the process will yield the information that is being sought. However, humility is also important as meaning is crafted and impressions are shared. Rather than being oppositional, confident humility can synthesize effectively during shared data analysis.

■ Forming the Data Analysis Team

Although academic researchers are usually the research methods and process experts, their skill is not considered more or less important than community members who are the content and context experts. Shared data analysis draws extensively on both types of expertise in a cyclical pattern that reciprocally expands the capacity of both expert types. Additionally, a wide array of research methods, content, and context experts often yields an expanded view of the evolving pattern of the whole.

With this in mind, the research partnership group needs to deliberate carefully about who should be represented on the data analysis team. For example, community members who were involved in defining the research question may be invited back into the research process to help with analysis. In some instances, critical friends who were consulted during research design may be queried again for advice on who should be included on the team. In other situations, asking research participants to be part of the data analysis team is appropriate to the research question and subsequent action plan. For example, describing research on Aboriginal health worker practices, Genat (2009) identified a "critical reference group" (CRG)—a term coined by Wadsworth (1997) to indicate a particular group whose experiences and knowledge are unknown or marginalized. In Genat's research, Aboriginal health workers were considered the CRG, and a CRG subset became his data analysis partners. According to Genat, the key to selecting a CRG subset is finding "a group of participants to whom the research project is highly significant, to the point of being interested enough to prompt their ongoing engagement as 'participant researchers'" (p. 106). These participants not only shared their own experiences (which became data), but also analyzed, interpreted, and constructed meaning from the entire data set. Similarly, in a CBCAR study on quality nursing care, a nursing management team could partner with former patients and practicing nurses as the CRGs to conceptualize the question, design the method, collect and analyze data, and plan the changes needed to improve quality care.

Active engagement in the process of analyzing and making meaning from data is potentially transformative for all members of the data analysis team. Therefore, as the research team considers composition of the data analysis team, we suggest a brief mapping exercise to determine various groups of people who are potentially and primarily influenced by and influential in the change process. For example, since social and/or organizational change is the intended outcome of CBCAR and that change is most likely required within a certain arena, identifying all groups who are in the social or perhaps healthcare arena of the population being studied (as the arena pertains to the research question) might be helpful. Try placing the research question(s) and particular population in the center of a blank sheet of paper, and then, in the surrounding area, add all groups who interface with the population and have a significant relationship to the research question(s). The result will probably resemble an ecological map as described by Green and Kreuter (2005) or the "social worlds/arena maps" as identified by Clarke (2005, p. 86). This mapping process offers the opportunity for thoughtful dialogue about social actors, institutions, and discourses that pertain to the experiences being researched. Additionally, mapping provides a visual depiction of who should be represented during the data analysis process.

Some action-based researchers suggest that only research participants should make meaning of their experiences, and while the interpretation of research participants about their own situation provides important insights, we suggest a more inclusive approach that results in more diverse perspectives on data analysis teams. The process of attending to and creating diverse perspectives about experiential data often reveals pathways to deeper understandings of human experiences as well as the context in which these experiences occur. One example of diverse team analysis was illustrated by Burgos and Foster (2009) who, in the Dominican Republic, partnered with nurses and community members to research why women with obstetric complications delayed accessing hospital care. During data analysis, a group of community members and a group of nurses separately analyzed the same data set. Interestingly, different perspectives and patterns emerged from each subgroup, which then offered an opportunity for all group members in dialogue with each other to further explore meaning in differences and expand contextual understandings of delayed care. Analyzing the meaning inherent in these very different perspectives offered new insights into community patterns that delayed access to obstetrical care.

Although the number of team members generally correlates with the amount of data being analyzed, ideally the collaborative analysis team should be composed of 5 to 12 people (Bray, Lee, Smith, & Yorks, 2000). This size allows for diversity, democracy, and efficiency. Commenting on focus group discussions, Krueger and Casey (2000) claimed that groups discussing complex topics should be smaller, ideally 6 to 8 people. This size allows for deeper engagement in dialogue yet also offers diversity of thought. If a research study is quite large, and data suggest subcategories, such as the topic of "barriers to care" within a research study about quality nursing care across several patient care units in a hospital, then more than one data analysis team may form to analyze specific sections of research data. The key idea is to be intentional and inclusive, yet keep data analysis teams workable. If the collaborative becomes too large, then the work of shared analysis might become too cumbersome to work effectively. Additionally, group dynamics change when people want to participate but are not able because of group size (Bray et al., 2000). Boredom and disengagement among members are sometimes observed in larger groups (Kreuger & Casey, 2000; Bray et al., 2000).

In summary, although a perfect formula does not exist for data analysis team composition, we suggest that research teams consider their research question(s) as well as draw on populations who are most affected or previously silenced, and people who are potentially influential in promoting change. Some general suggestions surface such as the following:

- Both method experts (academic or field researchers) and content–context experts (community, organization, or group members) should be included and their ideas blended.

- Representatives from the population being studied should be invited to participate in data analysis.

- When people who have the capacity to create systems change at the structural level are involved in data analysis and interpretation, they often comprehend the issue more fully and can become champions for meaningful change.

- Some members of the original research partnership group should be represented and act as the conveners and organizers of early data analysis sessions. However, their leadership will subsequently fade as group members adjust to collaborative data analysis, and leadership responsibilities circulate among the entire group.

- Heterogeneous teams can potentially offer more diverse perspectives; however all team members should have in common an interest in the research question(s) and a commitment to systems change.

- People who suffer most from the issue under study and people who have been marginalized from previous discussions on the research topic should be represented on the team (Abma, Nierse, & Widdershoven, 2009).
- Teams should be small enough for everyone to have the opportunity to make meaningful contributions and yet large enough to provide diverse perspectives.

Prior to securing a commitment from those who have been contacted about participating in the data analysis team, conveners should hold some information sessions. As potential team members gather, information about the research project such as origin, goals, and progress thus far needs to be shared. Specific tasks, expected responsibilities, and anticipated time commitment should also be discussed. Dialogue about the intensity and complexity of data analysis work should be included. Multidirectional learning opportunities must also be emphasized. In other words, all group members are viewed as both teachers and learners within the data analysis process. Stringer (2007) described research as a perpetual and interactive learning process, and therefore, data analysis team members should be encouraged to see themselves as part of a collaborative learning group.

Differences between typical working meetings and data analysis meetings should also be emphasized (Bray et al., 2000). For example, most people are accustomed to working meetings where interactions are more structured and usually focused on decision making or problem solving. However, data analysis meetings are less task oriented, more dialectic, and often leaderless since all group members participate equitably. Adequate time for discussion of questions and concerns must also be included. These information sessions are important so group members are realistic about whether they can commit to the time and work required for data analysis.

■ Orienting Toward Teamwork

Once the data analysis team has assembled, group members need to consider ways to effectively work together. Several suggestions pertain. First, group process norms that support equitable and efficient working relationships should be established. These "operating norms should be a living, breathing and dynamic document that can be revised based on team process evaluations and periodic review" (Palermo, McGranaghan, & Travers, 2006, para. 1). Operating norms facilitate open communication, decrease conflict risk, and promote task accomplishment. However, these norms cannot be imposed. Instead, team members create and periodically revise their own operating norms. To accomplish this, Bray et al. (2000) suggested that group members quietly reflect on the statement, "Regarding collaborative work, I assume that . . ." (p. 73). Each member then creates a list of assumptions about the collaborative analysis work, which is subsequently shared with the group. For example, an assumption might be "I assume that everyone will have the opportunity to share their perspectives." All assumptions are displayed, and group members then combine similar assumptions and create a final list of working norms that are acceptable to everyone. Alternatively, group members may be asked to share their worst group experiences and then create a list of working norms that could prevent those negative group experiences from occurring. See **Box 6-2** for sample operating norms.

Second, open dialogue about capacity is important. All members should consider and discuss their level of confidence and readiness to examine the research topic, conduct data

---

Box 6-2 Sample Group Operating Norms

- Mutual respect
- Equitable participation of all group members
- Open and honest communication
- Agreeing to disagree
- Avoiding interrupting
- Valuing diverse perspectives
- Starting and concluding meetings on time

analysis, and explore community or organizational context. In CBCAR, capacity building must be viewed as consistently multidirectional (Genat, 2009). For example, depending on the degree of familiarity among team members with the research setting, community members as content–context experts should share pertinent historical, sociocultural, and political information. Depending on the degree of research experience among team members, academic researchers as methods–process experts should share information that expands the team's research capacity. Whether instructional or conversational, reciprocal capacity building and knowledge sharing equalize relationships among group members, develop cohesiveness, and facilitate effectiveness.

Third, the importance of validating each other's knowledge and expertise especially in early phases cannot be overlooked. For example, patients who were research partners in a series of health-related research studies in the Netherlands described how being respected and validated by others on the research team increased their confidence and sense of empowerment (Abma et al., 2009). Openly discussing means for respecting, validating, and encouraging each other during difficult work is helpful.

Fourth, these early dialogue sessions usually spark questions, contentions, problems, and creative solutions about anticipated data analysis concerns. Maintaining an early log of these analytic considerations provides an opportunity for the group to warm toward each other and the task at hand as well as anticipate ways to embrace rather than stifle different viewpoints. Additionally, team members are encouraged to continually reflect on the origin and reasons for their emerging perspectives and insights. These reflections enhance the integrity and quality of data analysis.

Finally, efficiently organizing for work is important. A person may be designated to arrange and disseminate information about meeting locations. Even though team situations may vary, we suggest that members assemble where they can separate themselves from outside responsibilities and meet in settings that provide a secure, relaxed, relatively quiet, and comfortable space for gathering. Recordkeeping is also important; the group should devise effective means of documenting group decisions during data analysis. Keeping track of individual statements is not as significant as tracking team decisions, especially as the group coalesces and assumes collective ownership of ideas. Some teams audio-record and transcribe their sessions as a method of recordkeeping, and others visually diagram or chart their analysis process. Groups are encouraged to find ways of organizing their work for maximum effectiveness, efficiency, and productivity.

■ Becoming Reflexive

Inhabiting a particular social world, each group member has a particular perspective on the focus of inquiry that is important to understand and reveal (Coenen & Khonraad, 2003; Genat, 2009). Therefore, prior to qualitative data analysis, team members need time to reflect on their positions or standpoints regarding the research phenomenon. Lincoln and Guba (2000) identified reflexivity as the "process of reflecting critically on the self as researcher, the human as instrument . . . as the one coming to know the self within the processes of research itself" (p. 183). Therefore, we encourage team members to individually record about their understandings regarding the research phenomenon. As noted by Behar (1996), "That [acknowledgement] doesn't require a full-length auto-biography but it does require a keen understanding of the most important filters through which one perceives the world and, more particularly, the topic being studied" (p. 13). Acknowledging one's pre-understandings about the topic being studied and developing a healthy caution about one's perspectives facilitate being more open to messages in the data (Gadamer, 1960/1995) and multiple perspectives on the data. Haraway (1988) claimed that qualitative researchers examine themselves as part of their analysis "for the sake of connections and unexpected openings [that] situated knowledges make possible" (p. 590).

These views on reflexivity assume that researchers are part of the social world they study and analyze. By becoming more aware of their own perspectives and data interpretations, data analysis team members produce "better representations" of the reality being described (Wasserfall, 1997, p. 152). In addition, "reflexive knowledge makes visible and critiques relations of power operating in social relations and structures" (Kirkham, Baumbusch, Schultz, & Anderson, 2007, p. 37). Reflexive dialogue about social position and situated perspectives is an important component of the CBCAR process.

The processes of reflecting on the data and being reflexive about data interpretations merge to deepen understanding about the research phenomenon being studied. According to Wasserfall (1997), reflexivity implies a simultaneous distance and unity with participants' descriptions and provides an opportunity to learn more deeply about "our own lives in the process of grasping how the lives of others could teach us something about all lives" (p. 154). Therefore, all team members as researchers should develop the habit of tracing and being transparent about origins of their perspectives—not only prior to but also during data analysis.

Some authors recommend the use of self-reflexive journals in analyzing researchers' influence on the research process and findings (Adamson & Donovan, 2002; Ahern, 1999; Rodgers & Cowles, 1993; Stearns, 1998; Sword, 1999). Additionally, many of these authors suggest that researchers bracket or deliberately harness their own assumptions about the research phenomena while analyzing data (Ahern, 1999; Dahlberg, Drew, & Nystrom, 2001). For example, as an outside academic researcher working in partnership with Congolese refugee women to study their health experiences, I (CP) needed to be aware of my own health experiences, context, and assumptions. My overall goal during data reading was to ground myself in the words that participants used to describe their experiences and contexts—and not mix in my own experiences to interpret their text. Therefore, during shared analysis with Congolese women, I kept a reflexive journal that encouraged me to question how I was examining data, what I was seeing, and why impressions were forming. Leading to new insights, these questions encouraged me to examine participants' descriptions separately from myself and my own health assumptions. I simply became more open to shared dialogue about meaning in the research text without hasty assumptions about meaning, and consequently posed more questions to the Congolese women who were the content and context experts on the data analysis team.

However, sometimes pursuing a more interpretive stance is appropriate for the research team. If, for example, nurse researchers are teaming with oncology nurses to study system barriers to palliative care, nurses on the data analysis team, although still aware of their own perceptions and experiences, may choose to be more interpretive and allow their own experiences and background to deepen meaning making during data analysis. Deepening awareness and being transparent about social positions in relation to the research phenomenon are the key aspects of reflexivity.

■ Appreciating Diversity

During data analysis as team members share their understandings about the data with one another, differences will emerge. Learning to recognize and appreciate the value of multiple and diverse perceptions is important. We offer a few suggestions. First, diversity as potential for synergistic energy and connected thinking should be celebrated. By adopting an open attitude to diversity and exploring a range of perspectives, group members often discover interesting connections and insights about the data. Searching for connections rather than commonalities in multiple and diverse ideas becomes the focus of team meetings. In this way, ideas about the data are enlightened, enlarged, and enriched by individual differences. Second, to more fully understand personal patterns, team members can take personality inventories, learning style assessments, or decision-making typologies. Sharing results provide opportunities to learn about one another and understand as well as appreciate individual differences (Bray et al., 2000). Third, rather than trying to convince team members that one way of looking at the data is better than another, Walkerdine, Lucey, and Melody (2002) suggested that group members "explore [different] interpretations in terms of the unconscious dynamics created [during] the encounter [with research data]" (p. 191). This highlights, once again, the importance of reflexivity. Furthermore, we suggest

that group members avoid saying, "I agree with your statements" or "I disagree." These and similar statements tend to establish unnecessary binaries during analysis. Instead, group
members should adopt the strategy of saying, "I have a similar/
different perspective on that point." Another strategy to avoid
binaries includes encouraging group members to say, "Yes,
and . . ." rather than, "Yes, but . . ." These subtle shifts in tone
encourage the group to explore a range of expressions rather
than negotiate between agreements and disagreements which
tend to suggest right and wrong perspectives.

Stewart (1994) cautioned researchers to avoid searching for
a unified voice and instead explore the possibilities that arise
from multiplicities, differences, and complexities. Silencing
voices and quelling differences, Stewart warns "always leaves us
without knowledge. Listening will leave us with more" (p. 30).

■ Planning the Collaboration

Collaborative data analysis is a complex set of cognitive and relational processes that "can be both exhilarating and painful"
(Bray et al., 2000, p. 11). Summoning persistence in the presence of difficulty and complexity can be challenging. As a con-
sequence, collaborative efforts sometimes disassemble during
data analysis with "participation work [being] diluted in favor
of analysis by outside [researchers]" (Pretty, Guijt, Thompson,
& Scoones, 2002, p. 66). In fact, little is known about the conditions and challenges of collaborative data analysis (Abma et
al., 2009). As part of a large systematic literature review, researchers at the Agency for Healthcare Research and Quality
(Viswanathan, Ammerman, Eng, Gartlehner, Lohr, & Griggith,
2004) examined 60 studies on community-based participatory
research (CBPR) and queried how CBPR is being implemented
regarding research methodology and community involvement.
Reviewers found little mention of community involvement in
the data analysis and interpretation phase. This finding could illustrate the challenges inherent in shared data analysis—particularly regarding time commitment, available resources, and
varying research capacities. The work of Viswanathan et al.,

(2004) illustrates the importance of defining *community-based* as more than just where the research takes place and *participatory* as more than community members simply being participants who provide data for the study.

Regardless of how the team chooses to work together, deliberately, clearly, and jointly planning the unfolding collaborative process is important. Although planning an emerging process sounds paradoxical, being organized and intentional about collaborative work is actually part of being systematic and rigorous during data analysis. However, rather than rigidly structuring the process, the team should consider the plan a map with general routing information that could change as the journey unfolds (Bray et al., 2000). The key is to build fluidity and flexibility into the planned structure.

Ideally the whole data analysis team makes most or all of the decisions that are required during data analysis. However, depending on time and resource constraints, decision making might need to be distributed to various team members or subgroups. For example, when resources are limited or confidentiality is an issue, academic researchers might preliminarily examine data to construct a coding schema or draft early data patterns. Subsequently, other data analysis team members can review the research text that has been stripped of identifiers and critique and expand on emerging patterns. For example, in a CBCAR project to better understand the high rate of "uncontrolled" diabetes for African-American women, the advisory council, which consisted of community members, community health clinic providers and administrators, and university researchers and students, directed the data collections process (Pierre-Louis, Akoh, White, & Pharris, in press). The advisory council partnered with university researchers to collect data from women in the population of concern. Researchers worked within a unitary perspective using Newman's (1994, 2008) method of data collection to understand where the experience of diabetes fit into the entirety of women's lives. The resulting narratives, even if the usual identifiers such as name and location were stripped, included women's stories that might have identified them given the close-knit nature of the community. Therefore, data were analyzed by a small team of university researchers and a nurse on the clinic's healthcare team. Once the essential concepts were identified in the women's stories, a nursing student on the research team worked with Mrs. Nothando Zulu of the Black Storytellers Alliance to weave the data into a spoken-word performance by seven women. To preserve patient confidentiality, data were presented in such a way that each woman's story was spoken by several different performers. A DVD of the performance was used to engage community members in dialogue about how to reduce incidence and disability of diabetes for African-American women. Essential aspects of this process included deciding up-front who would analyze the data and who would be involved in data dissemination and action planning.

Clarifying which decisions will be made by individuals, subgroups, and the entire team is an important component of the analytic plan (Zimmerman, Tilly, Cohen, & Love, 2009). In a community-based participatory study that examined medication administration in long-term care, the academic–community partnership coined the term "decision-point," which was defined as a "key decision that requires input from all partners" (Zimmerman et al., p. 60). The authors claimed that some decisions can be anticipated during planning while other decisions emerge in the course of data analysis. To avoid confusion during subsequent steps, these authors emphasized the importance of early identification and prompt discussion about key decision-points.

The data analysis team can use a variety of methods to detail their collaboration and determine key decision-points. Three examples are offered. First, as described in Chapter 4, the Memorandum of Understanding (MOU) which is the overarching, formal agreement between organizations can be revisited and revised to guide group decision making (see Boxes 4-2 and 4-3). Second, a Scope of Work (SOW) is similar but usually more detailed and task-oriented than an MOU. An SOW outlines each member's responsibilities, delineates expected outcomes, and establishes a detailed timeline (see **Box 6-3**). Finally, a Task and Timeline Contract (TTC) can be crafted and signed by members to visually depict the anticipated chronology of work details and accomplishments (see **Table 6-2**). A detailed visual graphic is often very effective—especially if subgroups have formed. TTCs track the work of all subgroups and details overall team progress with data analysis. Using written plans

Box 6-3 Sample Scope of Work

Purpose

Collaborate with local community health workers to develop materials for disseminating health and human rights information.

Specific Tasks

Collaboratively develop and field test activities for a health and human rights learning program (could be 2.5 days for half the group and then repeated for the second half of the group or could be 5 half-days for the first group and 5 half-days for the second group).

Program planners and community health workers will:

- Discuss preliminary findings on human rights research.
- Analyze human rights documents: African Charter on Human and People's Rights, Rwanda Constitution, Protocol for the Rights of Women in Africa, and Universal Declaration of Human Rights.
- Identify consistencies and conflicts in various human rights perspectives.
- Describe meaningful patterns in data and documents.
- Translate meaningful patterns into essential lessons for people's health and well-being.
- Create an action plan for spreading awareness about intersections between health/well-being and human rights/responsibilities.
- Develop community-based activities to disseminate essential lessons.
- Field test and subsequently revise activities.
- Explore ways to integrate health and human rights information into existing community activities and programs.

Duration

Two preparation days, 5 working days, and 3 follow-up days are required to implement this project on-site. Community organization will determine the most effective timeline for implementing these tasks.

Expected Outcomes

Participants will learn more about health and human rights as well as individual and community responsibilities in advancing human well-being and social justice. Furthermore, ways to disseminate health and human rights information will be developed—including ways to integrate human rights concepts and principles into existing community programs.

Table 6-2 Example of a Task and Timeline Table

Project tasks	Jan–Feb	March–April	May	June–Oct	Nov–Dec
Inviting the data analysis team					
• Contact potential members	X				
• Hold information sessions	X				
• Confirm team members		X			
• Schedule first meeting		X			
Gathering the data analysis team					
• Set up a means of communication		X			
• Introduce all team members		X			
• Conduct team building activities		X			
• Establish group norms		X			
Orienting to analytic teamwork					
• Build interacting capacities on research context and processes		X			
• Share reflexive stances on research topic		X			
Planning the collaboration					
• Assign roles and responsibilities		X			
• Structure tasks and establish timeline		X			
• Determine decision points		X			
Constructing an analytic pathway					
• Review entire data set; determine analytic pathway			X		
• Apply criteria to analysis plan; review tasks and responsibilities			X		
Conducting data analysis				X	
Summarizing the data					X
Re-presenting the findings					X

such as the MOU, SOW, or TTC tends to channel the group's attention and solidify members' commitment to the complex work of collaborative data analysis. Alternatively, if the group prefers a more informal style of partnering data analysis, simply reviewing goals, accomplishments, and group process prior to and at the conclusion of each working session can be sufficient. In this way, a collaborative plan unfolds gradually as the analytic process flows forward. Detailed notes in the form of a data analysis audit trail (see section on criteria in this chapter) help to maintain this unfolding process as systematic and methodical. Although collaborative data analysis can be operationalized in many ways, being transparent, deliberate, and clear about the collaborative process during data analysis is important.

■ Constructing an Analytic Pathway

After orienting toward teamwork and planning the collaboration, the team members begin to review the data set, consider analytic options, and construct an analytic pathway. Creating a flexible and workable plan is the key to collaboratively constructing an analytic pathway. We suggest researchers keep two general pathways in mind when constructing their plan (see **Figure 6-1**). One analytic pathway emerges from the chosen method in the research design. Following this pathway, researchers use their selected method to frame and guide data analysis. For example, if the research partnership group designed an ethnographic study to examine sociopolitical structures and cultural health beliefs, the data analysis team would then use analytic techniques consistent with ethnography (Roper & Shapira, 2000). In **Table 6-3**, we summarize data analysis techniques that are specific to phenomenology, narrative inquiry, grounded theory, and ethnography. Although some commonalities and analytic techniques exist, unique features for each design also apply. Therefore, CBCAR researchers should study method-specific analytic techniques further and seek mentors as needed.

The second analytic pathway is more controversial, and yet, perhaps more appropriate for an evolving and collaborative

Figure 6-1   Two Analytic Pathways: Emergent and Methods-Specific

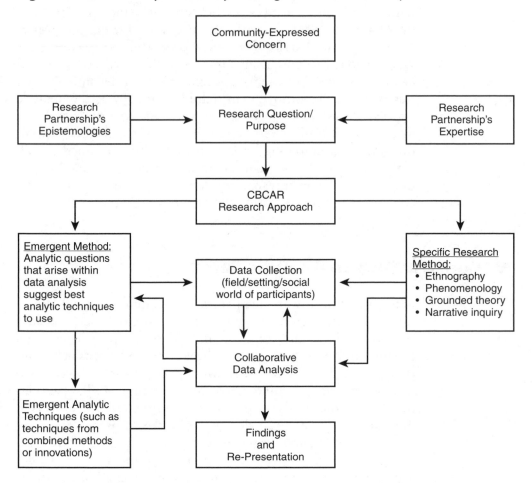

process. With this pathway, researchers allow analytic questions that arise during the shared analysis process to reveal the best techniques for examining the data. In other words, in the quest for "as complex an appreciation of [human] experience as possible" (Rapport, 2004b, p. 102), the most appropriate ways to answer the original and emerging research questions often reveal themselves in the analytic process itself. This pathway is "particularly well suited for studying uncharted, contingent, or dynamic phenomena" (Charmaz, 2008, p. 155). Therefore, researchers must be attentive, flexible, and comfortable with an-

Table 6-3 Four Methods Available for Shared Qualitative Data Analysis Within a CBCAR Framework

Research methods	Purpose(s)	Sample analytic techniques
Phenomenological study	Discover structures and meanings of lived experiences (Lopez & Willis, 2004; Munhall, 2007).	Dwell with description of phenomenon; return to participants for elaboration on ambiguous areas; identify meaning units; identify themes from participants' language; identify focal themes (moving description to researchers' language); synthesize general description of phenomenon (Giorgi, 1970).
		Identify common elements of phenomenon; eliminate expressions unrelated to phenomenon; formulate hypothetical definition; check hypothetical definition with original descriptions; specify structural definition (Van Kaam, 1966).
		Extract significant statements about the phenomenon; formulate meanings; cluster themes for each description; develop an exhaustive description; validate findings with participants; incorporate information from validating interviews into final description of phenomenon (Colaizzi, 1978).
Narrative study	Discover meaning in stories of everyday living through linguistic form analysis and/or theme analysis (Lieblich, Tuval-Mashiach, & Zilber, 1998; Reissman, 1993).	Examine stories that are grounded in context and reveal meaning; dialogue with stories (examine structure, linguistic form, discourse themes, and/or content); detect patterns across stories; identify common themes and core plots (or plot structures) in stories; interpret core plots to describe or explain life experiences or events.
Grounded theory study	Discover social theory by systematically gathering and analyzing data, and developing and verifying distinct hypotheses about relationships between concepts (Glaser & Strauss, 1967).	Code data (open, axial, and selective coding or open and focused coding); allow insights to develop throughout the study; use insights to determine what data is needed next and where to find it (theoretical sampling); continue to code;

(continues)

Table 6-3 Four Methods Available for Shared Qualitative Data Analysis Within a CBCAR Framework *(continued)*

Research methods	Purpose(s)	Sample analytic techniques
	Explain perspectives and actions of multiple respondents by clarifying patterns of action and interaction between and among various types of social units (Strauss & Corbin, 1994).	constantly compare codes; write analytic memos that construct conceptual and theoretical explanations; sample further as needed; refine evolving theoretical ideas, and construct theoretical framework (Charmaz, 2000).
	Interpret understanding of social processes by seeking meaning with respondents and defining "conditional statements that interpret how respondents construct their realities" (Charmaz, 2000, p. 524; Charmaz, 2006).	Charmaz (2006, 2008) encourages researchers to code for "actions and theoretical potential" (2008, p. 163) rather than coding for concepts, themes, or topics. Coding with gerunds helps to define what is happening; researchers can then memo about what it may mean.
Ethnographic study	Discover meanings that cultural groups attach to life experiences (Bhattacharya, 2008; Roper & Shapira, 2000).	Data collection and analysis often simultaneous; coding data for descriptive labels; comparing and sorting descriptions to find patterns; develop themes that fit the patterns; themes can fit together into more abstract networks.

alytic diversity. For example, a research partnership may have designed a CBCAR study to investigate nurses' palliative care practices by interviewing families about their experiences, and upon data review, the data analysis team discovers multiple narrations of palliative care stories. Therefore, the team may decide to extract all palliative care stories that are embedded in the research data and use one or a combination of narrative analysis techniques to develop deeper understandings about families' palliative care experiences. Furthermore, perhaps the data analysis team discovers that participants provided multiple descriptions of communication breakdown associated with palliative care. Therefore, by using a critical incident technique (Flanagan, 1954; Kemppainen, 2000; Schluter, Seaton & Chaboyer, 2007), the team could develop a categorical structure of factors influencing communication in palliative care. Analytic diversity works in part because analytic induction is a common feature of most qualitative analysis techniques (Jones, 2004). In other words, researchers examine data parts and then reason inductively toward creating deeper understandings about patterns of an ever-emerging whole.

At times in the data analysis process, the data reveal potential answers to new, emerging questions. Emergent analysis pursues the most appropriate techniques for developing insights on the original and evolving research questions. Consequently, on this pathway, CBCAR researchers avoid prescriptive analytic techniques. Instead, researchers review the entire data set, listen carefully to data messages, and determine which analytic techniques are appropriate to the original and emerging research questions. With this pathway, researchers need to be cognizant of differences between research methods and their related methodologies and analytic techniques before adapting, combining, or creating analytic strategies. The original and emerging research questions should be the researchers' guide for increasingly complex analysis. This pathway is similar to constructivist and emergent perspectives on grounded theory as proposed by Charmaz (2000, 2008). The keys to analytic flexibility include being knowledgeable about a variety of research methods and data analysis techniques, searching for and being open to analytic questions that emerge from data analysis, and consulting with research methods experts as needed.

No matter which analytic pathway is selected, the data analysis team must adhere to the rigors of a well-planned and executed study (Rapport, 2004a). In fact, decision making during this phase is often assisted by considering criteria for rigor in qualitative analysis. For example, all knowledge claims must be supported by clear explanations of the methods and standards used to produce research findings. Veering away from quantitative methods' criteria of generalizability and altering the face of validity and reliability, qualitative analysis generally employs five criteria for evaluating whether a rigorous and systematic process was followed and resulted in trustworthy findings (Kvale, 1996; Lincoln & Guba, 1985; Morse & Field, 1995; Patton, 2002; Sandelowski, 1986; Stringer, 2007):

■ *Credibility* is comparable to validity and indicates that the research topic was accurately identified and described such that patterns are consistent with the data collected and recognizable and understood by people in the study population. Thorne (2008) encouraged researchers to show consistency between their knowledge claims and the study participants such that findings are appropriately ascribed. Techniques that enhance credibility include data triangulation such as multiple data sources, shared data analysis, and mixed methods research; familiarity with the study context or research setting; verification with community members (often called member-checking); being grounded in research participants' language and descriptions rather than theoretical abstractions; and examination of diverse cases (including negative cases) as a way of including a broader data pattern.

■ *Transferability*, sometimes referred to as applicability, indicates that aspects of the research can be applied to other situations. Specific research findings are rarely transferable in their pure form from one context to another because unique features are found in all settings. However, insights can still be gleaned if the data analysis team provides a detailed description of the research context including study setting, history, sociopolitical patterns, participant characteristics, and data collection and analysis methods. People who were not involved in the study (i.e., research consumers) can then make accurate decisions about whether their situations are sufficiently similar to the research setting for the findings to be cautiously transferred. The ultimate decision on transferability is made by the research consumer whose decision is largely based on how clear and detailed the original study context is described. Therefore, the primary technique to enhance transferability is for the data analysis team to provide clear, detailed, and accurate descriptions of the setting and population being studied.

■ *Dependability* is often compared to reliability and sometimes referred to as analytic logic. Dependability requires team members to carefully adhere to a systematic process during data collection and analysis. Furthermore, rational and logical decision making to determine findings and draw conclusions must be evident. Team members must be knowledgeable about pertinent research methods and data collection and analysis techniques in order to claim dependability. The primary techniques to enhance dependability include designing a sound analytic pathway, and as analyses progresses, carefully documenting all research activities in a research audit trail. All revisions, decisions, and actions of team members are detailed in the log (Coenen & Khonraad, 2003; Lincoln & Guba, 1985; Rodgers & Cowles, 1993). Lincoln and Guba (1985) identified six aspects to the audit trail, which include research instruments (e.g., interview guides), raw data (e.g., documents, transcripts), data reduction and analysis procedures (e.g., code lists, working notes or memos on emerging themes and patterns), data displays (e.g., diagrams, matrices), process notes (e.g., summaries of team meetings), and researcher reflections (e.g., personal notes on motives, expectations, perspectives, biases). All aspects of the audit trail should be meticulously gathered and maintained in a secure location.

■ *Confirmability*, sometimes labeled neutrality, emphasizes that study procedures actually took place, and research findings are verifiable in participants' data. This criterion includes attention to researcher reflexivity and awareness of personal perspectives and how they influence the unfolding meanings. Primary techniques to enhance confirmability are maintaining a research audit trail as described in the previous item and incorporating opportunities for researcher reflexivity. Team members should be able to accurately describe their trail of decisions and verify that conclusions are grounded in research data, particularly during the steps of data analysis.

■ *Pragmatic utility* indicates the extent to which a research study guides future work (Kvale, 1996; Reissman, 1993; Thorne, 2008). Rather than being generalized to a larger population, qualitative research findings deepen understandings of specific contexts. Study findings can lead to transformed ways of practicing and can serve as the basis for context-sensitive policies, programs, and social practices. Researchers should consider whether pragmatic utility is a significant criterion for their study and build translation of findings into their process.

Even though the above criteria are considered the mainstay of evaluating rigor in qualitative data analysis, additional criteria could pertain to CBCAR (see **Table 6-4**). For example, calling for action-oriented research in this era of profound inequities and resource scarcity, Lincoln (1998) suggested three criteria for monitoring quality in action research. Additionally, Waterman (1998) proposed three types of validity to incorporate into action research. Coenen and Khonraad (2003) de-

Table 6-4 Additional Criteria for Rigor in Action Research

Reference	Suggested criteria for rigor
Lincoln, 1998	Criteria for quality in research for action • Community as arbiter of quality—community develops own standards for evaluating whether research has been useful in promoting positive change. • Positionality—social positions of knowledge producers are made visible. • Reciprocity—mutual exchange of knowledge between knowledge producers is evident.
Waterman, 1998	Criteria for evaluating validity in action research • Dialectic validity • Sources, evolution, and outcome of differences and tensions in perspectives are reported. • Movement between theory and practice is evident. • Iterative movement in the action research process is visible. • Critical validity • Active participation by community members is apparent. • Analytic discussions about action to improve people's lives are overt. • Reflexive validity • Analysis of potential for researchers' influences on project is made clear.

Table 6-4 Additional Criteria for Rigor in Action Research *(continued)*

Reference	Suggested criteria for rigor

Coenen & Khonraad, 2003	Criteria proposed for exemplarian action research
	• Reciprocal adequacy
	  • Knowledge production results from the joint efforts of researchers and participants.
	    • Mutual trust
	    • Democratic engagement
	  • Mutual relationship between scientific knowledge and common sense knowledge is evident.
	    • Findings in context of people's everyday language and lives
	• Explicitness
	  • Research process is precisely detailed.
	  • Critical examination of researchers' assumptions (reflexivity) is transparent.

Lincoln & Guba, 1986	Criteria for authenticity
	• Fairness
	  • Democratic processes are evident in research process.
	  • Viewpoints of participants represented (including variety and minority viewpoints).
	• Ontological authenticity
	  • Increased awareness among participants of the complexities in the issues being studied is evident.
	• Educative authenticity
	  • Increased appreciation for sources of alternative perspectives around the question (reflexivity) is evident.
	• Catalytic authenticity
	  • Participants provide reports of changed actions and decisions as a result of inquiry.

scribed exemplar-based action research and suggested that researchers and participants examine problematic situations and explore the most central phenomenon that has problem-solving potential. The authors offered two additional criteria for CBCAR researchers to consider. Finally, researchers might find Lincoln and Guba's (1986) authenticity standards helpful while planning collaborative analysis. By deliberately considering which evaluation criteria most clearly pertain to their research design and keeping particular criteria in mind *while* constructing the analytic pathway, data analysis teams can remain flexible within established boundaries that maintain a rigorous and systematic research process.

■ Uncovering Patterns Through Qualitative Data Analysis

Qualitative data analysis is complex work. In this section, we outline a wide array of qualitative data analysis processes. Bray et al. (2000) described qualitative analysis as a "discovery-oriented form of inquiry" in which "meaning arises and submerges, is tacit and articulated . . . with periods of clarity followed by confusion and then more clarity" (p. 89). There is no ideal way to conduct qualitative analysis (Saldaña, 2009). In this section, we offer ideas on how teams might work to extract meaning from research text. However, teams should consider these guidelines rather than rules as they map their own pathways to uncover data patterns.

Maxwell and Miller (2008) identified two general strategies for qualitative analysis. First, researchers make comparisons—examining data parts for similarities and differences and comparing data segments to an evolving pattern of the whole. Applying codes and sorting data into categories are the primary analytic strategies when using comparison. Second, researchers search for connections—examining data within the context of setting, time, and relationships. For example, narrative and case study analyses that tend to be holistic, interpretive, and process-oriented exemplify connecting strategies. Interpretive hermeneutics, which is often associated with phenomenology (Benner, 1994; Palmer, 1969; van Manen, 2001), also uses connecting strategies (see **Box 6-4**). Researchers examine data for meaning units, repeating patterns, and connections between data parts and whole.

Comparing and connecting strategies can also be combined. For example, researchers using narrative structural analysis can code and categorize research text according to plot, scene, conflict, and resolution before applying connecting strategies to cre-

Box 6-4 Sample Steps in Hermeneutic Interpretive Analysis

1. Reflect on the research topic. What current understandings do you have about the topic? What values and assumptions underlie those understandings? Where do those values and assumptions come from? Consider writing these thoughts down on paper and attempt to set aside (bracket) your ideas as you open yourself completely to the research text (i.e., without preconceived notions).

2. Enter the lifeworld of participants by immersing yourself in all data. Initiate dialogue with the text; be open to the text's meaning. As you read and re-read, you might think about "external supports" (such as theories) that arise during the reading. Note theories as they may arise but remain close and connected to the narrative text.

3. Write a preliminary interpretation of the text. Think critically here: does your interpretation reflect your openness to the text or have your pre-understandings been too influential?

4. Begin a new dialogue with the text in search of deeper, underlying, and sometimes hidden meaning. Look for ideas and messages in the text that might not be evident at first. Interpretation may arise from participants' explanations or from analysts' theory base. However, avoid using theory to impose meaning; instead connect yourself to data and allow theory to emerge from people's descriptions.

5. Construct a new whole, a "main interpretation" that incorporates earlier, preliminary interpretation.

6. Test the interpretation—does the interpretation illuminate the textual data?

ate a description of narrative themes (Lieblich, Tuval-Mashiach, & Zilber, 1998). Grounded theory methods also combine comparing and connecting strategies by first using open coding and constant comparison and then proceeding to connecting strategies when examining theoretical relationships between concepts and categories (Charmaz, 2000; Clarke, 2005).

Whether comparing, connecting, or combining strategies during data analysis, researchers iteratively shift through five intellectually-demanding processes—data reading, labeling, reducing, sorting, and displaying (Maxwell & Miller, 2008; Miles & Huberman, 1994; Stringer, 2007; Ulin, Robinson, & Tolley, 2005). If a specific research method such as grounded theory was chosen, then the team will work through these five intellectual processes within the framework of the selected method. If the team is following an emergent analytic pathway, these five processes still apply but in a more inductive fashion. Even though these five processes might appear as steps, we emphasize that data analysis is dynamic and iterative rather than linear. Detailing movement among these five steps during data analysis in a thorough data audit trail is very important.

Reading and Absorbing Data

Mind-immersion in the whole data set is important. Each research team member must become very familiar with participants' words—preferably reading the entire text the first time without a pen or highlighter to distract attention. Arranging uninterrupted time and working in a quiet space allow the mind to absorb words and subtle flavors contained within research narrations. Group members should avoid the temptation to quickly label or question or highlight. Data immersion and absorption are the key activities. There will be subsequent opportunities to label, question, and sort. This first reading is an opportunity to encourage the mind to flow freely with the data as if listening to a fascinating dialogue without the need to interrupt or contribute. Subsequent data readings allow plenty of opportunity for conversing with the data. After reading all data, team members might choose to write freely and reflectively about early data impressions that can be shared during subsequent group meetings.

Next, read data again and this time use various techniques such as highlighting, margin-writing, or color-coded commenting. In addition, we often circle words and phrases that require more attention when we return to data during a third read. Sometimes creating a trail of topics is helpful during the second reading. For example, when working transculturally, we often work descriptively to avoid introducing our own cultural interpretations to the data. Therefore, we stay very close to participants' words and note in the margin specific topics that participants describe. This technique is sometimes labeled descriptive coding (Miles & Huberman, 1994; Saldaña, 2009); however, we prefer to separate this process from subsequent coding and simply list topics and their sequence within each interview (see **Table 6-5**). Team members could work separately during this phase and create their own trail of topics to later share with other team members. Examining the trail of topics sometimes provides clues about next steps for data analysis. For example, topics that are raised repeatedly or are accompanied by strong feelings might become categories that require subsequent, deeper analysis.

A preliminary category list may be started at this point; however, it is important to note that these categories are not themes or patterns. Instead, at this point, categories offer a preliminary, descriptive framework in which to begin arranging or classifying data. These categories might correlate to the guide that was used to collect data or could emerge from data readings. For example, during a human rights research study, a category that was suggested by the interview guide included community factors that facilitated human rights realization (Pavlish & Ho, 2009). However, the trail of topics revealed that participants repeatedly raised the issue of human rights violations—even though the interview guide did not ask for that data. Therefore, we generated a category for human rights violations and sorted all research text that mentioned rights violations into that category. We then coded data within the human rights violation category to develop deeper understandings about rights violations.

Some research teams may choose not to identify a trail of topics and instead use second-step data reading as an opportunity to initiate coding. Allowing the data to suggest analytic steps corresponds to the emergent nature of qualitative analysis. As suggested previously, the research team should remain flexible yet logical and transparent about all of their decisions regarding analysis. Keeping research purpose and criteria for rigor in mind, the team can make reasoned decisions about what analytic steps the data is suggesting. Recording these decisions in the audit trail is important.

Table 6-5 Participant Demographics, Interview Topic Trail, and Primary Issues

Woman	Age	Marital status	Years of school	Number of children	Trail of topics (discussed by participant)	Issue (researcher analysis)
A	38	Married	0	8	Poverty Background/children Poverty (past/present) Worry about daughters Poverty Women forced to do sex Beatings Poverty Women's work Need equality for women	Gender roles Sexual exploitation Domestic violence Poverty Social pressure on girls and women
C	36	Widow	5	6	Marriage and husband's death Difficulty of caring for sick husband and parenting; God and friends help Loneliness Difficulty of mothering alone Poverty Widows not respected Pressure from men Section chief refuses house repairs Poverty and children Worries for her daughters Poverty—wants a job Women's work, men's work Poverty Loneliness; shame Worries and hopes for her daughters	Sexual exploitation Corruption Grieving and loneliness Safety Poverty and informal sector work Worry for daughters

In summary, early data readings allow the mind to absorb and appreciate the whole data set whereas subsequent readings create space for examining specific aspects of the data and provide an opportunity to delve more deeply into participants' realities, perspectives, actions, and situations. Deeper readings of the data prepare researchers to apply labels to their research text.

Labeling Data—Coding and Categorizing

Coding is the most common technique for examining aspects of the data in qualitative analysis (Maxwell & Miller, 2008; Miles & Huberman, 1994; Ryan & Bernard, 2000; Saldaña, 2009). In fact, Miles and Huberman (1994) claim that coding *is* analysis (p. 56). Saldaña (2009) defines coding as ascribing "a word or short phrase that symbolically assigns a summative, salient, essence-capturing, and/or evocative attribute for a portion of language-based or visual data" (p. 3). Researchers can code at different specificity levels including words, phrases, sentences, incidents, or paragraphs in written texts. Single actions or a series of activities can be the labeling unit in visual texts.

Early reads of the entire data set help data analysis team members decide on the best approach to coding. We present two general approaches to consider (see **Figure 6-2**). First, if researchers gain the sense that the entire data set is falling into large chunks of similar data, then proceeding to unitize or categorize data before in-depth coding makes sense (Stringer, 2007). For example, when reading the human rights research text, large topics seemed to fall out of the data, and therefore, all data were sorted into these categories before coding within each category (see **Box 6-5**).

Alternatively, research team members may initiate in-depth coding without chunking data into categories. For example, in narrative research on women's health concerns, all responses were coded; codes were compared and then connected into patterns as analysis proceeded. Focused coding (Charmaz, 2006) often follows initial coding. Researchers sometimes use the most significant or frequently occurring codes that emerged

Figure 6-2 Approaches to Coding

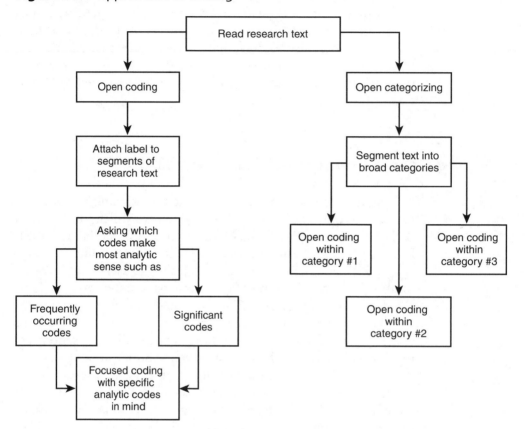

from initial coding to form more focused analytic codes. Research text is then recoded with these analytic codes in mind.

Both coding approaches are considered inductive since researchers allow both categories and codes to emerge from their data. The data analysis team should discuss coding options and then determine which coding strategy seems most appropriate to their data set.

Sometimes a code may indicate what is missing in the data. For example, in an exploration of the experiences of African-American women with diabetes, a community member who reviewed the data after identifiers were stripped observed that each participant described numerous energy drains but identified no energy sources other than food. This was coded as a *lack of sis-*

Box 6-5 Categories of Human Rights Descriptions

Meanings of human rights

- Incidents of human rights violations
- Men's human rights descriptions
- Women's human rights descriptions
- Community structures involved in human rights
- Human rights facilitators
- Human rights barriers
- Human rights metaphors

---

ter friends which was strongly evident when the team reread the narratives. This code also resonated deeply with the African-American women with diabetes who engaged in dissemination and action planning strategies (Pierre-Louis et al., in press).

Word choices for codes emerge from the analysts' readings, questioning, and in-depth thinking about the text. Some questions that researchers could apply to the text as they code include:

- What is happening and what does it mean?
- What are people trying to accomplish?
- How do people interpret events as they unfold in descriptions?
- What assumptions are participants making in their descriptions?
- What is meaningful to participants as they describe events?
- What seems to be missing; what is not being said?

As coding occurs, we suggest that the data analysis team create a code list that identifies all codes and cross-references where the same or similar codes appear in text. Eventually, through analysis, codes in the original code list will gradually be arranged into a coding schema that offers a structural picture of how codes fit together to shape the view of evolving and expanding patterns of the whole.

Coding is both strategic and inductive. Most CBCAR research groups will code inductively to gain an in-depth view of the phenomena being researched. The primary goal is to capture the essence(s) that exist within participants' narratives to gain a deeper understanding from their perspectives. This is usually completed in an open, questioning manner without a priori theory in mind. However, in some cases, researchers might allow theory to guide their coding (i.e., code deductively).

Coding can be done manually with labels and notes sketched in the margins of research text or electronically with an insert comment function. Additionally, several computer software programs are available for qualitative analysis (see **Box 6-6**). However, remember that computers do not actually code data, research teams do. Computers assist researchers with code storing, sorting, and organizing, which can save many hours of manually sorting research text according to codes. While the process of computer coding breaks narratives into data parts, other functions provide opportunities to see connections between data parts that perhaps might not have been evident when sorting codes manually. In addition, when working collaboratively, researchers can use the computer to share and merge codes, compare analytic memos, cross-reference and link codes, and create coding families. Computers also assist researchers to track coding frequencies, ranges, and co-occurrences. However, some researchers claim that computers distance researchers from the text (Ulin et al., 2005). The time and cost of equipment and training must also be considered. Computers are certainly not appropriate for all CBCAR projects, especially when working with team members who have limited access to technology.

After all members of the data analysis team have read and coded the text, the entire team gathers to compare coding impressions and code lists. During these discussions, provocative questions emerge that lead to new and richer codes—especially as the team works expansively instead of competitively. As the team's codes begin to merge, a master code list is generated that guides further work. Sometimes at this point, assigning one per-

---

Box 6-6   Software for Qualitative Data Analysis

- Atlas.ti
- HyperQual
- QSR N6/NUDIST
- Ethnograph
- MAXQDA
- NVivo
- AnSWR*
- CDC EZ-Text*
- Epi-info*

*Available on the Centers for Disease Control and Prevention website at http://www.cdcnpin.org/scripts/tools/software.asp.

---

son as the "codebook editor" is helpful (MacQueen, McLellan-Lemal, Bartholow, & Milstein, 2008, p. 132). As an alternative, data analysis teams may read and collaboratively code research text. If time is limited, subgroups could form to code different portions of the text.

Many excellent resources exist on the mechanics of coding, and we suggest that readers explore some of these readings as they initiate and conduct their coding (Charmaz, 2006; Ellsberg & Heise, 2005; MacQueen et al., 2008; Miles & Huberman, 1994; Patton, 2002; Robson, 2002; Roper & Shapira, 2000; Ryan & Bernard, 2000; Saldaña, 2009; Schreiber & Stern, 2001; Stringer, 2007; Thorne, 2008; Ulin et al., 2005). Different levels of coding, such as line-by-line or focused coding, and various types of coding, such as attribute, gerund, or in vivo coding are also presented in these references.

Albeit interesting, the work of coding is detailed, tedious, intense, and time consuming. Charmaz (2006) and Saldaña (2009) cautioned researchers about potential coding problems such as coding at too general a level, overlooking context when coding, forcing new findings into existing codes instead of adding codes, coding too finely such that unifying concepts are missed, and attending to researchers' rather than participants' concerns. To avoid these common coding errors, Saldaña identified several attributes that researchers need, such as being organized, flexible, comfortable with ambiguity, persistent, creative, and ethical. We believe that engaging in collaborative coding allows members of the data analysis team to help one another further develop these capabilities. Taking time periodically to assess the group's capabilities and acknowledge one another as these attributes develop is important to effective teamwork.

Reducing, Comparing, Sorting Data

Once the team is satisfied with a temporary code list, the group is ready to move toward reducing and sorting data. This phase includes:

- Analyzing which codes seem to fit together to create deeper understandings about the emerging patterns of the whole
- Determining what aspects of the data seem most significant to the research purpose

Setting aside less significant data segments allows the mind to focus on the more fertile data segments. However, never discard data segments. They may become very useful as analysis progresses and further questions emerge.

Code sorts can be completed manually with highlighters and cut-and-paste techniques or computer-assisted with simple word-processing programs and qualitative research software. However, when moving text segments during code sorts, be sure to indicate the original location of each text segment. Otherwise, valuable time is lost trying to locate the original file when returning to the whole data set. At this point, researchers are generally applying constant comparison and moving among data segments and between segments and the whole data set. This ongoing sorting, swirling, and spiraling between data parts and whole eventually allows researchers to develop themes that can progress further into descriptive patterns of the whole. For example, to facilitate the process of tracking data sources in a

CBCAR project that sought to understand the interplay of racism, health, and well-being for women and girls of color, data were read and coded in teams organized by ethnicity (Amaikwu-Rushing, Fitzgerald, Wilson, Smith, Irwin, & Pharris, 2005). In other words, African-American women analyzed data gathered from African-American participants; Latina women analyzed data from Latina participants and so forth. Data from each ethnicity were printed on paper of the same color. When all data analysis teams met to develop a master code list and determine salient quotes for data presentation, each team cut and pasted data onto large scrolls of paper to create patterns of the whole. Because data were color-coded, data sources could easily be tracked.

Whether working together or separately during code sorts, team members should record (written or voice) their process in a series of analytic memos. These memos trace an individual's or group's thinking as sorting progresses (see **Box 6-7**). A series of analytic memos tell the story of how and why certain codes fit together or provide contrasts. Additionally, memos contain early hunches about how code groups point toward broader concepts, themes, or patterns of a larger whole. For example, in a human rights research study, certain codes such as respecting everyone equally, distributing materials unevenly, discriminating against girls, and favoring certain community members were linked, so data were re-sorted according to these code groups. The re-sorted data contributed to deeper understandings about how equity/fairness fit into the community's emerging description of human rights. Analytic memos were written to describe our code-sort rationale, pertinent human rights literature, and persistent questions.

Teams may choose to organize their sorting work in various ways. For example, if a team decides to perform code sorts individually, then group members can subsequently gather to discuss their data sorts and analytic memos. Alternatively, teams might assign sorting to a subgroup or one person who can then perform data sorting and initiate analytic memoing. The team can then meet to review and revise the data sorting and expand and deepen analytic memos. With this model, the key assumption is that any preliminary work done by one person or subgroup is evolving and requires the entire group to breathe new life and sustenance into its existence.

Box 6-7 Writing Analytic Memos

- Separate coding (descriptive data labeling) from analytic memoing (interpreting data meanings).
- Record current thoughts and ideas about data and code meanings.
- Push yourselves to think reflectively and expansively.
- Incorporate insights related to theory and practice experience into memos.
- Note questions and hunches related to data meanings and relationships.
- Be specific and connect analytic memos to particular data segments, codes, or code groups.
- Distinguish (with different colors or fonts) between *analytic memos* which represent deeper thinking about data from *data analysis audit trail* which records specific steps and decisions about data analysis; creating one on-going log of both results in a more complete written record of data analysis activities. Date all entries.
- In initial analytic memos, compare data parts such as codes, experiences, categories.
- Periodically review analytic memos to spark deeper insights and find interesting parallels and intersections between data segments.
- Consider drawing or diagramming your data in analytic memos. Add to these diagrams as analysis progresses. Patterns become larger as later memos represent the synthesis of data parts.
- Consider audio-taping memos and transcribing to share ideas during team meetings.

(Adapted from Charmz, 2006; Saldaña, 2009)

Sorting data involves constant circling between data segments and the whole data set. There is no map with a specified route to research findings. Periods of clarity oscillate with periods of confusion, and what seemed a certain fit one day may not fit so well later. We urge data analysis teams to read, reflect, write, dialogue, experiment, and listen, listen, listen—not only to one another but to research participants' descriptions in the research text. Meaning is present in their words, actions, explorations, reflections, reported consequences, relationships, key events, and contexts. However, meaning needs to be extracted, questioned, understood, re-fit, pulled apart, compared to the whole, requestioned, and understood again. Tracking it all in an audit trail is essential to good science.

As the group works with various code sorts, combinations, and linkages, group members will gradually see more abstract concepts, patterns, themes, or relationships emerge from their analytic work. What the group actually searches for at this point will depend partially on the research method. For example, if grounded theory method is being used within the CBCAR approach, then researchers will see core concepts and possible relationships. If ethnography is being utilized, then researchers will probably see cultural and contextual themes and patterns emerging from the code sorts. If groups are using emergent methods, then members have to be especially tuned into whatever elements the data sorting has yielded. Regardless of what elements emerge, they should be traceable back to the research text and offer insight on the research question. Members can then transition into the next step of creating displays to enrich analysis.

Displaying Data

Data displays offer researchers an opportunity to view research data from different angles and in various contexts and relationships. Displays are particularly helpful during collaborative analysis since visual depictions of data often spark new dialogue and expanded insights. Revealing new information on what is happening, displays also offer ideas for corrective action (Miles & Huberman, 1994). In addition, preparing and analyzing data displays allow researchers an opportunity to develop some distinctions between major and minor concepts or themes and subthemes and see patterns in the whole (Ellsberg & Heise, 2005). Data displays assemble a significant amount of data and present that information in various visual forms including matrices, decision trees, taxonomies, timelines, maps, and diagrams. However, it is important to keep in mind that data displays are a form of data analysis and not simply a method for showcasing data (Miles & Huberman, 1994).

Consequently analytic memos should accompany each display. A few data display techniques are described.

Matrices assist researchers to make comparisons and identify trends and patterns in the data that might not otherwise be apparent (Marsh, 1990). Although matrices can be displayed in various forms, generally one of two formats is used (Payne, 1999). The first is a category-by-text format that compares a selected category to a text reference number. Particularly pertinent or interesting categories are selected and analyzed according to a reference number that usually indicates a specific population, location, time period, or other observation unit. For example, since so many women described sadness in a women's health research, the team analyzed the context of sadness according to participant (see **Table 6-6**). In a different study on immigrant women's health, the team constructed 2 matrices to compare women's health descriptions to healthcare professionals' categorical descriptions of immigrant women's health. This type of grid usually reveals clusters of data and provides information about across-case patterns that are not always evident in narrative form alone.

The second type of matrix illustrates a category-by-category comparison that identifies when categories intersect or co-occur. Researchers use their intimate knowledge of the data to determine which categories might be most appropriate for analysis. For example, in an early indicators of ethical dilemmas research study, the team wondered whether respondents described various ethical principles in certain contexts. Specific respondents were assigned a code number, and if they described patient preferences at end of life, then the participant's code number was entered into the box that intersected autonomy and end of life (see **Table 6-7**). Code numbers were inserted every time categories intersected in participants' descriptions. In category-by-category matrices, researchers extract pertinent aspects of the data (i.e., categories) that seem to relate and test whether these aspects co-occur in participants' descriptions. The more times that two categories co-occur, the stronger or more frequent the relationship. This type of grid permits comparisons across cases and categories and offers information on subtle relationships that are not always evident in narrative data until examined more closely.

Table 6-6   Category-by-Text Matrix: Context of Struggles

Subject	Life is very bad when . . .	What I do . . .	I get sad when . . .	What helps . . .
A	I don't have a job. I can't give money to my daughter. Husband can't give me what I need. I can't get food for children. No equality for women.	Get food from UNHCR. Worry. Ask neighbor for loan. Just want to fall down. Work hard.	Women have to do sex for money.	Survive. Cares about us. Watches us. Only God helps us.
B	UNHCR decreases food. Girls have no jobs so go to Kigali. Women work so hard. You don't feel free.	Worry. Work. Go to friend. Try to take it easy.	I can't give my kids food and clothes. I think about my life before.	Nothing.
C	No one assists me. I have no food for my children. I get no respect from others.	Pray. Borrow from someone. Ask chief for house repairs.	I run out of food.	God takes care of me when I suffer.

(continues)

Table 6-6 Category-by-Text Matrix: Context of Struggles *(continued)*

Subject	Life is very bad when . . .	What I do . . .	I get sad when . . .	What helps . . .
D	I have to give my husband food. When I pray and it doesn't help. When I think about my life.	I have no choices; just take it. Just stay at home and not go anywhere.	Think about what my husband did to me.	God sometimes makes me strong.
L	I don't have anyone to assist me. There is war in the house The husband takes money to drink.	Pray to Mary to be strong.		Pray to Mary. God keeps me strong.
N	Husband goes to other women. You don't get enough food.	I get so annoyed that I fight.		I go to church, but it's the same thing [nothing changes].

Table 6-7 Category-by-Category Matrix: Ethical Issues

	Patient autonomy	Resource allocation (justice)	Risk/benefit ratio (nonmaleficence & beneficence)	Equitable treatment (justice)	Privacy/ confidentiality	Provider, patient, family conflict	End-of-life care
Patient autonomy	X	13, 36, 61, 65	2, 7, 18, 33, 45, 63	4, 12	10, 19, 25, 31	1, 3, 5, 11, 15, 21, 24, 34, 52, 64	6, 8, 10, 14, 16, 18, 22, 24, 28, 30, 31, 35, 38, 39, 43, 47, 48, 51, 55, 59
Resource allocation (justice)	X	X	7, 11, 39, 50	12	11, 50	39	10, 18, 51, 59
Risk/benefit ratio (nonmaleficence & beneficence)	X	X	X	33, 59	22, 37, 45, 54	9, 13, 27, 29, 33, 34, 51, 55, 60, 63	3, 5, 6, 9, 11, 13, 15, 17, 22, 27, 29, 31, 34, 38, 42, 43, 57
Equitable treatment (justice)	X	X	X	X	22	17, 39	2, 23, 37, 57
Privacy/ confidentiality	X	X	X	X	X	3, 9, 12, 15, 23, 60	12, 15, 18, 20, 21, 26, 31, 39, 42, 55
Provider, patient, family conflict	X	X	X	X	X	X	3, 6, 7, 16, 17, 23, 29, 41, 44, 60
End-of-life care	X	X	X	X	X	X	X

X = redundant matrix box
Number = particular participant/case

Networks that contain nodes and links are another type of data display. For example, contextual maps can be constructed to develop deeper understandings about complex situations. When analyzing interview data on refugee women's lives, the team mapped factors that were mentioned to influence violence against women (see **Figure 6-3**). This map was constructed with pictures and words and then displayed for data analysis team members to examine and discuss. Our dialogue about the map raised the questions about power balance in gender relationships. The team then returned to the research text to analyze the degree of agency women experienced in their gender relationships and the power dynamics that were implied.

Clarke (2005) offers three types of networks that help teams visualize and analyze specific situations. First, *situational*

Figure 6-3   Factors Contributing to Violence Against Women

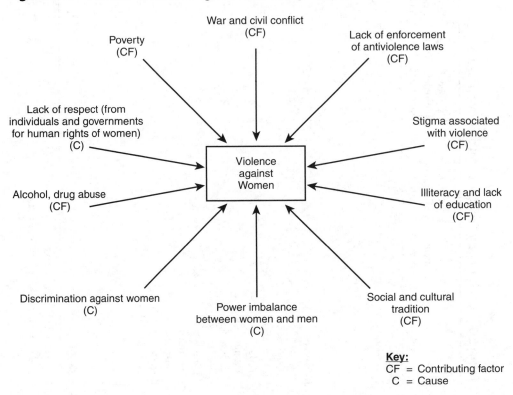

maps illustrate the major conditions that pertain to the situation that is being investigated. Researchers ask themselves, "Who and what matters in this situation?" (p. 87). After capturing the major elements, researchers then focus on how each element relates to all other elements that are depicted in the map. Analyzing data in this way encourages team members to view the study population and situation within a broader contextual setting. Second, *social arena maps* depict participants' descriptions of the primary social elements with and within which they interact in their lived realities. Individuals, agencies, organizations, social movements, and work groups are just a few examples of elements to capture in social arena maps. Analyzing these maps, team members gain expanded insights into larger sociopolitical structures that impact participants' situations. Third, *positional maps* display "the major positions taken in the data on major discursive issues therein" (Clarke, 2005, p. 126). Therefore, team members consider how participants describe conflicts, struggles, controversies, and relative social positions in the narrated data. Illustrating these positions on a map offers team members an opportunity to further analyze relationships and fluctuating power dynamics in participants' situations. All three types of situational maps lead to more in-depth and powerful analyses than if team members were only examining narrated data for themes and patterns (Clarke, 2005). Additionally, situational maps assist researchers to consider the social change required to improve people's lives and encourage human flourishing.

Other interesting mapping techniques are also available. For example, when exploring perspectives on how neighborhood factors influence women's experiences of intimate partner violence, public health researchers combined concept mapping with sorting-and-rating sessions (Burke, O'Campo, Peak, Gielen, McDonnell, & Trochim, 2005). First, research participants in dialogue with one another generated a list of neighborhood factors that they believed pertained to intimate partner violence. Then each participant was asked to sort the factors into "piles that make sense" and subsequently label each pile (p. 1398). The various sorts were entered into a concept-mapping software program. Additionally, participants were asked to rate each item on the list in terms of importance to violence prevalence, severity, perpetration, and cessation. Once these data were added to the computer program, a map that depicted the degree of similarity between factors resulted. Similar factors formed a cluster and were named by participants. The map also revealed the relative importance of each cluster to prevalence, severity, perpetration, and cessation. Finally, participants analyzed the visual maps and through small group dialogue, interpreted meaning for follow-up action. Social maps (Kumar, 2002) and neighborhood maps (Aronson, Wallis, O'Campo, & Schafer, 2007) also provide valuable visual displays for teams to analyze and for communities to consider in action planning.

Data displays offer specific ways to examine relationships in narrated data that have already been reviewed, labeled or coded, sorted, and reduced. The keys to successfully constructing data displays include:

- Considering the original research question(s) as well as the questions that have emerged during analysis
- Selecting the most important categories for further analysis in a display
- Seeking possible relationships in the data
- Moving beyond data descriptions and interpretations toward explanation

Once data displays are constructed, team members need time to absorb, query, and discuss them. Remember that data displays are part of the data analysis process, and therefore, should not be seen as the final analytic product. Data displays should provide ideas for action as well as new avenues to explore in the current research data or in future research studies.

Interpreting Data Meanings

Even though meaning making permeates all data analysis phases, team members need time at this point to consider the entire data set and core messages. Using knowledge gleaned from the study along with their knowledge of context and theory, group members enter into summative dialogue to construct key lessons regarding the research question(s). Rather than compartmentalizing data, the team concentrates on constructing new and wiser explanations about people's circumstances. Once again, different interpretations may surface. Making differences visible, engaging in purposeful and respectful dialogue, and being inclusive about interpretations are important processes during these summative sessions. For example, rather than solely focusing on common, similar, or repetitious patterns in findings, the team might decide to explore incongruencies, tensions, silences, and multiple interpretations. Dialogue on what contributes to distinct and different interpretations, and what these differences may signify could ensue.

Circling back to incorporate criteria for trustworthiness in these summative sessions is critical. Discussing appropriate knowledge claims and refraining from tangential theorizing are also important to keep in mind. In addition, summative dialogue sessions explore modes of representing research findings and offers some initial insights on what circumstances need to change to correct inequities, enhance quality of care, and encourage human health and flourishing.

■ Summary of Qualitative Data Analysis

Qualitative research methods provide analytic techniques that circulate through people's descriptions of life experiences. A variety of analytic techniques are available—some of which are closely connected to the research design and others that are more emergent and linked to the analytic questions that unfold as the analysis proceeds. However, recognizing that many of the techniques are complementary, we suggested that team members be flexible as they consider various analytic options, and then be intentional and rigorous once within the selected technique. Generally during data analysis, CBCAR researchers simultaneously segment descriptions and construct new understandings of the whole in an effort to highlight recurrent, important, and previously unexplored or marginalized aspects of people's realities. Iteratively and collaboratively moving between the tasks of data reading, coding or labeling, sorting, reducing, and displaying, team members engage with the data and each other to reach deeper understandings about the research question(s). These new insights are usually shared with a broader community—a task we turn to next.

■ Reflecting the Patterns

Once the data analysis team has summarized their findings, a process for re-presenting the findings back to the greater community is developed. Traditionally research findings have been encapsulated as formal academic and technical reports; however, these communication media often silence participants' voices and mask their daily realities (Denzin & Lincoln, 2000; Stringer, 2007). More recently, some researchers have recommended weaving research results into dramatic performances, songs, videos, artwork, interactive theater, or another medium that engages communities in holistic reflection and dialogue about findings (Bhattacharya, 2008; Denzin, 1997; Denzin & Lincoln, 2000; Sandelowski & Barroso, 2001). These media are powerful ways to portray multiple perspectives and make social positions, power dynamics, and situational contexts more visible.

The methods that researchers select to present what was seen and heard in the data carry as much ethical responsibility for authenticity and accuracy as does the process of implementing the research design (Newton, 2009). However, researchers often do not pay adequate attention to design issues in re-presenting findings (Newton). Design becomes especially significant for CBCAR researchers since research re-presentation often launches dialogue and sparks ideas for social action and change. This process inherently traverses complex political landscapes since problems with current social structures and arrangements are revealed and often critiqued (Ospina, Dodge, Foldy, & Hofmann-Pinilla, 2008). Fine, Weiss, Weseen, and Wong (2000) described a "triple representational problem" when considering how to present findings (p. 120). First, research team members must consider themselves and how accurately their voices have choreographed participants' experiences in the research findings. Second, narrators' voices need to effectively convey research findings to the community—findings which often uncover system ineffectiveness and social injustices. Third, the objects and subjects of social critique must also be re-presented to the community in a form that encourages nondefensive reflection, respectful interaction, and productive dialogue about social change. CBCAR's complex social and political landscapes must be considered as data analysis team members design appropriate forms in which to re-present findings.

We offer some principles to guide CBCAR researchers as they design ways to re-present findings to audiences—who may be involved in subsequent steps of action planning:

- Connect re-presentation design to the purpose of the research and the intended audience (Sandelowski, 1998). Considering research purpose and audience can assist design decisions. Additionally, closely examine how you are shaping the representations and why you have chosen to re-present the findings in the selected ways. An audit trail should detail these re-presentation decisions (Mantzoukas, 2004).

- Present findings as "close approximations" of people's realities (Newton, 2009, p. 357). Findings emerge as negotiated and sometimes contested text between participants' narrations, researchers' depictions, and audiences' responses (Cheek, 1996; Mantzoukas, 2004; Ospina et al., 2008). An open and humble attitude is appropriate when designing re-presentation of findings.

- Focus on participants' voices and experiences without excessive analysis and interpretation. Re-presenting participants' experiences in a descriptive manner helps to release "smothered voices" (Fine et al., 2000, p. 120) and shifts attention away from theoretical abstractions and toward pragmatic understandings and solutions.

- Re-present findings about daily experiences not only in terms of differences and conflicts but also in terms of the similar and mundane. A "quilt of stories" more accurately portrays the multiplicities and complexities inherent in social realities addressed by CBCAR projects (Fine et al., 2000, p. 119).

■ Build dialogue into re-presentation such that communities are invited into conversations about findings. Audience responses can be considered part of the evolving pattern of the whole as deeper understandings are revealed and action planning ensues.

Several significant decisions are required while designing the plan for re-presentation of findings. Additionally, as data analysis teams consider various presentation forms, they must also keep the next step of action planning in mind—a step in the CBCAR process to which we turn next.

■ Summary—Moving Toward Action

Returning to our study of a tree trunk with its multiple channels, delicate intersections, and complex patterns, we find many ways to carve meaning from our observations. Examining the trunk from both the inside and outside, we learn much more about its complexities. Similarly, CBCAR provides opportunities to examine data from multiple perspectives. We encourage those who are interested in CBCAR to view data analysis from a wide lens and appreciate the possibilities in quantitative, qualitative, and mixed-methods strategies as these techniques are implemented within a fixed or emergent research design. Central to data analysis is a sharp focus on the research question(s) that guided the research endeavor. Analytic questions may emerge and new ideas for examining data may unfold; however, the original research question(s) must remain the fulcrum around which all analytic techniques revolve. Additionally, because CBCAR projects tend to ask community-based questions about multidimensional phenomena and for which multiple voices are required, a partnered and team-based approach provides the necessary width and depth in data analysis. Specific criteria for scientific rigor guide teams toward common pathways and goals. Additionally, data analysis audit trails detail the multiple analytic decisions and construct the story of finding meaning in data and appreciating the wonder of connections. Returning the story to the community and engaging in dialogue about appropriate actions reveal the true power of CBCAR to design better futures and build communities that advance people's health and construct systems that improve quality of care.

■ References

Abma, T., Nierse, C., & Widdershoven, G. (2009). Patients as partners in responsive research: Methodological notions for collaborations in mixed research teams. *Qualitative Health Research, 19,* 401–415.

Adamson, J., & Donovan, J. (2002). Research in black and white. *Qualitative Health Research, 12,* 816–825.

Ahern, K. (1999). Ten tips for reflexive bracketing. *Qualitative Health Research, 9,* 407–411.

Amaikwu-Rushing, L., Fitzgerald, D., Wilson, C., Smith, K., Irwin, D., & Pharris, M. (2005, February). Health, well being, and racism. *Minnesota Monthly,* 28–31, 41.

Aronson, R., Wallis, A., O'Campo, P., & Schafer, P. (2007). Neighborhood mapping and evaluation: A methodology for participatory community health initiatives. *Maternal Child Health Journal, 11,* 373–383.

Behar, R. (1996). *The vulnerable observer: Anthropology that breaks your heart.* Boston, MA: Beacon.

Benner, P. (1994). The tradition and skill of interpretive phenomenology in studying health, illness, and caring practices. In P. Benner (Ed.), *Interpretive phenomenology: Embodiment, caring, and ethics in health and illness* (pp. 99–127). Thousand Oaks, CA: Sage.

Bhattacharya, H. (2008). New critical collaborative ethnography. In S. Hesse-Biber & P. Leavy (Eds.), *Handbook of emergent methods* (pp. 303–322). New York, NY: Guilford.

Bray, J., Lee, J., Smith, L., & Yorks, L. (2000). *Collaborative inquiry in practice: Action, reflection, and making meaning.* Thousand Oaks, CA: Sage.

Burgos, R., & Foster, J. (2009, July). Quality improvement and community-based participatory research in the Dominican Republic. Paper presented at the International Council of Nurses conference, Durban, South Africa.

Burke, J., O'Campo, P., Peak, G., Gielen, A., McDonnell, K., & Trochim, W. (2005). An introduction to concept mapping as a participatory public health research method. *Qualitative Health Research, 15,* 1392–1410.

Charmaz, K. (2000). Grounded theory: Objectivist and constructivist methods. In N. Denzin & Y. Lincoln (Eds.), *Handbook of qualitative research* (pp. 509–535). Thousand Oaks, CA: Sage.

Charmaz, K. (2006). *Constructing grounded theory: A practical guide through qualitative analysis.* Thousand Oaks, CA: Sage.

Charmaz, K. (2008). Grounded theory as an emergent method. In S. Hesse-Biber & P. Leavy (Eds.), *Handbook of emergent methods* (pp. 155–170). New York, NY: Guilford.

Cheek, J. (1996). Taking a view: Qualitative research as representation. *Qualitative Health Research, 6,* 492–505.

Clarke, A. (2005). *Situational analysis: Grounded theory after the post-modern turn.* Thousand Oaks, CA: Sage.

Coenen, H., & Khonraad, S. (2003). Inspirations and aspirations of exemplarian action research. *Journal of Community and Applied Social Psychology, 13,* 439–450.

Colaizzi, P. (1978). Psychological research as the phenomenologist views it. In R. Valle & M. King (Eds.), *Existential phenomenological alternatives for psychology* (pp. 48–71). New York, NY: Oxford University Press.

Dahlberg, K., Drew, N., & Nystrom, M. (2001). *Reflective lifeworld research.* Sweden: Studentlitteratur.

Denzin, N. (1989). *Interpretive interactionism.* Newbury Park, CA: Sage.

Denzin, N. (1997). *Interpretive ethnography.* Thousand Oaks, CA: Sage.

Denzin, N. & Lincoln, Y. (2000). Introduction: The discipline and practice of qualitative research. In N. Denzin & Y. Lincoln (Eds.), *Handbook of qualitative research* (pp. 1–28). Thousand Oaks, CA: Sage.

Ellsberg, M., & Heise, L. (2005). *Researching violence against women: A practical guide for researchers and activists.* Geneva, Switzerland: World Health Organization.

Fine, M., Weis, L., Weseen, S., & Wong, L. (2000). For whom? Qualitative research, representations, and social responsibilities. In N. Denzin & Y. Lincoln (Eds.), *Handbook of qualitative research* (pp. 107–131). Thousand Oaks, CA: Sage.

Flanagan, J. (1954). The critical incident technique. *Psychological Bulletin, 51,* 327–358.

Gadamer, H. G. (1995). *Truth and method.* (J. Weinsheimer & D. Marshall, Trans.). New York, NY: Continuum Publishing (Original work published 1960).

Geertz, C. (1973). *The interpretation of cultures.* New York, NY: Basic Books.

Genat, B. (2009). Building emergent situated knowledges in participatory action research. *Action Research, 7,* 101–115.

Giorgi, A. (1970). *Psychology as a human science: A phenomenologically based approach.* New York, NY: Harper & Row.

Glaser, B., & Strauss, A. (1967). *The discovery of grounded theory.* Chicago, IL: Aldine.

Green, L., & Kreuter, M. (2005). *Health program planning: An educational and ecological approach.* New York, NY: McGraw-Hill.

Grove, S., & Burns, N. (2008). *The practice of nursing research: Appraisal, synthesis, and generation of evidence.* St. Louis, MO: Elsevier Saunders.

Haraway, D. (1998). Situated knowledges: The science question in feminism and the privilege of partical perspectives. *Feminist Studies, 14,* 575–599.

Hesse-Biber, S., & Leavy, P. (2008). Pushing on the methodological boundaries: The growing need for emergent methods within and across disciplines. In S. Hesse-Biber & P. Leavy (Eds.), *Handbook of emergent methods* (pp. 1–15). New York, NY: Guilford.

Jones, K. (2004). The turn to a narrative knowing of persons. In F. Rapport (Ed.), *New qualitative methodologies in health and social care research* (pp. 35–54). New York, NY: Routledge.

Kemppainen, J. (2000). The critical incident technique and nursing care quality research. *Journal of Advanced Nursing, 32,* 1264–1271.

Kirkham, S., Baumbusch, J., Schultz, A., & Anderson, J. (2007). Knowledge development and evidence-based practice: Insights and opportunities from a postcolonial feminist perspective for transformative nursing practice. *Advances in Nursing Science, 30,* 26–40.

Kreuger, R., & Casey M. (2000). *Focus groups: A practical guide for applied research.* Thousand Oaks, CA: Sage.

Kumar, S. (2002). *Methods for community participation: A complete guide for practitioners.* London, UK: ITDG.

Kvale, S. (1996). *InterViews: An introduction to qualitative research interviewing.* Thousand Oaks, CA: Sage.

Lawler, S. (2002). Narrative in social research. In T. May (Ed.), *Qualitative research in action* (pp. 242–258). Thousand Oaks, CA: Sage.

Lieblich, A., Tuval-Mashiach, R., & Zilber, T. (1998). *Narrative research: Reading, analysis, and interpretation.* Thousand Oaks, CA: Sage.

Lincoln, Y. (1998). From understanding to action: New imperatives, new criteria, new methods for interpretive researchers. *Theory and Research in Social Education, 26,* 12–29.

Lincoln, Y., & Guba, E. (1985). *Naturalistic inquiry.* Thousand Oaks, CA: Sage.

Lincoln, Y., & Guba, E. (1986). But is it rigorous? Trustworthiness and authenticity in naturalistic evaluation. In D. Williams (Ed.), *Naturalistic evaluation* (pp. 73–84). San Francisco, CA: Jossey-Bass.

Lincoln, Y., & Guba, E. (2000). Paradigmatic controversies, contradictions, and emerging confluences. In N. Denzin & Y. Lincoln (Eds.), *Handbook of qualitative research* (pp. 163–188). Thousand Oaks, CA: Sage.

Lopez, K., & Willis, D. (2004). Descriptive versus interpretive phenomenology: Their contributions to nursing knowledge. *Qualitative Health Research, 14,* 726–735.

MacQueen, K., McLellan-Lemal, E., Bartholow, K., & Milstein, B. (2008). Team-based codebook development: Structure, process and agreement. In G. Guest & K. MacQueen (Eds.), *Handbook for team-based qualitative research* (pp. 119–135). Lanham, MD: AltaMira.

Mantzoukas, S. (2004). Issues in representation within qualitative inquiry. *Qualitative Health Research, 14,* 994–1007.

Marsh, G. (1990). Refining an emergent life-style: Change theory through matrix analysis. *Advances in Nursing Science, 12,* 41–52.

Maxwell, J., & Miller, B. (2008). Categorizing and connecting strategies in qualitative data analysis. In S. Hesse-Biber & P. Leavy (Eds.), *Handbook of emergent methods* (pp. 461–477). New York, NY: Guilford.

Mertens, D. (2005). *Research and evaluation in education and psychology: Integrating diversity with quantitative, qualitative, and mixed methods.* Thousand Oaks, CA: Sage.

Miles, M., & Huberman, A. M. (1994). *Qualitative data analysis: An expanded sourcebook.* Thousand Oaks, CA: Sage.

Morse, J. (1999). Qualitative methods: The state of the art. *Qualitative Health Research, 9,* 393–406.

Morse, J., & Field, P. (1995). *Qualitative research methods for health professionals.* Thousand Oaks, CA: Sage.

Munhall, P. (2007). Phenomenology: The method. In P. Munhall (Ed.), *Nursing research: A qualitative perspective* (pp. 145–210). Sudbury, MA: Jones and Bartlett.

Munro, B. H. (2004). *Statistical methods for healthcare research.* Philadelphia, PA: Lippincott Williams & Wilkins.

Newman, M. A. (1994). *Health as expanding consciousness.* Boston, MA: Jones and Bartlett.

Newman, M. A. (2008). *Transforming presence: The difference nurses make.* Philadelphia, PA: F. A. Davis.

Newton, J. (2009). Visual representation of people and information. In D. Mertens & P. Ginsberg (Eds.), *The handbook of social research ethics* (pp. 353–372). Thousand Oaks, CA: Sage.

Ospina, S., Dodge, J., Foldy, E., & Hofmann-Pinilla, A. (2008). Taking the action turn: Lessons from bringing participation to qualitative research. In P. Reason & H. Bradbury (Eds.), *The Sage handbook of action research: Participative inquiry and practice* (pp. 420–434). Thousand Oaks, CA: Sage.

Palermo, A., McGranaghan, R., & Travers, R. (2006). Unit 3: Developing a CBPR partnership: Creating the "glue." In The Examining Community-Institutional Partnerships for Prevention Research Group (Eds.), *Developing and sustaining community-based participatory partnerships: A skill-building curriculum.* Retrieved from http://depts.washington.edu/ccph/cbpr/u3/u35.php.

Palmer, R. (1969). *Hermeneutics: Interpretation theory in Schleiermacher, Dilthey, Heidegger, and Gadamer.* Evanston, IL: Northwestern University Press.

Patton, M. (2002). *Qualitative research and evaluation methods.* Thousand Oaks, CA: Sage.

Pavlish, C., & Ho, A. (2009). Pathway to social justice: Research on human rights and gender-based violence in a Rwandan refugee camp. *Advances in Nursing Science, 32,* 144–157.

Payne, J. (1999). *Researching health needs: A community-based approach.* Thousand Oaks, CA: Sage.

Pierre-Louis, B., Akoh, Z., White, P., & Pharris, M. (in press). Patterns in the lives of African-American women with diabetes. *Nursing Science Quarterly.*

Polit, D., & Beck, C. (2008). *Nursing research: Principles and methods.* Philadelphia, PA: Lippincott, Williams, & Wilkins.

Pretty, J., Guijt, I., Scoones, I., & Thompson, J. (2002). *Participatory learning and action.* London, UK: International Institute for Environment and Development.

Rapport, F. (2004a). Shifting sands in qualitative methodology. In F. Rapport (Ed.), *New qualitative methodologies in health and social care research* (pp. 1–17). New York, NY: Routledge.

Rapport, F. (2004b). From the porter's point of view: Participant observation by the interpretive phenomenologist in the hospital. In F. Rapport (Ed.), *New qualitative methodologies in health and social care research* (pp. 99–122). New York, NY: Routledge.

Reissman, C. (1993). *Narrative analysis.* Newbury Park, CA: Sage.

Robson, C. (2002). *Real world research.* Malden, MA: Blackwell.

Rodgers, B., & Cowles, K. (1993). The qualitative research audit trail: A complex collection of documentation. *Research in Nursing and Health, 16,* 219–226.

Roper, J., & Shapira, J. (2000). *Ethnography in nursing research.* Thousand Oaks, CA: Sage.

Ryan, G., & Bernard, H. R. (2000). Data management and analysis methods. In N. Denzin & Y. Lincoln (Eds.), *Handbook of qualitative research* (pp. 769–802). Thousand Oaks, CA: Sage.

Saldaña, J. (2009). *The coding manual for qualitative researchers.* Los Angeles, CA: Sage.

Sandelowski, M. (1986). The problem of rigor in qualitative research. *Advances in Nursing Science, 8,* 27–37.

Sandelowski, M. (1998). Writing a good read: Strategies for representing qualitative data. *Research in Nursing and Health, 21,* 375–382.

Sandelowski, M., & Barroso, J. (2001). Finding the findings in qualitative studies. *Journal of Nursing Scholarship, 34,* 213–219.

Schluter, J., Seaton, P., & Chaboyer, W. (2007). Critical incident technique: A user's guide for nurse researchers. *Journal of Advanced Nursing, 61,* 107–114.

Schreiber, R., & Stern, P. (2001). *Using grounded theory in nursing.* New York, NY: Springer.

Stearns, G. (1998). Reflexivity and moral agency: Restoring possibility of life history research. *Frontiers: A Journal of Women's Studies, 19,* 58–71.

Stewart, A. (1994). Toward a feminist strategy for studying women's lives. In C. Franz & A. Stewart (Eds.), *Women creating lives: Identities, resilience, and resistance* (pp. 11–35). San Francisco, CA: Westview.

Strauss, A., & Corbin, J. (1994). Grounded theory methodology: An overview. In N. Denzin & Y. Lincoln (Eds.), *Handbook of qualitative research* (pp. 273–285). Thousand Oaks, CA: Sage.

Stringer, E. (2007). *Action research.* Los Angeles, CA: Sage.

Sword, W. (1999). Accounting for presence of self: Reflections on doing qualitative research. *Qualitative Health Research, 9,* 270–278.

Thorne, S. (2008). *Interpretive description.* Walnut Creek, CA: Left Coast Press.

Ulin, P., Robinson, E., & Tolley, E. (2005). *Qualitative methods in public health: A field guide for applied research.* San Francisco, CA: Jossey-Bass.

Van Kaam, A. (1966). *Existential foundations of psychology.* Pittsburgh, PA: Duquesne University Press.

van Manen (2001). *Researching lived experience.* Ontario, Canada: Althouse.

Viswanathan, M., Ammerman, A., Eng, E., Gartlehner, G., Lohr, K., & Griggith, D. (2004). *Community-based participatory research:*

Assessing the evidence. Evidence Report/Technology Assessment No. 99 (No. AHRQ Publicaton 04-E022-2). Rockville, MD: Agency for Healthcare Research and Quality. Retrieved from http://www.ahrq.org

Wadsworth, Y. (1997). *Everyday evaluation on the run.* Crows Nest, Australia: Allen & Unwin.

Walkerdine, V., Lucey, H., & Melody, J. (2002). Subjectivity and qualitative method. In T. May (Ed.), *Qualitative research in action* (pp. 179–196). Thousand Oaks, CA: Sage.

Wasserfall, R. (1997). Reflexivity, feminism, and difference. In R. Hertz (Ed.), *Reflexivity and voice* (pp. 150–168). Thousand Oaks, CA: Sage.

Waterman, H. (1998). Embracing ambiguities and valuing ourselves: Issues of validity in action research. *Journal of Advanced Nursing, 28,* 101–105.

Zimmerman, S., Tilly, J., Cohen, L., & Love, K. (2009). *A manual for community-based participatory research: Using research to improve practice and inform policy in assisted living.* Retrieved from http://www.shepscenter.unc.edu/research_programs/aging/publications/CEAL-UNC%20Manual%20for%20Community-Based%20Participatory%20Research-1.pdf.

Chapter 7

Engaging in Action Planning and Envisioning Future Studies

You planted this cherry tree 3 years ago and finally it looks like there will be enough cherries for a good harvest. You remember the afternoon you brought the tree home and were tempted to simply plant it, but you resisted that urge. You did some research on how to prepare the root ball, how big to dig the hole, what mulch and fertilizer to use to prepare the ground to receive and nurture the tree's roots, and where this little tree should be planted to best thrive. You gathered just the right group of friends to help—a neighbor who is a master gardener, a strong teenager from next door, and a community Elder who brought good spirit to the effort. The four of you gently patted down the soil, bidding the little tree to grow strong. It was an act of hope in the future.

This spring the cherry tree's branches were engorged with white flowers, even before the leaves were visible—a sign of a plentiful harvest. And now, here you are looking at this beautiful, bountiful tree, thinking about what to do with the cherries. The Elder has passed on. The teen is no longer a teen and is living overseas (but the last Internet message made mention of how nice a package containing a jar of cherry jam might be). The master gardener and you talk about what to do with all of the cherries. Jam is definitely in the mix, but you have a group of family and friends coming in a few weeks and you would like to prepare a dessert from this tree for them—cherry pie?—cherry oatmeal walnut cobbler? A simple bowl of cherries would perhaps be more nutritious, but not as tasty. All good options, but WAIT!

You cannot just simply make this decision at *this* point—you don't know what kind of cherries these are—how sweet or tart they are—and you have not taken into consideration the preferences or sensitivities of your guests. If the cherries are sweet, jam and pie are out of the mix. If the cherries are too tart, you cannot serve them fresh in a bowl. You think of your guests and realize that Anastasia, Martín, Malaika, Amalia, Chuck, Ellisa, Tim, Elizabeth, Nikolas, Chanh, and Bill are all pretty much indiscriminate eaters—they would love the pie—even more with ice cream, but would also like the cobbler. Maya and Randall both have diabetes and a family history of heart disease, so they would be challenged by the pie, so maybe the cherry oatmeal walnut cobbler is the best choice. Then you realize that Lisa has a severe nut allergy. Obviously, your decision about what to bake with the cherries is going to be based on the most vulnerable first—walnuts are out. You have to think about Lisa first and foremost to avoid an anaphylactic reaction. You will be sure that all substances containing nuts are out of the house before she arrives. Then there are also Maya and Randall. You want everyone to be safe, healthy, satisfied, and feel fully included, so you decide on an oatmeal cherry cobbler, without walnuts and minimal sugar.

And so it is with action planning in community-based collaborative action research (CBCAR). You cannot decide how the data will be presented to the wider community or what actions should follow until you know what the nature of the findings are, and until you are clear about who your audience is—what they are hungry for and what their sensitivities and vulnerabilities are. You should hold the well-being of the most vulnerable close to your heart and central to your plan.

■ Visioning the Change and Crafting Solutions

In CBCAR, the research process does not stop when data are analyzed and presented. This is only the beginning of an important phase in the process aimed at promoting health, shaping healthier systems, and enacting social justice. Once the data have been analyzed and woven into a format for presentation, the wider community is engaged in the action planning process, which begins with discerning the meaning of the data.

For example, in an *Envisioning Educational Equity* CBCAR project aimed at identifying factors behind the disproportionately low percentage of African-American students graduating from a school of nursing, concerned nurse educators engaged a team of educators, students, and staff from various student service departments within the university to better understand and address this inequality. Applying a CBCAR process, they envisioned and planned their data collection and analysis strategies. In order to visualize the flow of African-American students through the university system, the data collection team first gathered demographic data from university records about admission to the university, entrance to the school of nursing, and retention to graduation for African-American students. To understand students' experiences, they conducted focus group and individual interviews with students and faculty. They also conducted a systematic assessment of the university's physical pattern—from who was pictured on the walls, in faculty photos, in university publications, and in educational materials, to what sort of skin and hair care products were sold in the university student center market. These three data collection efforts provided insight into the pattern of student and university interactions. After the work of the data analysis team was completed, the CBCAR team constructed a diagram to illustrate where the flow of African-American students into and through the school of nursing was constricted and needed attention. They found constrictions in what they called "the pipeline" into the university, in interpersonal relationships within the university, in coping with stresses during the first 2 years of university, in the test-taking process, and in the general university environment. A community action planning meeting was called and advertised. Key stakeholders—nursing faculty, students, and administrative and support personnel from all departments concerned with the education and well-being of students—were personally invited through phone calls and meetings to describe the importance of the project and their presence at the action planning meeting. The group followed the process outlined in **Figure 7-1** to move toward the development of an action plan.

Data Presentation and Community Dialogue: The Heart of the Matter

The action planning meeting started with a dramatic reading of a poem by a senior nursing student to center the group in an emotive, creative, and open stance. Two members of the CBCAR team introduced the process that would be used to reflect on the data presentation. They introduced the group to the principles of dialogue (as presented in Chapter 4) and gave an overview of the unfolding CBCAR process that brought them to this point. The data presentation team then showed colorful graphs and flow charts that depicted the pipeline and flow of students into and through the university and school of nursing. The patterns began to come into focus. The environmental factors were depicted with a photo slide show set to music, which clearly showed unequal and unwelcoming conditions. The patterns became clearer. The relational experiences of students and faculty, as revealed in the focus group and individual interviews, were then presented through two spoken-word narrative performances—one centered on the students' experience and the other on the experience of faculty. The audience quickly un-

Figure 7-1 Overview of Action Planning

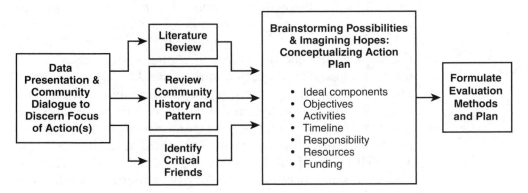

derstood on a deep level the complex mix of pain, resilience, anger, and confusion experienced by African-American students, as well as the feelings, desires, fears, and struggles experienced by faculty who were trying to act in such a way that discrimination and bias were recognized and quickly managed. The pattern was vivid and clear. Those present were encouraged to take 15 minutes to write what they were feeling and what insights arose as they reflected on the data from the CBCAR study. The group was then engaged in a dialogue to discern what actions needed to be taken.

Discerning Action Focus

The process of discerning action steps is a spirited, creative process. It is important to have ample large sheets of paper on the wall, bold markers, and attentive recorders. A comfortable, inviting room and a colorful array of nutritious yet delicious food help set the stage for good action planning. A circle process is often used to ensure that all voices are equally heard. During the *Envisioning Educational Equity* community action planning dialogue, several concerns arose over and over, and from various university perspectives. It became clear that (1) there was little being done to recruit African-American high school students into the university and the nursing program; (2) African-American students were experiencing discrimination, hurtful comments, stereotyping by professors, and stereotypical threats, which led to disproportionate disengagement, lower grades, and dropouts before and after entering the nursing program—a trajectory that was mitigated for some students by supportive staff and faculty; and (3) a pervasive, dominant culture of privilege was being expressed through much of the campus, in classrooms, and in many textbooks. There was clearly much work to be done. In CBCAR action planning, it is more inspiriting to work toward a vision of a just and loving community than to simply work on problems to combat injustices.

As problems are identified through data presentation and dialogue in the CBCAR process, it is helpful to rephrase the problem into statements that express the ideal components of the action plan. Ludema and Fry (2008) encouraged action researchers to move into a practice of appreciative inquiry, which they defined as "the study and exploration of what gives life to human systems when they function at their best." They went on to state that appreciative inquiry "is based on the assumption that every living system has a hidden and under-utilized core of strengths—its positive core—which, when revealed and tapped, provides a sustainable source of positive energy for both personal and organizational transformation" (p. 282). The aim of appreciative inquiry is to: (1) discover the best of what is, (2) dream to imagine what could be, (3) design what will be, and (4) enact change, learning to become what we most hope for. Problem statements are transformed into a vision of what is hoped for and what is believed to be ideal. The resulting action plan is thus expressed as ideal components, which are broad statements that provide an image of where and how the community ideally wants to be (see the first column of **Table 7-1**).

Ideal components of an action plan paint a picture of human flourishing in a just community. These statements are the main focus and final products of the first action planning meeting, along with determining when the community will reconvene and identifying who will seek more information so that specific action objectives and activities can be formulated. Decisions that shape the specific action plan need to be based on the fullest and best knowledge available. At this point, if the group is large enough, it is wise to formulate work teams to review the literature, assess what has been and is currently being done related to the topic, and identify critical friends to challenge and thus strengthen the action plan.

The literature review team searches for information on any new topics that have arisen, such as stereotypical threat. They also determine what is known to be best practice in the areas of action. They then critique and synthesize what they have learned so it can be presented clearly, accurately, powerfully, and succinctly to the larger group. The pattern recognition team explores what has historically been done in this community related to this issue and what the current pattern of action is—who is doing what to work toward the stated vision and who should be invited to join in the CBCAR actions. The third team works on identifying and engaging critical friends who are

Table 7-1 Action Plan for *Envisioning Educational Equity*

Pipeline

Ideal components	Objectives	Activities	Timeline	Responsibility
Strong relationships are built with local high schools that serve the African-American community. African-American nursing students are supported to be role models for high-school students interested in the health professions. Faculty are engaged in health fairs and education courses.	To ensure that high-school students are fully informed on nursing as a career option and see themselves as potential university students	1. Individual/Community: Collaborate with students at North and Central High Schools to conduct annual health fairs and regular health education programs. 2. Structural: Provide community work and learning funding for 2 African-American students to work in the high schools doing health education and shadowing school nurses. 3. Structural: African-American nursing faculty given one course load to support high-school programming and meet with nursing student every two weeks to review their leadership goals and objectives.	September to May	Dean of Nursing to assure funding and support of program, nursing students, nursing faculty
Students come to campus and are engaged in campus community and programs that help them discern college choices. There is excitement over the possibility of becoming a nurse.	To expose high-school juniors and seniors to college life and healthcare careers and facilitate enrollment at the university	1. Structural: Secure scholarships for 20 African-American H.S. juniors and seniors to attend First Step program. 2. Structural: Organize First Step program to include leadership development and exposure to a variety of programs. 3. Individual: Teach students health education topics. 4. Individual: Teach basic skills in nursing lab. 5. Individual: Arrange visits to interesting nursing sites. 6. Structural: Secure scholarship funds.	August	Multicultural Student Service staff, development office, community health nursing coordinator, nursing students, community nurses, and lab instructor

(continues)

Table 7-1 Action Plan for *Envisioning Educational Equity* (continued)

Relationships and Stereotypical Threat

Ideal components	Objectives	Activities	Timeline	Responsibility
Faculty understand the historical and social constructs of racism, as well as the dynamics of stereotypical threat. They feel comfortable and sure of their ability to create an inclusive educational environment in the classroom and clinical settings.	Faculty are aware of the dynamics behind racism and how to mitigate its effects through the creation of an inclusive nursing education environment.	1 Community: Convene monthly faculty circles to study and reflect on the history and dynamics of racism and how it is manifest in the educational environment. 2. Structural: Create teaching scenarios that deal directly with situations involving discrimination (overt and covert). 3. Structural: Develop a statement for all syllabi encouraging anyone to call a moment of consideration when they notice a stereotypical or discriminatory comment has been made—normalize this critical reflection.	September–May	Action team will facilitate faculty circles. Nursing faculty will develop pedagogical approaches.
Stereotypical threat is understood by students and they are able to employ strategies to mitigate its effects on exam performance. Students enter exams with confidence in their knowledge and test-taking ability. African-American students confidently excel to reach their goals at graduation and beyond.	African-American students improve exam performance and report decreased stereotypical threat.	1. Individual: Meet with Admissions Dept staff to assure accurate and consistent demographic data collection. 2. Individual: Pair first-year African-American students who declare nursing as a major with a mentor and invite to African American Student Nurse Association 3. Individual: Educate African-American nursing students about stereotypical threat 4. Community: Pair African-American nursing students with African-American high-school students to teach them about stereotypical threat and its effects, as well as how to eliminate them. 5. Structural: Track goals and achievement at entry to university, entry to nursing school, and 1 and 5 years postgrad.	October–November (consider ongoing)	Action team and Multicultural Student Services staff at university, nursing faculty, African American Student Nurse Association, Black Nurses Association, H.S. counselors, alum office

Ideal components	Objectives	Activities	Timeline	Responsibility
African-American students have a confidential contact person with whom they can discuss situations involving stereotypes, bias, discrimination and threats. They feel supported. This service is well known to all students and the administrative personnel are known to respond quickly and effectively.	African-American students are aware of who to contact to discuss concerns related to discrimination and express confidence in administrative commitment to respond appropriately.	1. <u>Structural</u>: Create brochure that details who to contact if students experience or witness bias, stereotyping, discrimination, or threat, and assures confidentiality. 2. <u>Community</u>: Provide brochures and information about the African American Student Association during orientation. 3. <u>Structural</u>: Assure that brochures are available in the multicultural student room and around campus. 4. <u>Structural</u>: Spot check system every semester. 5. <u>Structural</u>: Audit complaints to assess campus climate concerns.	September–January and yearly assessment	Senior Vice President of university, Dean of Student Services and Multicultural Affairs, Action team

Campus and Classroom Environment

Ideal components	Objectives	Activities	Timeline	Responsibility
African-American students see themselves reflected in the photos of the campus community, faculty, classroom materials, and student activities.	All aspects of campus environment reflect the community the university serves.	1. <u>Structural</u>: Systematically analyze all campus publications and educational materials; assure representational equity. 2. <u>Structural</u>: Set up system to monitor and analyze faculty hiring and promotion trends to assure equity. 3. <u>Structural</u>: Conduct an audit of all course materials and texts to assure equity of representation and no stereotypes.	September–May year II	Action team, nursing education graduate students, Multicultural Student Services staff, Human Resource staff, & Marketing
Student services respond equitably to all students and are caring and welcoming.	All student services equitably serve needs of African-American students.	1. <u>Structural</u>: Train student life and student services staff on conducting racial equity audits, which are done in the fall of every year.	September–Oct & yearly audit	Dean of Student Services, Student Life staff, action team

experts in the area of concern, and can be consulted to critique the action plan once formulated and as it proceeds. At this stage, it is also helpful to engage critical friends who are evaluation experts. Alternately, identifying critical friends can be done by the entire group prior to adjourning, with the intent that all participants would think about others who should be invited to the next meeting so that they can lend their energy and insights to plan effective actions. In this phase, CBCAR project members are constantly thinking about who within the larger community needs to be invited into the action project.

Conceptualizing the Action Plan

When the CBCAR group gathers again, it may be a larger group because more interested members will have been identified to help with the important work at hand. The action conceptualization meeting(s) involve a creative process of brainstorming and imagining new hope for the community. An engaging process should be used to elicit insights as the literature review team reports what they have learned about the new topics that had been identified, and about what is known to be best practice in the action focus area(s). It is important for the community to dialogue about how what has been identified as best practices elsewhere might need to be adapted to be applicable in this community.

The people who have done pattern recognition report on the community's history related to the issue at hand, and what is currently being done within the community to address the issue and by whom. For example, if there was a previous grant-funded effort to address the issue, it is important to analyze the extent to which those efforts were successful, and what challenges to sustainability were experienced. An analysis of the current community structure will add to the context-specific knowledge for the action plan conceptualization. Ideally, interested stakeholders are present at this stage of action conceptualization; efforts to expand representation from the critical reference group (Wadsworth, 1997), policy makers, and potential funders serve to strengthen the project. At this point, the specific components of the action plan will be determined.

If there are two or more foci to the action plan and the group is large, it may be helpful to break into action teams, one for each action focus. If the group is small and has limited resources, the action plans may need to be prioritized and the most important chosen for the first action cycle. The decision of how to prioritize the work is based on principles of social justice.

In order to conceptualize each component of the action plan, a series of questions are asked (see **Box 7-1**). These questions assist in creatively brainstorming to envision the ideal components of a transformed community, as well as determining objectives, specific activities, and a timeline to address each ideal component and to specify who will be responsible for en-

---

Box 7-1   Questions for Creative Brainstorming

Why? Naming the inequities, injustices, and concerns that must be addressed

What? Imagining the ideal situation and stating objectives to get there

How? Determining the sequence of tasks and steps for each objective

Who? Calling forth the specific people who will assume responsibility for each activity

Where? Envisioning the place where the activities will take place

When? Developing a timeline for when the activities will be initiated and completed

Funding? Engaging existing resources and identifying potential sources of funds

Process? Deciding on a way to assure our process is equitable, just, and on target

Effects? Discerning how, when we reach the end of the project, we will know that we have done what we set out to do—that we have improved the lives of the critical reference group

(Inspired by Stringer & Genet, 2004)

suring that the activities are carried out. So that everyone has a clear idea about what has been decided, it is extremely helpful to create an action planning grid as depicted in Table 7-1.

Drawing on the socioecological perspective of health (Brofenfenbrenner, 1979; Flood, 2006; Green & Kreuter, 2005), a significant principle to keep in mind when action-planning is that multiple, multilevel strategies are more effective in addressing social inequities and injustices than interventions targeting only individual knowledge, behavior, or perceptions (Aronson, Lovelace, Hatch, & Whitehead, 2006; Best, Stokols, Green, Leischow, Holmes, & Buchholz, 2003; Cohen, Scribrier, & Farley, 2000; McLaren & Hawe, 2005; Sallis, Cervero, Ascher, Henderson, Kraft, & Kerr, 2006). Moreover, multilevel and multipronged actions geared toward health determinants help to prevent structural perpetuation of these disparities (Commission for the Social Determinants of Health, 2008; Committee on Health and Behavior, 2001; Lane et al., 2004; Semenza & Maty, 2007).

This is also a time to brainstorm about what resources are available and to identify potential sources of funding for the larger aspects of the project. Another brainstorming activity is for the action planning team to create a dream map—several varieties exist (Kumar, 2002). For example, team members can consider the data that describe the present status and then brainstorm aspirations—listing all their hopes for a better future regarding the issue at hand. These ideas are then collated and listed as ideal components for an action plan. Team members can analyze each component by considering community assets, vulnerabilities, and opportunities. Out of that discussion emerge pragmatic actions that are firmly connected to ideal aspirations. Further planning regarding implementation, such as required resources and tasks, can then occur.

Just as in the early phases of the CBCAR process, teams continue to ask critical questions, such as—Will our actions make significant structural changes to improve the lives of the people in the critical reference group, i.e., the people most affected by the research topic? Is there equity in our process? Are all voices being heard and honored? Is the cost to some greater than the cost to others? Who is at the margins of our work and how can we erase the margins? Who are the best people to do this work? Who else might we invite in? Do we have sufficient resources? Is the funding stream adequate? Are current funders placing unrealistic expectations on this project and are the funders' requirements taking us off task? How will we know we have done well when we are done? Who should benefit from our actions and how? How will we monitor our process to assure it is just, equitable, and on target? All actions are held to the standards of the CBCAR guiding principles.

As new responsibilities are assumed, a new memorandum of understanding (see Chapter 4, Boxes 4-2 & 4-3) may need to be developed to outline the new constellation of partnerships, responsibilities, and commitments. When deciding who will do what, it is important to keep in mind principles of equity, fairness, and democratic participation. For example, students, people who have limited incomes, or people who are caregivers with limited resources may not be able to contribute as much as people who have comfortable salaries and fewer mandatory responsibilities. On the other hand, people who are actively engaged in the work oftentimes end up making more of the decisions, which can marginalize those who are less involved. This is something that needs to be openly discussed and frequently assessed. There may be a need to put the project on hold until adequate funds can be obtained to compensate those who could not otherwise be involved.

Stringer (2007) stressed that the heart of action research is not "the techniques and procedures that guide action but the sense of unity that holds people to a collective vision of their world and inspires them to work together for the common good" (p. 132). Groups should be intentional about building unity and remaining unified throughout the action planning process. Stringer (2007) recommended linking partners in networks of support so that they have people to draw on if they need consultation or assistance. This is a way for people who do not have the time or resources to be actively doing the work to contribute in a significant way. This network stimulates a (comm)unity-building process and generates energy to sustain the partnership (2007).

As actions are being implemented, it is important to set regular intervals at which the teams will report back to the larger CBCAR group so that they can evaluate progress, revise the plan as needed, and celebrate accomplishments. Stringer (2007) pointed out that most action plans start out with a flourish, but people need to check back in to make sure their activities are in line with the collective track and to be reenergized. It is wise to acknowledge one another for work well done and provide honest feedback for improvements still needed. Assigning a research facilitator may help keep projects on track and assure that essential communication is flowing. This person can attend to logistical details such as arranging meeting rooms, collecting items for agendas, and maintaining essential documents. The process of maintaining a decision audit and easily accessible meeting minutes, which was started earlier in the CBCAR planning phase, is just as important in the action planning and implementation phases.

■ Acting Imaginatively

Conceptualizing the action plan is a creative process in which community insights are mined and compared to best practices identified in the literature; both are rigorously scrutinized as teams consider what the most relevant action is for the local context. Successful action plans are those that resonate widely within the community. Action planning holds open the possibility for community transformation. Smith (1997) drew on the work of Freire (1985) to point out that when we engage in action with a critical consciousness and realize new insights, we have the opportunity to "break the echo" of simply repeating the realities of the dominant culture—"comprehension shifts and deepens . . . rendering the inner self more complex" (1997, p. 195). On a collective level, community relationships deepen, heads are held higher, relational bonds become stronger, community spirit becomes more vibrant, and a sense of shared purpose to make the community more just and whole abounds. A new possibility arises when people come together to systematically research their reality, engage in dialogue about the meaning of their findings, and plan and carry out actions to create a new ideal for the community.

Researchers and data collection and data analysis team members are often tempted to jump ahead as they uncover new information, discover new patterns, and reach new insights during the discovery process. They need to be firmly committed to presenting the data, while at the same time honoring the fact that the best actions rise up from the larger community. This is why data presentation to the wider community needs to be carried out with rigor and careful attention. Discerning actions involves a democratic process that provides fertile ground from which collective wisdom can spring forth. Making this point, Mary Law (1997) described a participatory research process in Ontario, Canada in which she, as a university researcher, was collaborating with parents of children with physical disabilities. The parents had experienced isolation from others in a small town. Law described using "intentional nudging" throughout the process to encourage parents to take control of the research process and findings (p. 45). After conducting a series of focus groups, the researchers and parents gathered to discern potential actions inspired by the data that were presented. In her write-up of this process, Law stressed the importance of researchers resisting the temptation to manipulate the process by promoting participants' suggestions that favor researchers' ideas (p. 45). Law wrote:

> As a researcher, I found this aspect to be one of the most difficult. Once a participant had suggested that a parent support group be formed, I recognized that this would be an exciting result of the study process. For such a group to be successful, it had to be suggested and supported by a number of participants. The participatory action-research process would be ineffective if I, as a researcher, unduly pushed or influenced any decision-making about organizing a support group. (p. 46)

If the actions are going to be relevant to the community and sustainable, it is important that they not be imposed from the outside and that there be widespread excitement over their potential.

If, after attentive dialogue and careful discernment, the action that is conceptualized is a construction created through the collective insights of the group, and no similar projects have been reported in the literature, it may be advisable to pilot the action before initiating it on a large scale. For example, in the *Health, Well-Being, and Racism* CBCAR project described in Chapter 1, one of the action steps was to conduct groups for African-American teens to learn about the dynamics of racism and how to effectively manage the incidents without internalizing racism's negative effects. Since evidence about the effects of such groups was lacking in the literature, the women's advisory council decided to create and conduct a small group session over 6 weeks, evaluate it, revise the program, conduct a second session, and then do a second evaluation before developing the final curriculum to be disseminated to the wider community.

Incorporating Empirically Supported Initiatives in Action Plans

Horowitz, Robinson, and Seifer (2009) made the point that healthcare providers are painfully aware that what has been determined to be true in randomized clinical trials, does not always help them serve their patients. This is because these studies could not and did not control for the unique and complex challenges the healthcare providers' patients face in their daily lives. These social determinants of health contribute significantly to health problems. Many of these determinants, such as environmental exposures and "living in a neighborhood with poorer safety, walkability, social cohesion, and food availability," are outside of the control of the individual (Horowitz et al., p. 2634). The factors that are the fundamental causes of diseases worldwide are macrosocial, necessitating structural level interventions (Semenza & Maty, 2007). Randomized clinical trials tend to look at individual-level factors rather than social structures that significantly alter the health of individuals. Horowitz et al. (2009) claimed new approaches are needed to translate research findings from clinical trials for improved outcomes. They pointed out that community-based participatory research "may be the ultimate form of translational research, moving discoveries bidirectionally from bench to bedside to *el barrio* (the community) to organizations and policy makers" (p. 2634).

Becker, Stice, Shaw, and Woda (2009) also called for participatory approaches to empirically supported intervention (ESI) designs and suggested that community-partnered research enhances the dissemination process and intervention effect. These authors reviewed how the application of ESIs can be strengthened through a community-researcher partnership, although they cautioned that working to disseminate ESIs in communities requires considerable time that "extends outside the boundaries of traditional research grants and our own research interests" (p. 267).

When deciding whether to incorporate an ESI in an action step, the CBCAR partnership should draw on the insight of diverse voices to discern whether the ESI is appropriate. Whether evidence-based practices are incorporated into the local community should be judged by the nature of the CBCAR research findings and the unique community contextual factors. Just as a banana tree planted in Canada would not be expected to thrive, so too, some well-tested interventions may not work in particular communities. As stressed in Chapter 3, knowledge for health resides in the community. Through critical dialogue, community members can discern what will work in their context. Academic research partners impart essential knowledge and expertise when teaching communities how to critique empirical studies and judge to what extent specific ESIs might apply to the local context. If an ESI from the literature is being considered, its authors could be invited as critical friends in the action planning, implementation, evaluation, and dissemination phases of the CBCAR project.

Clinical Trials as Action Plans

Although most actions will involve creating new programs, revising protocols, or engaging in organizational change, another possible way to follow up CBCAR research results with action steps is to plan a community-designed clinical trial. For example, a CBCAR partnership might decide to implement a clinical trial in response to a particularly prominent issue that emerged during earlier steps in the CBCAR research process. Clinical trials would also pertain to CBCAR interventions that have the potential for impact beyond the immediate context (Leykum, Pugh, Lanham, Harmon, & McDaniel, 2009). So if a CBCAR partnership believes that a particular action step has the potential for benefitting people in other communities or practice groups, then a clinical trial might be considered. For example, during an ethnographic study on human rights, participants emphasized the prevalence of human rights violations experienced by marginalized groups. Participants identified orphaned children, widows, adolescent girls, people living with HIV/AIDS, people living in extreme poverty, and people with special needs such as those who lived with mental illness as the groups most affected. A community-wide human rights awareness campaign with particular activities was planned. One of the action steps, a human rights learning program, was developed by the action planning group and is now being refined in preparation for a clinical trial (see **Box 7-2**). The clinical trial seeks to examine the effects of a culturally-appropriate *Ubuntu and Human Rights Learning and Advocacy Program* on social interactions, satisfaction with relationships, and interpersonal violence. Ubuntu is an African ethic that upholds the fact that we are who we are in relationship with others, and that our actions should enhance community well-being (Chilisa, 2009). The action team for this project will be well aware that the insights gained during the data collection process might significantly alter the way the program is delivered and what the possible outcome measures might be.

The key in using a clinical trial approach for CBCAR action planning is to ensure that the plan is a result of community dialogue and discernment of appropriate actions to meet pressing needs. Community members should be fully engaged in the planning and implementation processes. The dilemma for CBCAR clinical trials is how to design an intervention trial that is flexible enough to be developed and implemented locally, and yet, also has enough controls to be able to judge the generalizability of the findings with some degree of precision (Leykum et al., 2009). Leykum and colleagues (2009) called for new, community-created approaches to designing interventions and determining appropriate outcome measures. Creative and con-

Box 7-2 Sample Action Plan with a Clinical Trial

UHAKI (Harmony): Ubuntu-Human Rights Learning and Advocacy Program

- Develop a community advisory group with young adults (ages 19–25), teachers, community leaders, and human rights experts.

- In a community-based formative design, conduct focus groups with the following:

  - Community young adults to assess their knowledge and beliefs about ubuntu and human rights, relationships, and responsibilities; strengths and challenges of incorporating ubuntu and human rights into their daily lives; and community resources for human rights

  - Representatives of schools, community-based organizations, and community leaders to assess how they teach youth about ubuntu and human rights, relationships, and responsibilities; community mechanisms for ubuntu/human rights; and community facilitators and barriers for ubuntu/human rights programs

- Based on focus group findings, develop with assistance of community partners and participants, a culturally-appropriate Ubuntu and Human Rights Learning and Advocacy Program and outcome measures.

- Assess acceptability and feasibility of the Ubuntu and Human Rights Learning and Advocacy Program and cultural-appropriateness of selected impact measures in 2 focus group sessions with young adults and 20 one-on-one interviews with young adults (N = 10 for each gender) and 6 one-on-one interviews with community leaders (N = 3 for each gender). Revise program accordingly.

- Conduct a randomized intervention pilot study to assess the outcomes of 30 young adults (age 19–25) who participated in the Ubuntu-Human Rights Learning and Advocacy Program at 6-month follow-up, as compared with a similar number of young adults who had just the formal human rights curriculum in school (usual care program) in terms of the following outcomes:

  - Improvement in knowledge about ubuntu and human rights principles

  - Empowerment in social interactions

  - Satisfaction with self in relationships

  - Reduction in number of reported violence incidents in schools trolled designs are being developed for CBCAR intervention studies. The Agency for Healthcare Research and Quality (AHRQ) reported four clinical trials using a participatory approach (Viswanathan et al., 2004) and, more recently, listed several community-based participatory research projects that they funded, some of which were intervention studies (AHRQ, 2009).

■ Evaluating the Impacts

The unitary-transformative and participatory theoretical perspectives (Cowling, 1999, 2007; Heron & Reason, 1997; Newman, 1994, 2008; Reason 1998; Skolimowski, 1994) at the root of CBCAR propose that change is a construction of the CBCAR process and cannot be predetermined. The true impact of a project can only be fully appreciated in retrospect, which makes traditional evaluation methods difficult. If research teams are not certain what the outcome measures might be, they will not know with any degree of certainty which baseline measures to collect. Yet, in CBCAR projects people come together to promote human health and flourishing and to address inequities; a plan can be made to envision what that *may* look like and thus, what factors might change as the action plan is carried out. Capturing unfolding community patterns enables us to be good stewards of community resources and people's time and energies; ideally evaluation efforts assist in this process. CBCAR, with its social justice, unitary-transformative, and participatory roots calls for theoretically consistent evaluation methods.

The evaluation process can play a key role in sharpening the focus of the action plan and enhancing accountability for all involved. In larger projects that receive outside support, funders most often ask for a detailed list of outcomes their investment will yield. While this is a reasonable request, the agenda of funders can take action research projects away from what the project team finds to be most important. Increasingly funders are realizing the power and potential of community-based action research efforts and are willing to invest their money in established partnerships with sound action research plans (AHRQ, 2009; Horowitz et al., 2009). They invest in the process and trust that a sound and equitable collaborative effort will yield strong results.

Choosing an Evaluation Method

There are various schools of thought regarding the best methods for evaluating the action steps of community-based participatory and collaborative action research. **Figure 7-2** presents a continuum of evaluation methods. Additionally, Patton (2011) has presented a process of developmental evaluation to enhance innovation development in complex environments. Small project collaborators will choose appropriate indicators and measurements for each action strategy and determine the best means to collect indicator data. These indicators should be trended over the course of the action project so necessary adjustments can be made. If the action project is completed, the group can evaluate its process and outcomes. When the action is expected to have significant effects, it may be advantageous to collect baseline data for indicators that might measure the change. In some intervention testing designs, baseline measures of essential indicators must be collected. In this way, the indicators can be trended throughout the project to monitor possible program interaction and impact. New indicators of interest that emerge during the action steps as the project unfolds are also trended. In this way, evaluation captures changing patterns over time.

Larger projects with external funding typically include an external evaluation team in the budget. The availability of funding does not necessarily dictate the type of evaluation used. Projects that do not have funding for evaluation would do well to seek people skilled in participatory or empowerment evaluation theory and methods as critical friends. CBCAR evaluators—whether consultants, critical friends, or project team—must be able to engage stakeholders, particularly members of the critical reference group, in planning and implementing the evaluation. Besides creating a better evaluation plan,

Figure 7-2 A Continuum of Evaluation Methods

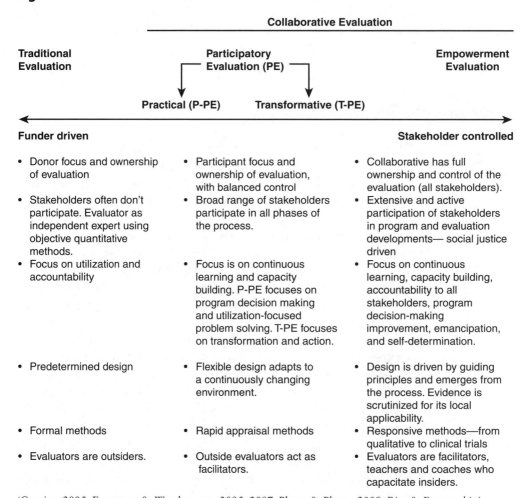

(Cousins, 2005; Fetterman & Wandersman, 2005, 2007; Plottu & Plottu, 2009; Rice & Franceschini, 2007; Suárez-Herrera, Springett & Kagan, 2009; USAID, 1996)

this inclusive approach also builds democratic evaluation capacity. In CBCAR projects, evaluation teams serve as skilled and committed teachers, critics, facilitators, mentors, and coaches—people who competently work their way to the sidelines as the entire group becomes skilled in evaluation. Consistent with the theoretical underpinnings of CBCAR, evaluation should be created by people in the collaborative—not just some of the people or partners, and certainly not just created by outside evaluators. Evaluation is an unfolding and participatory process.

There are varying perspectives in the evaluation community as to what extent and in which ways collaborative, participatory, empowerment, and developmental evaluation differ. All of these methods seek to shape a collaborative effort between evaluators, researchers, and community members to shape an evaluation that is responsive to the local context, draws on the knowledge of key stakeholders, embraces the contributions of critical reference group perspectives, and develops a sense of ownership, new skills, and confidence in improving the quality of decisions.

Participatory Evaluation

Rice and Franceschini (2007) made the point that participatory research has no fixed predetermined outcomes and its evaluation requires the following:

- Participation of key stakeholders in all phases of the process
- Negotiation and consensus about what to evaluate and how results will be interpreted and utilized
- Continuous learning that results in capacity building and incorporation of lessons learned in the decision-making process
- Flexibility to adapt to a continuously changing environment (p. 68)

Of the participatory methods, practical-participatory evaluation (P-PE) is seen to be more utilization-focused. It encourages stakeholders, including the critical reference group, to take control of decision making and to develop problem-solving skills in order to increase the usefulness of the knowledge gained in the evaluation process (Suárez-Herrera, Springett, & Kagan, 2009). Parkinson (2009) made the point that P-PE is "more broadly practiced in countries of the global North, whereas transformative-participatory evaluation (T-PE) is more explicitly focused on social justice and empowerment of the marginalized and has its roots in practice and theory founded in the global South" (p. 230)—referring to the work of Freire

(1970), among others. T-PE is seen to be more ideological and action-oriented. It reaches out to involve the marginalized in order to more fully democratize social change processes. This type of evaluation also presumes that the most useful knowledge is in the community and uses critical reflection to unlock that knowledge. "Both streams [of evaluation] stimulate a process of collective production of knowledge through communicative actions and supportive partnerships" (Suárez-Herrera, Springett, & Kagan, 2009, p. 330).

Empowerment Evaluation

Empowerment evaluation is guided by principles to a greater extent than strict methods of evaluation. Fetterman and Wandersman (2005) presented several principles of empowerment evaluation: improvement, community ownership, inclusion, democratic participation, social justice, community knowledge, evidence-based strategies, capacity building, organization learning, and accountability. **Table 7-2** draws on the work of Fetterman and Wandersman (2005) to outline how each principle guides evaluators, community members, and funders. To clarify the concept of empowerment, Fetterman and Wandersman (2007) stated "No one empowers anyone—including empowerment evaluators—people empower themselves. Empowerment evaluators help create an environment conducive to the development of empowerment" (p. 182). These authors pointed out that empowerment evaluation can be practical and/or transformative; it just depends on the task at hand and what is more pertinent in the particular situation and context. Self-determination and building the capacity for self-evaluation are central to empowerment evaluation; both foster improvement. Wandersman et al. (2005) defined empowerment evaluation as:

> An evaluation approach that aims to increase the probability of achieving program success by (1) providing program stakeholders with tools for assessing the planning, implementation, and self-evaluation of their program, and (2) mainstreaming evaluation as part of the planning and management of the program/organization. (p. 28)

Table 7-2 Roles in Empowerment Evaluation by Practice Principles

Principle	Evaluator	Community	Funder
Improvement	Helps community build on strengths and design improvement-oriented goals. Suggests appropriate tools to measure change over time. Helps community internalize evaluation logic.	Assumes responsibility for direction and implementation of evaluation and uses evaluator to help keep process organized and rigorous. Uses the tools designed to monitor change and data to improve program.	Respects community's right to govern itself and make its own program and evaluation decisions. Provides sufficient funds for improvement-oriented evaluation. Participates in problem solving.
Community ownership	Communicates understanding of community ownership. Provides training, tools, encouragement and does not take over.	Actively engages in directing and implementing evaluation, using the evaluator expert as a teacher, coach, and mentor. Informs funder of progress and findings.	Encourages community ownership of the evaluation and supports opportunities that facilitates ownership and capacity. Supports development of a framework for ongoing use.
Inclusion	Studies the demographics of the community and encourages inclusion of all. Analyzes own biases and develops multicultural skills. Requests use of interpreters.	Constant analysis of margins to reach beyond for greater inclusion. Ensures all voices are heard. Critical reflection to address power differentials in decision making.	Encourages inclusion. Provides appropriate funding for interpretation and translation as needed. Explicitly expresses expectation of inclusion.
Democratic participation	Suggests frameworks for democratic participation in planning, implementation, and reporting of evaluation activities.	Critically reflects on the degree of democratic participation and ensures democratic processes for all activities. Allocates the time needed for all voices to be heard and included. Institutes formal way of monitoring and addressing concerns promptly.	Encourages democratic forms of participation and decision making.

(continues)

Table 7-2 Roles in Empowerment Evaluation by Practice Principles *(continued)*

Principle	Evaluator	Community	Funder
Social justice	Helps design processes that contribute to social justice. Contextualizes findings and decision within a social justice framework. Helps community select evaluation tools that accurately measure social justice outcomes and the potential consequences of the findings.	Actively seeks to work with people experiencing inequalities and frames work to include their voice and address their concerns. Focuses program on a social justice agenda and chooses evaluation tools to measure social justice outcomes. Uses findings to initiate structural change.	Funds programs aligned with a social justice agenda. Helps bring disenfranchised communities into the center of decision-making and in this way fosters self-determination rather than dependency.
Community knowledge	Respects, values, and encourages local community knowledge. Helps community develop strategies to combine community knowledge with evidence-based strategies.	Recognizes the value of its own knowledge and contribution to determining the applicability of evidence-based strategies and the potential of evaluation findings.	Respects community knowledge as essential for sound programming and meaningful change. Shares examples of community knowledge shaping outcomes for other projects.
Evidence-based strategies	Searches out and shares evidence-based strategies and helps community apply its knowledge to adapt to the local context. Suggests strategies for evaluation.	Analyzes and adapts evidence-based strategies to the community context and conditions. Solicits the assistance of evaluators and critical friends to critique evidence-based strategies. Rejects unsound/ unworkable plans.	Supports the community using evidence-based strategies with the caveat that they should adapt rather than adopt them if they do not fit the local context. Respects community decisions.
Capacity building	Trains community in all aspects of evaluation from logic to instrument development. Finds ways to internalize and institutionalize evaluation.	Assumes responsibility for oversight and direction of evaluation—including data collection, analysis, and reporting activities. Organizes training as needed. Works with evaluation mentors as needed.	Supports capacity building as essential part of the evaluation. Provides funds for capacity building and models by sharing funder management skills with community.

Organizational learning	Creates workshops and training experiences that set the stage for organizational learning. Helps create learning organization feedback loops to inform decision making.	Commits to an organizational learning paradigm and creates an atmosphere conducive to taking calculated risks, sharing successes and failures, and feedback loops. Makes decision making transparent. Values engagement of all.	Supports organizational learning with funding for activities, training, and staff support and tracking mechanisms.
Accountability	Places evaluation in the hands of the community and holds funder accountable for agreements with community related to community control of the evaluation. Serves as coach, not director.	Creates a culture in which each person values and assumes accountability for the program and evaluation. Holds evaluator accountable to be coach and critical friend who does not dominate the process.	Holds the community for project results and evaluator accountable for having done adequate capacity building. Critically reflects on the adequacy of its support for capacity building, inclusivity, adaptation and application of evidence-based strategies related to effective program development and evaluation.

Adapted from Fetterman and Wandersman (2005)

Empowerment evaluation is geared toward assisting groups to take stock, set goals, develop strategies, and document their progress in carrying out those strategies to meet their goals. Fetterman and Wandersman (2007) asserted that the principles evaluation guide rather than mandate specific methods. They stated, "Evaluation approaches need to be adapted (with quality)—not adopted by communities" (p. 187) and presented two approaches for communities to use—the *three-step approach* and the ten-step *Getting to Outcomes (GTO)*. It is important to note that these processes are part of the action planning process, not separated from it.

Three-Step Approach to Empowerment Evaluation

In the three-step approach, the evaluation team helps the group to:

1. Establish their mission or purpose
2. Take stock or assess their current state of affairs using a 1 (low) to 10 (high) rating scale of current program goals
3. Plan for future (specifying goals, strategies to achieve goals, and credible evidence) (Fetterman & Wandersman, 2007, p. 187)

The second step, *taking stock*, will help the group to determine their baseline measures. The third step, *plans for the future*, is actually the action step of CBCAR with the addition of determining what the exact measurable indicators will be to discern that strategies have been successfully completed. A wide range of evaluation tools are used to determine whether the strategies selected during action planning have been met, including surveys, focus groups, interviews, demographic data collection, process audits, and clinical trials or comparison groups. As baseline measures are trended and process reflections are done, those strategies that are not working are replaced with strategies that better meet the stated goals and bring the community closer to their stated ideal components. Routine taking-stock sessions are completed at decided intervals in the course of the action step to document changes from baseline, monitor the group's progress and process, inform decision making, and foster group learning.

Ten-Step Getting to Outcomes (GTO) with Empowerment Evaluation

Fetterman and Wandersman (2007) presented a second approach to empowerment evaluation, which is a results-based accountability method involving a process of answering the following 10 accountability questions:

1. What are the needs and resources in the collaborative? (needs assessment; resource assessment)

2. What are the goals, target population, and desired outcomes (objectives) of your action plan?

3. How does the action plan incorporate knowledge of science and best practices in the area of interest?

4. How does the action plan fit with other efforts in the community? (collaboration, cultural competence)

5. What capacities do you need to put this action into place with quality? (capacity building)

6. How will this action plan be carried out? (planning)

7. How will the quality of implementation be assessed? (process evaluation)

8. How well did the action plan work? (outcome and impact evaluation)

9. How will continuous quality improvement strategies be incorporated? (CQI)

10. If the action plan is successful, how will the action and the collaborative be sustained? (sustainability) (adapted to CBCAR from Fetterman & Wandersman, 2007)

The process of answering these 10 questions will foster the collaborative's skills in planning, implementing, and evaluating action steps. To further describe this process, Chinman, Imm, and Wandersman (2004) have published a Rand Report manual and worksheets on the GTO methodology, which are available for free download from the Web.

Developmental Evaluation

In the 1990s, organization development and program evaluation expert, Michael Quinn Patton (2011), responded to the expressed needs of a rural Minnesota community leadership program that contracted him as a project evaluator. The contract included 2.5 years of formative evaluation and 2.5 years of summative evaluation. When the time came to switch from formative to summative evaluation, community members protested and clearly stated they did not want a fixed model, but rather felt they needed to continue to adapt their program in response to a changing environment. It was at that moment that Quinn conceptualized developmental evaluation, which "tracks and attempts to make sense of what emerges under conditions of complexity, documenting and interpreting the dynamics, interactions, and interdependencies that occur as innovations unfold" (2011, p. 7). Developmental evaluation supports exploration and innovation for program development and supports ongoing program adaptation in the context of complex and changing environments. Developmental evaluation's "systems-and-complexity-based interactive design" involves rapid assessment and rapid feedback (p. 46). Common techniques used in developmental evaluation include ongoing environmental scanning and outcomes monitoring, continual reflecting, network analyzing, and systems change mapping (i.e., drawing pictures or diagrams of the system's pattern over time). Developmental evaluation honors the history of the community and the issue at hand in order to know what to monitor and expect going forward. In the process of developmental evaluation, the action planning group engages in on-going assessment of whether emerging innovations are ready for more formal implementation as pilot programs, and thus, might be ready for formative evaluation. As programs are improved and perfected, summative evaluation informs decisions related to dissemination as a best-practice model. Like other participatory evaluation methods, developmental evaluation draws on an overarching collaborative framework to engage all major stakeholders in "reality testing about what is being developed—and what difference is being made" (Patton, 2011, p. 245)

Since the intent of CBCAR is to improve systems and enhance life for all involved, and particularly for the most marginalized stakeholders in the project, no matter which evaluation method is utilized, the entire group engages in critical reflection on whether their work is improving systems and making life better for the most marginalized stakeholders. It may help to draw a diagram outlining who has benefited from the entire CBCAR project, in what way, and to what extent. All evaluation methods should be rooted in the principles of social justice (Mertens, 2009).

Considering Baseline Measures

Extreme care must be taken when asked to define outcome measures for a project that has not yet started. We give the example of an agricultural development project in Guatemala. In the 1990s, an external development agency came into a community in the highlands of Guatemala to improve the income of very poor farmers in the region. The outcome measures for this farming development project were determined by the development agency to be crop yield and income. Before the project started, the men in the region worked in the fields, which they tended with their hands and hoes. The women did back-strap weaving and produced fine colorful tablecloths, hangings, and clothing, which they sold for money that they invested in their children's educational supplies, food, and healthcare expenses. The development agency brought in farm machinery, seeds, and education on how to increase crop yield.

By the end of the first year, the crop yield and family income had risen dramatically. However, part of the increase was due to the addition of the women working in the fields with their husbands. The women no longer had the time to weave and thus, no longer had income to support the health, education, and nutritional needs of their children. After a while, the children were also working in the fields with their parents. The men controlled the income from the farm, which they primarily spent on alcohol and additional machinery. Within 3 years, family income doubled and the development agency deemed the project a huge success. Unfortunately, the development agency failed to measure children's educational level, health data, and mortality rates at baseline and completion—all of which were adversely affected by the project. Emotional well-being of the women, cultural connectedness, relationship with the land, and alcoholism were also not included in the baseline or outcome measures. This is all to say that we only see what we measure, and people from the critical reference group must be engaged in deciding what is important to them and what they see as important outcomes. The people in the development agency did not intend to cause harm; they promised wealth, as promoted by media images. People who are poor may be silent when talking with "educated" and "wealthy" people— out of respect and an often-internalized message that the "educated" and the "rich" know what they are doing. Engaging the critical reference group in a dialogue to determine their views on important baseline and outcome indicators is essential. It mobilizes the wisdom of indigenous knowledge and averts potential disaster. For example, had child mortality, and health education level status been monitored over the course of the farm development project in Guatemala, and a participatory or collaborative evaluation process used, the farmers and their families could have reflected on the community's changing patterns and controlled the project's trajectory.

Evaluation from the Perspective of the Critical Reference Group

When brainstorming potential indicators to be measured at baseline, it is wise to do so cautiously, widely, and in respectful focused attention to the words, lives, and situations of those most affected by the project. How do *they* define human flourishing? How might this be measured? Perspective taking is an essential aspect of this work. We get a glimpse of the whole from each person's experience. Saville Kushner (2000) made the point that projects and programs are best evaluated through the lens of the people whose lives the programs intend to impact. As a metaphor, Kushner presented the example of a hologram, which is a piece of glass that reflects a three-dimensional image. If the hologram is shattered, each piece still holds a view of the whole, but from its own unique perspective. For example, if you look head-on at the bottom center piece, you see only the bottom center of the image; however, if you tilt the piece and look from the lower edge, you can see a view of the whole image as if looking at it from below. So too, the upper-right hand corner piece reveals the whole viewed from the right side of its top. The whole is in the parts; you need simply look from various angles to grasp it. A skilled evaluation team develops this ability to see programs through the perspective of people in the critical reference group. In their evaluation of community-based participatory programs that address cancer disparities, Scarinci, Johnson, Hardy, Marron, and Partridge (2009) made the point that often people from the academy and people from the community have strikingly different views of what desirable outcomes are and use different "tools" to measure "success" (p. 222).

Parkinson (2009) stressed this point in a report on a participatory monitoring and evaluation (PM&E) project that measured the effectiveness of a farming program in Uganda. Very few farmers participated in the evaluation (14–19%). What evaluators intended to be a community-driven evaluation process was perceived by the farmers, many of whom were barely literate, as a process that was too complicated (13-page forms to fill out), and required too much time and effort. Farmers consistently expressed their belief that the PM&E was a tool of the program managers for their own purposes, not something that would benefit farmers (Parkinson, 2009). In her critique of the PM&E process in this project, Parkinson concluded that the "tendency towards an official 'power blindness' is fairly common in development literature," and it results in "a distorted form of consensus, because of the different positions and perspectives of stakeholders" (p. 237). In this case, the requirement of literacy to be fully involved gave more responsibility and control to the educated farmers while provoking distrust on the part of the farmers who could not read (Parkinson, 2009). Yet, PM&E was originally developed to address the unequal power distribution by incorporating the perspective of project beneficiaries and providing the opportunity for shared understanding and cooperative learning. In this aspect, PM&E would follow its roots, which are in transformative participatory evaluation (T-PE).

Cultural Appreciation and Inclusion

CBCAR evaluation involves cultural appreciation and inclusion. Hansberger (2010) made the point that evaluators need to have multicultural awareness to be able to evaluate projects that represent multicultural interests and efforts. Hansberger built on the work of SenGupta, Hopson, and Thompson-Robinson (2004) to broadly define multicultural competence in evaluation as:

> A systematic, responsive inquiry that is well-informed by the cultural norms of the majority and minority cultures involved and of different notions of multiculturalism as well as the context in which the evaluation takes place; that frames and articulates the epistemology of the evaluative endeavour; that employs multiculturally valid and contextually appropriate methodology; and that uses stakeholder-generated, interpretive means to arrive at the results and further use of the findings. The evaluator needs competence to negotiate and promote a dialogue across cultural borders. (p. 183)

Hansberger stressed the importance of an appreciative attitude for the cultural context within which projects are situated, yet cautioned against cultural appreciation that does not protect individuals' basic human rights. Specifically, evaluators should assess whether the CBCAR action plan looks at the problem from different cultural perspectives, illuminates power relationships, and creates its ideal components in a way that incorporates the vision of all aspects of the community. Evaluators assess whether the program is steered and shaped predominantly by the dominant culture (or academia, health department, nongovernmental organization) and whether the CBCAR collective has considered the cultural implications of the program. In terms of program implementation, evaluators would look for evidence of critical reflection to unearth cultural biases and insensitivities. Furthermore, evaluators examine whether an appreciative attitude for all cultures existed throughout all efforts, and whether all cultures have been equitably included, without requiring assimilation to the dominant culture. Overall, multiculturally aware programs promote diversity and enhance tolerance in society (Hansberger, 2010).

■ Documenting Outcomes and Disseminating Results

During action and evaluation planning—which should both occur simultaneously—the specific indicators and their measures are determined. These data are then pulled together at the end of the project and documented in a format that can best speak to their audience. For example, funders may have specific forms or formats that need to be filled out and followed. Funders also benefit from attractive presentations of the evaluation findings. For example, *Racism and How It Affects Our Health* curriculum guides were artfully done and included two DVDs of forum content. Various funders have commented on the quality of this work. Quality documentation lays the groundwork for future funding and should highlight the strength of the partnerships and the extensive involvement of diverse stakeholders in all aspects of the project.

Other audiences might include the wider community, media, policy makers, specific organizations and agencies in the community, administrators, clients, collaborating organizations and staff, students, and professional review communities. The documentation modalities should speak concisely and powerfully to these varied interest groups. Fetterman (2001) advocated the creation of videos, claiming their face validity and power to document effects. This can be done for the CBCAR research process and repeated at the end of the action steps to evaluate the process from various perspectives as it evolves. Care must be taken to represent who was truly involved in the project. An exercise that is also helpful is to collectively come up with a 30-second statement that summarizes the impact and quality of the project—the traditional elevator speech in which the message can be delivered between floors. This is a way to have fun while creating the group rendition of the essence of the important collective work that was done. It is like gathering together and presenting a beautiful bouquet from a garden collectively planted.

Not only do the CBCAR research and process findings need to be documented and disseminated, but the evaluation findings may also be pertinent for dissemination. The first act of dissemination is the presentation of the CBCAR research findings to the community for action planning. This may be a time to also involve the local media, and thus engage the wider community in what has been learned. We have used media to recruit the wider community into action planning efforts and to disseminate our findings. Dissemination of research findings is an action step in and of itself and occurs at various phases in the CBCAR process. When people absorb the wisdom of the CBCAR process findings, they are often inspired to take action. An example is given in **Box 7-3**.

An important focus of dissemination involves carefully targeting findings to people who can help create structural change—change that brings about more just, equitable, and healthy social and organizational conditions. This is the core of the CBCAR process; all actions should be strategically directed to promote the health of people and systems. One strategy for assuring structural change to address inequalities is to develop ongoing relationships with policy makers and their staff. Seifer (2006) recommends that groups create and disseminate policy briefs that explain the key issues, findings, and recommendations for action.

Partners, funders, and policy makers will benefit from an attractive and engaging presentation of what the project meant to those most profoundly impacted. With very little funding, we have presented research findings through videos, DVDs of spoken-word performances, CDs of hip-hop music, and monographs with artistic graphics and ample color photos. As pointed out in Chapter 4, decisions about dissemination are made at the onset of the partnership. Who is going to take the lead on publications, how organization names will be listed, and how funders will be credited in documents and productions should be decided and documented prior to beginning the work (see Chapter 4, Boxes 4-2 & 4-3).

Decisions about where to aim professional publications may also change. Even though academics are rewarded in the

---

Box 7-3 Dissemination of Actions Through Data Presentation and Pattern Recognition

At a community forum action planning meeting where a hip-hop rendition of data from teens was being presented, community members broke down into small dialogue circles to discern needed actions. The health center and university staff, who were responsible for seeking funds for action planning, were becoming increasingly nervous when the groups began generating dozens and dozens of action steps. When the groups reconvened it was interesting to note that each person had discerned several things they could do to promote community health. The actions ranged from grandmothers deciding to dedicate more time to their grandchildren to the person responsible for the school lunch menu deciding to initiate nutritional changes to teens deciding that they will be more active in challenging friends engaged in unhealthy behaviors. The hip-hop words and music touched people deeply, and each person was motivated to decide what she or he personally was going to do. The university and health center staff did not have to take responsibility for initiating officially funded actions, the community was charging ahead. When careful attention is paid to presenting the pattern of research findings, actions flow out like ripples in a pond.

---

promotional process for publishing their work in refereed journals, the findings may benefit the community more if they are aimed elsewhere. For example, in the *Health, Well-Being, and Racism* project described in Chapter 1, the women's advisory council decided physicians were their target audience and therefore chose to publish their findings in *Minnesota Medicine,* a publication distributed widely to Minnesota physicians. The guiding principle for dissemination is that impact counts, and it should ultimately serve the most vulnerable in the community whenever possible. For this reason, it is helpful to discern which structures need to be changed and aim the dissemination of findings to maximize structural change. Another guiding principle—mutuality is a must—leads CBCAR partners who are skilled at publishing and writing to teach those skills to others who can then take the lead in publications. In the same manner, partners who are skilled in visual media productions and working with policy makers and the press can capacitate others by teaching these dissemination skills.

Although CBCAR findings should definitely be disseminated in various venues, perhaps it is more important to disseminate the lessons learned and the process used, which might be more generalizable and interesting to others. Seifer (2006) pointed out that action researchers should also disseminate information about barriers, challenges, and other pressing issues. Sommer (2009) recommended that specific and substantive articles be aimed toward technical journals or venues to reach people interested in the topic, while methodological and reflective articles be aimed toward journals designed to address and improve the practice of action research. Within academia, a case needs to be made to stress that appearing on a TV show, publishing in a local newspaper, or producing a community organizing DVD can be profound scholarly work from an action research perspective. To aide in this effort, Community Engaged Scholarship for Health (www.ces4health.info) provides a peer review process for multimedia action research dissemination products. Addressing mentorship of graduate students, Sommer (2009) pointed out that, ". . . it is important to tell them that for most positions in government agencies, non-profits, and higher education, non-journal publication is valued" (p. 234).

In an engaging three-act play published in a refereed journal, Fisher and Phelps (2006) presented tensions and incongruities graduate students face between the conventions for writing traditional theses and the principles of action research. They stated that the written presentation of this work should move people to action and reflection, and therefore must be more of a performance and less of a recipe to be followed. A more creative and honest approach often involves the mixing of actors' and authors' voices where bylines are difficult to claim. Greenwood, Brydon-Miller, and Shafer (2006) presented several issues related to intellectual property and action research. For example, if a doctoral student is working with a clinical practice group on an action research project, whose name should be attached to the findings chapter of the thesis? If a few people in a 40-person collaborative write about a project, and all 40 collaborated on the work, how many names belong on the manuscript and who decides? While talking openly and having decisions in writing are helpful, the quality of the relationships within the collaborative is most important. Open and honest conversations have to occur through all steps of the CBCAR process in order for collaborating members to make just and transparent decisions as the project unfolds.

The dissemination of research findings, CBCAR insights, innovative action plans, and evaluation findings is important— not only to advance knowledge on content but also to advance the science of the CBCAR process. There are various avenues for dissemination. The most important avenues lead to structural transformation and process improvements to promote human health and flourishing. To this end, the dissemination process is strategically focused.

■ Sustaining the Partnership

One of the major criticisms people in communities express about academics and graduate students is that they arrive in a community, gather data, publish their findings, and then are never seen again in the community, where conditions have not improved. In CBCAR, the control of the research direction and the research question is reversed—it is community defined and controlled. The end result is action. This is a tremendously fulfilling process for all involved. It is a great change for academics who are skilled at traditional research methods; they can now connect in a meaningful way with the beneficiaries of their research. Sustaining CBCAR partnerships takes time and careful attention.

Israel et al. (2006) analyzed the factors that sustain partnerships in Centers for Disease Control-funded Urban Research Centers in three large US cities and found the following to be essential: commitment to relationships; maintenance of knowledge, capacity, and values generated by the partnership; and stable funding, staff, programs, and policy changes. They found that challenges are magnified when the core funding ended. Challenges to sustaining relationships and commitments revolved around lack of time and resources, need to share reduced resources, and maintaining morale and energy. They found that to overcome these challenges, having and adhering to shared principles, the existence of structured yet flexible governance rules, "having the right people around the table" over the long term, and jointly serving a clear community benefit helped to sustain the partnership (p. 1030). Challenges to sustaining knowledge, capacity, and values were mainly limited time and resources and partners not being fully aware of the community-based research process. These challenges were mitigated through critical self-reflection, organizational affiliation and commitment to the partnership, centering several projects within the partnership, and recognizing the fact that communities possess essential knowledge and skills. These researchers found that funding of the community-based research infrastructure and unrestricted program funds helped to sustain partnerships that previously had insufficient time to reach the translation cycle of their research. The Urban Research Center initiatives were large projects with primarily organizational, rather than individual, relationships and with annual funding between $250,000 and $448,000 (Israel et al., 2006).

Smaller projects are more likely to be sustained by interpersonal relationships, shared values, and common meaningful work. For example, a practice group of nurses in a clinical setting engaged in action research without any outside funding might be more stable over the long run, particularly if they are held together by healthy relationships and the fulfillment of working collaboratively to improve patient outcomes and their work environment.

In CBCAR, trusting collaborative relationships and the common desire to promote human flourishing and human rights for all are at the center of the partnership. As collaborative work proceeds through research, action, and evaluation steps, new ideas constantly arise. A strong partnership will reach the end of a project only to realize that they are faced with a new burning issue and increased capacity to take it on.

■ Exploring New Questions

Readers are referred back to Figure I-1 to appreciate the cyclical nature of CBCAR. It began with a partnership and a research question being posed. Critical friends were invited in and a process was devised to create a healthy working collaborative where power differentials were quickly identified and leveled. Human flourishing was sought as a means and an end to the collaborative work. The group went through a process of data collection and analysis to better understand evolving patterns. The data were creatively organized and presented for the community to discern appropriate actions. More critical friends were invited in; the literature was searched for best practices; and the historical and baseline patterns were captured. Ideal components were visualized and distilled into goals and specific activities to reach those goals. Indicators were chosen to measure whether the activities had the intended impact. Once again, dialogue was centered on the meaning and value of the actions—and now, the collaborative finds itself once more on the threshold of a new question to be answered. For this new effort, new partners may surface or be called on; additional resources might need to be sought; and additional critical friends might need to be brought on board. It is again a time for dialogue.

■ Summary—Insights into Action

The cherry oatmeal cobbler was enjoyed by all. It was a satisfying dessert, and it did not distract in the least from the spirited conversations and laughter of the gathering. Everyone was able to be fully present. And so too it is with CBCAR; our attention is on setting the context for relationships to flourish. The wisdom of necessary actions lies within the community; our task is to create the context within which it can be revealed. When people come together to dialogue and reflect on the presented pattern of what is happening in the community, the collective wisdom gives rise to actions not previously seen. What has been demonstrated as best practice elsewhere can be scrutinized for its applicability in the local context. A new local product is branded and ready to be launched and tested.

■ References

Agency for Healthcare Research and Quality. (2009). *AHRQ activities using community-based participatory research to address health care disparities.* Retrieved from http://www.ahrq.gov/research/cbprbrief.pdf.

Aronson, R., Lovelace, K., Hatch, J., & Whitehead, T. (2006). Strengthening communities and the roles of individuals in community life. In B. Levy & V. Sidel (Eds.), *Social injustice and public health* (pp. 433–448). New York, NY: Oxford.

Becker, C., Stice, E., Shaw, H., & Woda, S. (2009). Use of empirically supported interventions for psychopathology: Can the participatory approach move us beyond the research-to-practice gap? *Behaviour Research and Therapy, 47,* 265–274.

Best, A., Stokols, D., Green, L., Leischow, S., Holmes, B., & Buchholz, K. (2003). An integrative framework for community partnering to translate theory into effective health promotion strategy. *American Journal of Health Promotion, 18,* 168–176.

Brofenfenbrenner, U. (1979). *The ecology of human development.* Cambridge, MA: Harvard.

Chilisa, B. (2009). Indigenous African-centered ethics: Contesting and complementing dominant models. In D. Mertens & P. Ginsberg (Eds.), *The handbook of social research ethics* (pp. 407–425). Los Angeles, CA: Sage.

Chinman, M., Imm, P., & Wandersman, A. (2004). *Getting to Outcomes 2004: Promoting accountability through methods and tools for planning, implementation, and evaluation* (TR-TR101). Santa Monica, CA: RAND. Retrieved from http://www.rand.org/publications/TR/TR101/.

Cohen, D., Scribrier, R., & Farley, T. (2000). A structural model of health behavior: A pragmatic approach to explain and influence health behaviors at the population level. *Preventive Medicine, 30,* 154–164.

Commission for the Social Determinants of Health. (2008). *Closing the gap in a generation: Health equity through action on the social determinants of health.* Retrieved from http://www.who.int/social_determinants/en.

Committee on Health and Behavior. (2001). *Health and behavior: The interplay of biological, behavioral, and societal influences.* Washington, DC: National Academy of Sciences.

Cousins, J. B. (2005). Will the real empowerment evaluation please stand up? A critical friend perspective. In D. Fetterman & A. Wandersman (Eds.). *Empowerment evaluation principles in practice.* New York, NY: Guilford.

Cowling, W. R. (1999). A unitary-transformative nursing science: Potentials for transcending dichotomies. *Nursing Science Quarterly, 12*(2), 132–137.

Cowling, W. R. (2007). A unitary participatory vision of nursing knowledge. *Advances in Nursing Science, 30*(1), 61–70.

Fetterman, D. M. (2001). *Foundations of empowerment evaluation.* Thousand Oaks, CA: Sage.

Fetterman, D., & Wandersman, A. (2005). *Empowerment evaluation principles in practice.* New York, NY: Guilford.

Fetterman, D., & Wandersman, A. (2007). Empowerment evaluation: Yesterday, today, and tomorrow. *American Journal of Evaluation, 28*(2), 179–198.

Fisher, K., & Phelps, R. (2006). Recipe or performing art? Challenging conventions for writing action research theses. *Action Research, 4*(2), 143–164.

Flood, R. (2006). The relationship of "systems thinking" to action research. In P. Reason & H. Bradbury (Eds.), *Handbook of action research* (pp. 117–128). Thousand Oaks, CA: Sage.

Freire, P. (1970). *Pedagogy of the oppressed.* New York, NY: Continuum.

Freire, P. (1985). *The politics of education: Culture, power and liberation.* New York, NY: Bergin & Garvey.

Green, L., & Kreuter, M. (2005). *Health program planning: An educational and ecological approach.* Boston, MA: McGraw-Hill.

Greenwood, D. J., Brydon-Miller, M., & Shafer, C. (2006). Intellectual property and action research. *Action Research, 4*(91), 81–95.

Hansberger, A. (2010). Multicultural awareness in evaluation: Dilemmas and challenges. *Evaluation, 16*(2), 177–191.

Heron, J., & Reason, P. (1997). A participatory inquiry paradigm. *Qualitative Inquiry, 3*(3), 274–294.

Horowitz, C., Robinson, M., & Seifer, S. (2009). Community-based participatory research from the margin to the mainstream: Are researchers prepared? *Circulation, 119,* 2633–2642.

Israel, B. A., Krieger, J., Vlahov, S. C., Foley, M., Fortin, P., Guzman, J. R. . . . Tang, G. (2006). Challenges and facilitating factors in sustaining community-based participatory research partnerships:

Lessons learned from the Detroit, New York City and Seattle Urban Research Centers. *Journal of Urban Health: Bulletin of the New York Academy of Medicine, 83*(6), 1022–1040.

Kumar, S. (2002). *Methods for community participation: A complete guide for practitioners.* London, UK: ITDG.

Kushner, S. (2000). *Personalizing evaluation.* London, UK: Sage.

Lane, S., Rubinstein, R., Keefe, R., Webster, N., Cibula, D., Rosenthal, A., & Dowdell, M. (2004). Structural violence and racial disparity in HIV transmission. *Journal of Health Care for the Poor and Underserved, 15,* 319–335.

Law, M. (1997). Changing disabling environments through participatory action-research. In S. E. Smith, D. G. Willms, & N. A. Johnson (Eds.), *Nurtured by knowledge: Learning to do participatory action-research* (pp. 34–58). New York, NY: The Apex Press.

Leykum, L. K., Pugh, J. A., Lanham, J., Harmon, J., & McDaniel, R. (2009). Implementation research design: Integrating participatory action research into randomized controlled trials *Implementation Science 4,* 69–76. doi:10.1186/1748-5908-4-69

Ludema, J. D., & Fry, R. E. (2008). The practice of appreciative inquiry. In P. Reason & H. Bradbury (Eds.). *The SAGE handbook of action research: Participatory inquiry and practice* (2nd ed.), pp. 280–296. Thousand Oaks, CA: Sage.

McLaren, L., & Hawe, P. (2005). Ecological perspectives in health research. *Journal of Epidemiology and Community Health, 59,* 6–14.

Mertens, D. M. (2009). *Transformative research and evaluation.* New York, NY: The Guildford Press.

Newman, M. A. (1994). *Health as expanding consciousness* (2nd ed.). Boston, MA: Jones and Bartlett.

Newman, M. A. (2008). *Transforming presence: The difference nursing makes.* Philadelphia, PA: F. A. Davis.

Parkinson, S. (2009). Power and perception in participatory monitoring and evaluation. *Evaluation and Program Planning, 32,* 229–237.

Patton, M. Q. (2011). *Developmental evaluation: Applying complexity concepts to enhance innovation and use.* New York, NY: Guilford.

Plottu, B., & Plottu, E. (2009). Approaches to participation in evaluation: Some conditions for implementation. *Evaluation, 15*(13), 343–359. doi: 10.1177/1356389009106357

Reason, P. (1998). Three approaches to participatory inquiry. In N. Denzin & Y. Lincoln, (Eds.), *Strategies of qualitative inquiry.* Thousand Oaks, CA: Sage.

Rice, M., & Franceschini, M. C. (2007). Lessons learned from the application of a participatory evaluation methodology to Healthy Municipalities, Cities and Communities initiatives in selected countries in the Americas. *Promotion & Education, 14*, 68–73.

Sallis, J., Cervero, R., Ascher, W., Henderson, K., Kraft, M., & Kerr, J. (2006). An ecological approach to active living communities. *Annual Review of Public Health, 27*, 297–322.

Scarinci, I. C., Johnson, R. E., Hardy, C., Marron, J., & Partridge, E. E. (2009). Planning and implementation of a participatory evaluation strategy: A viable approach in the evaluation of community-based participatory programs addressing cancer disparities. *Evaluation and Program Planning, 32*, 221–228.

Seifer, S. D. (2006). Building and sustaining community-institutional partnerships for prevention research: Findings from a national collaborative. *Journal of Urban Health: Bulletin of the New York Academy of Medicine, 83*(6), 989–1003.

Semenza, J., & Maty, S. (2007). Acting upon the macrosocial environment to improve health: A framework for intervention. In S. Galea (Ed.), *Macrosocial determinants of population health* (pp. 443–461). New York, NY: Springer.

SenGupta, S., Hopson, R. K., & Thomson-Robinson, M. (2004). Cultural competence in evaluation: An overview. *New Directions for Evaluation, 104*, 5–19.

Skolimowski, H. (1994). *The participatory mind. A new theory of knowledge and of the universe.* London, UK: Penguin Books.

Smith, S. E. (1997). Deepening participatory action-research. In S. E. Smith, D. G. Willms, & N. A. Johnson (Eds.). *Nurtured by knowledge: Learning to do participatory action-research* (pp. 173–263). New York, NY: The Apex Press.

Sommer, R. (2009). Dissemination in action research. *Action Research, 7*(2), 227–236.

Stringer, E. T. (2007). *Action research* (3rd ed.). Thousand Oaks, CA: Sage.

Stringer, E. T., & Genet, W. J. (2004). *Action research in health.* Upper Saddle River, NJ: Pearson.

Suárez-Herrera, J. C., Springett, J., & Kagan, C. (2009). Critical connections between participatory evaluation, organizational learning and intentional change in pluralistic organizations. *Evaluation, 15*(13), 321–342. doi: 10.1177/1356389009105884

USAID Center for Development Information and Evaluation. (1996). Conducting a participatory evaluation. *Performance Monitoring and Evaluation TIPS, 1*, 1–4.

Viswanathan, M., Ammerman, A., Eng, E., Gartlehner, G., Lohr, K., Griffith, D. . . . Whitener, I. (2004). *Community-based participatory research: Assessing the evidence.* Retrieved from http://www.ahrq.gov/downloads/pub/evidence/pdf/cbpr/cbpr.pdf.

Wadsworth, Y. (1997). *Everyday evaluation on the run* (2nd ed.). Crows Nest, Australia: Allen & Unwin.

Wandersman, A., Snell-Hons, J., Lentz, B. E., Fetterman, D. M., Keener, D. C., Livet, M. . . . Flaspohler, P. (2005). The principles of empowerment evaluation. In D. M. Fetterman & A. Wandersman (Eds.). *Empowerment evaluation principles in practice,* (pp. 27–41). New York, NY: Guilford.

CHAPTER 8

CBCAR and a Relational Approach to Research Ethics

Anita Ho

After World War II, 23 German physicians and administrators were tried for their willing participation in crimes against humanity, including conducting medical experiments on thousands of concentration camp prisoners without their consent, leaving many of these involuntary subjects dead or permanently disabled. As a direct result of the military tribunal, the Nuremberg Code (1947) was enacted, making it the first international document to explicitly establish voluntary and informed consent as essential for ethical research involving human participants.[1] Although the Nuremberg Code is not a legally binding document, it has guided other international medical and scientific associations in establishing broad and comprehensive ethical documents and treatises to prevent similar transgressions in the name of science.

While such protective measures are often helpful in establishing side constraints on what researchers may do to research participants in their pursuit of knowledge, particularly those who are deemed vulnerable, this paper examines whether these paternalistic assumptions may also inadvertently reinforce power hierarchy. Informed by qualitative fieldwork experience and the concept of community-based collaborative action research (CBCAR), this paper argues that a relational approach to research ethics that attends to power relations, inclusivity, and reciprocity can better promote respect and autonomy of vulnerable populations than traditional protective approaches.

■ An Unlikely Prospective Research Participant

"Can she really provide voluntary consent?" was among the many concerns that unsettled us when the United Nations police advisors (UNPOL) brought a young woman, her mother-in-law, and her three small children out of a packed jail cell at a police station in a village in Southern Sudan. As a philosopher from a Canadian university, I was collaborating with Dr. Carol Pavlish, a nursing faculty member from the University of California, Los Angeles (UCLA), and the American Refugee Committee (ARC), an international nongovernment organization (NGO) that provides humanitarian assistance to this post-conflict region. Dr. Pavlish had previously conducted preliminary assessment with ARC and local residents regarding various struggles facing the community. The goal of the follow-up ethnographic study was to meet with multiple stakeholders at various levels and further investigate local perspectives on human rights and gender-related issues facing returnees from the civil war, so that we could bring community voices to our partnering organization and collaboratively develop sustainable programs that would be responsive to local priorities.[2] We had just finished conducting focus groups and key informant interviews on similar issues with Congolese refugees in Rwanda. Armed with translated consent forms and approval documents from the local agency and our respective universities' research ethics boards, we arrived at the police station with our Sudanese interpreter, who also works with the village residents on gender-related issues. We were there for a pre-arranged key-informant interview with the chief officer about the police's experience with human rights issues facing the community.

The poorly equipped police station was surprisingly crowded, with many people attempting to gain attention from the few officers, all of whom were busy with various matters. The UNPOL was there to train the local police on investigation techniques and other matters. A few meters behind the counter was a room with a couple of small, dark, damp, and full jail cells—women and men were not separated; neither were adults and children. We were greeted by a few UNPOL and local officers, who explained that the police chief was very busy and unfortunately would not be able to meet with us at that time. While we were trying to determine if we could return later, the officers brought two women and three children from one of the cramped jail cells. The youngest of the children, only 18 months old, was completely naked. The officers said that we should talk to this young mother, whose plight could shed light on community perspectives on human rights and gender relations in this postconflict region. A few days before, the woman's estranged husband, who was a lieutenant of the army and had reportedly abused her in the past, threw a grenade at the woman because he suspected her of infidelity and was angry about her attempt to divorce him. While she and the children escaped physical harm, the explosion killed a bystander and injured many others. The police detained the husband, but some relatives of the deceased/injured wanted to kill the husband's mother and take the children to replace the deceased. The village did not have a safe house to shield anyone from domestic or other kinds of violence, and the young mother did not have other resources or support network to relocate or seek refuge. So, for protection, the family stayed in the crowded jail cell with suspects of various crimes.

Part of our project design was to take direction from previous and current community informants and to continue collaborating with our local NGO partner to gather the village residents' perspectives regarding human rights and gender relationships. And from UNPOL's brief introduction to the family's situation, it appeared that the young mother would have much to contribute to this dialogue; her experience might be integral in assessing the community's needs and designing appropriate programs to address such unmet needs. But given her dire circumstances, should she be recruited to participate in the research?

■ Participant Recruitment and Protection in International Documents

Women in economically impoverished areas that are male-dominated, including this small village in Southern Sudan, often have few social and economic resources as well as limited educational and development opportunities (Pavlish & Ho, 2009a). While the Southern Sudan Interim Constitution (Government of Southern Sudan, 2007) promises to "enact laws to combat harmful customs and traditions which undermine the dignity and status of women" (p. 10), government and community infrastructures in this village are lacking, and women in our study lamented their vulnerability to violence, abandonment, and forced marriage (Pavlish & Ho, 2009a). The young mother we met was subjected to domestic violence and had no other means to protect herself and her family. Her reliance on the local police as the only source of basic protection made her a potential target for manipulation or even coercion to participate in the research, since a woman who could not leave the jail cell without risking personal and familial safety would unlikely feel free to decline UNPOL's request to meet with the researchers.

Concerns for involuntary research participation, particularly in the shadow of the Nazi atrocities, formed the basis for various domestic and international ethical guidelines for participant recruitment. The *Belmont Report* (United States National Commission for the Protection of Human Subjects of Biomedical and Behavioral Research, 1979), which was created in 1979, unequivocally establishes respect for participants, beneficence/nonmaleficence, and justice as the three unifying ethical principles for research using human subjects. According to this document, respect for persons requires treating individuals as "autonomous agents" and protecting those "with diminished autonomy." Focusing on one participant at a time, this principle demands that "subjects enter into the research voluntarily and with adequate information" (Part B.1, para. 5). The *Belmont Report* reminds researchers to take extra care when recruiting "vulnerable subjects," whose legal or sociocultural status reduces their relative power or ability to promote their own vital interests. Within the context of research ethics, conceptions of vulnerability center upon characteristics associated with particular groups. "Racial minorities, the economically disadvantaged, the very sick, and the institutionalized" are often considered vulnerable. Given "their dependent status and their frequently compromised capacity for free consent," the *Belmont Report* cautions that these individuals may be "easy to manipulate" and thus "should be protected against the danger of being involved in research solely for administrative convenience" (Part 3.3, para. 5).

Other international research ethics documents have also established guidelines on working with people who may be subject to giving consent under duress because of their vulnerability. The Declaration of Helsinki (World Medical Association, 2008), first enacted in 1964 and subsequently revised to address increasingly complex research arenas, explicitly states that populations that "cannot give or refuse consent for themselves" or are economically and medically disadvantaged, are vulnerable and "need special protection" (Section 9). Section 17 of the declaration asserts that recruitment of a disadvantaged or vulnerable population "is only justified if the research is responsive to the health needs and priorities of this population or community and if there is a reasonable likelihood that this population or community stands to benefit from the results of the research." The Council for International Organizations of Medical Sciences (CIOMS) (2002), which established its International Ethical Guidelines for Biomedical Research[3] and last revised it in 2002, also asks for "special justification" and strict application of rights/welfare protection when recruiting prospective participants who are relatively incapable of protecting their own interests. In its attempt to address the conditions and the needs of low-resource countries as well as the implications for multinational research in which they may be partners, CIOMS pays special attention to vast socioeconomic and political disparities in the global community.[4]

These protective considerations are in place to ensure that those who are in vulnerable positions, like the young mother in the Sudanese jail, will not be coerced into participating in research projects or exploited for the sake of researchers' benefits. While it is beyond our scope to provide a thorough analysis of these concepts, a brief discussion may be helpful here. The principle of autonomy requires that we respect the right of rational persons who have the capacity for self-determination, to take charge of their lives and act according to their values and goals, provided that their actions do not harm others. Coercion is thought to counter people's capacity for self-directed action. It generally involves an intentional and overt threat of harm one party uses to obtain compliance from another party to do or not do something, by making a certain choice irresistible, i.e., the options are so weighted that only one reasonable course of action remains open (Hawkins & Emanuel, 2005). In these cases, A's choices are *unfavorably* narrowed, or their baseline is made worse off by B, who is attempting to get A to do something they would not otherwise do if not for the threat. When such threat violates A's rights or fails to fulfill an obligation B has to A if the latter chooses noncompliance, and A has no reasonable alternative but to accept such proposal, coercion is illegitimate and invalidates the consent (Wertheimer & Miller, 2008). If UNPOL's ongoing protection for the woman was conditional on her willingness to talk with the researchers, that condition would be a clear form of coercion that would violate the young mother's right to determine if she wanted to participate in the research.

Exploitation, on the other hand, involves a more subtle form of undue pressure. It occurs when a person takes unfair advantage of another, particularly when the latter is in a comparatively disadvantaged situation (Wertheimer, 1999). Such exploitation violates the moral norm of protecting the vulnerable (Goodin, 1988). It involves treating the one in the relatively vulnerable position instrumentally, with less than full respect for their well-being and agency. In the research setting, exploitation may occur when the researcher, who stands in unequal power and relationship with prospective participants, takes advantage of the latter's poverty, powerlessness, or dependency to serve their research needs (Macklin, 2003). When those whose welfare or autonomy may be compromised are not likely to benefit from the research in ways *they* deem important, participants may feel exploited or wronged. It is worth noting that, under this understanding, exploitation can occur even when both parties benefit, as in cases where researchers and participants gain relative to a baseline of noncooperation, but where the distribution of the benefits is unfair to participants (Wertheimer, 1999). While some research studies may benefit all parties involved in the research, how the benefits are measured and distributed may affect the community's perception of fairness of the process and the real purpose behind conducting the research. If the young mother were to be recruited because she was a convenient participant who could not leave the station due to her security situation, and her contribution, albeit most relevant to the project at hand, was sought mainly for the sake of the researchers' academic pursuit rather than based on the woman's wishes and/or the community's priorities, such recruitment might be exploitative. Echoing concerns noted by Meredith Minkler (2004), some community members we met in both Rwanda and Southern Sudan voiced their general suspicions of foreign researchers. These outsiders are sometimes perceived as taking data from impoverished communities to serve their own academic or professional interests rather than local priorities. The community members' concerns signal their awareness of the inherent power relationship, worry about potential exploitation, and skepticism concerning meaningful benefit that some international research would bring to their community.

■ Vulnerability, Protection, and CBCAR

Certainly, assurance that research subjects are not coerced or manipulated into participation is a minimal requirement in respecting people's autonomy. Nonetheless, even as many international guidelines on research ethics provide a much needed framework for presenting coercion and exploitation, the nature of CBCAR raises questions of whether a blanket protective approach to restrict participation of vulnerable persons would indeed be the most effective means to promote or respect autonomy. Informed by a feminist research ethic (Ackerly & True, 2008), this section critically evaluates the protective approach in mainstream research ethics discussions. In considering epistemic and ethical reasons for including those who are most vulnerable in CBCAR, this section argues that a relational approach to research ethics that attends to power relations and inclusiveness is more appropriate for CBCAR in attending to vulnerability issues and finding culturally respectful ways to uphold our ethical requirements to promote participant autonomy, beneficence, and justice.

Ethical issues regarding recruitment and protection of vulnerable populations are particularly interesting for CBCAR, which is often carried out in a complex and multilayered sociopolitical context. This context raises questions of whether the standard ethical approaches to recruitment can address the complexities of CBCAR. In some respects, the issue of vulnerability likely arises more frequently in CBCAR than many other types of traditional research. The focus on community needs in CBCAR makes it probable that some prospective participants will come from impoverished backgrounds (Minkler, 2004), since these individuals are often the ones whose unmet needs are at the center of the study and who would be most affected by the results of the proposed projects. Such a focus on community needs renders it imperative for researchers to attend to power relations. Vulnerability is often a side constraint in conventional research, in the sense that it poses ethical boundaries on what researchers can legitimately study, who they can recruit as participants, and how they invite such participation. It is, however, often a significant component of CBCAR. In contrast to research projects that recruit vulnerable populations for administrative convenience for the researchers, CBCAR, by its very nature, considers participation of these populations necessary. A research project cannot be community-based if it does not include the voices of those who would be most affected, particularly the most vulnerable. Special problems regarding how to work with vulnerable participants, which are acknowledged in North American research guidelines (Canadian Institutes of Health Research, Natural Sciences and Engineering Research Council of Canada, & Social Sciences and Humanities Research Council of Canada, 1998; United States Department of Health and Human Services, 2009), are thus embedded in the nature of CBCAR. Given such "special justification" to involve those who are disadvantaged in the research process, including a commitment to equitable subjects selection (United States Department of Health and Human Services, 2009), the question becomes how we can guard against exploitation or attempt to mitigate the pernicious effects of power hierarchies throughout the whole research process.

The young mother's situation helps to illustrate the complexity of power when working with vulnerable participants and the importance of being self-reflective about how such issues affect the research process. The socioeconomic, cultural, and relational contexts surrounding the woman's plight raise questions of whether or not she may have the means to promote her vital interest. Our prior focus groups and key informant interviews in this village revealed that dire poverty, cultural ideologies, as well as lack of accessible information and protection mechanism make it difficult for women who are subjected to gendered-based violence to leave the abusive environment. Many women have no other financial and social means to support their livelihood or stay with their children if they leave their husband—they often endure various forms of violence as part of their reality. Those who manage to leave are often discriminated against or harassed by others in the community. Bearing in mind these general struggles for many women in the community, the young mother's exhaustion from having been in the jail cell for a few days, her emotional trauma from the latest attack, her standing in the community, and the context of protective custody only exacerbated her vulnerability.

Given her lack of resources to promote her personal and familial interests as well as the power dynamic surrounding her immediate situation, guidelines from aforementioned international documents would likely raise questions regarding this woman's ability to provide free consent. Since the young mother was asked by UNPOL to speak to the researchers, who clearly came from more resourceful backgrounds, her vulnerability to power or authority in the desperate situation could compromise her ability to make a truly voluntary decision (Miller and Wertheimer, 2007). However, a closer look at the research context reveals that while this position of "decisional soft paternalism" has intuitive appeal, decisions to include or exclude her participation are not so simple. When and how such paternalism can legitimately apply to a particular case will partly depend on careful, consistent, and reflective considerations of the type of research being conducted, the goal of such inquiry, the priorities of community members, resources available to enhance prospective participants' ability to make informed and voluntary decisions, and other contextual factors surrounding the research process.

It is interesting to note that discussions regarding conventional research often focus on whether it is ethical to *include* certain individuals or groups due to the imperative to protect. With much of research ethics literature focusing on issues of autonomy, there has been generally little attention on the ethics of *excluding* various populations from participation. Nonetheless, a closer look at the context of CBCAR and other justice questions would reveal that exclusion from research participation can sometimes be morally problematic. The young mother's vulnerability and the circumstances surrounding her plight, while morally significant factors that call for careful attention, should not *automatically* exclude her from participation. Rather, these factors may explain why a relational and collaborative approach to find culturally appropriate and safe ways to engage this woman and others in similarly vulnerable situations is *required*, both ethically and epistemically.

The considerations are two-fold. First, there are epistemic reasons to ensure inclusion of those who are most vulnerable. People whose needs are often unmet and whose voices are generally unheard are in a unique position to explain their struggles and concerns. Certainly, researchers would need to be mindful of how the woman's circumstances and the power dynamics between UNPOL and the woman may affect her decision-making process, particularly her ability to imagine refusing participation if she so desired. They also need to be self-reflective of how their own presence in the community as well as their economic and social privileges may exacerbate the power disparity and/or affect how prospective participants consider their research decisions. Nonetheless, given that community members of different backgrounds have varying experiences and perspectives, many or all of which can contribute to knowledge creation, CBCAR demands that researchers work with community stakeholders to inform their inquiry with a wide range of perspectives. Researchers need to recognize that there are many epistemological perspectives, each opening and foreclosing certain understandings of what it means to know and to contribute to shared knowledge (True & Ackerly, 2007). Suppressing the participation of this woman, even if out of a protective stance, may prevent insightful understanding of the broader context of gender-based violence in this village as well as various circumstances and barriers that led to her current situation. It may hinder the development of responsive programs and policies, such as safe houses and legal protection for people escaping domestic violence, separate jail cells for men and women, advocacy programs for vulnerable populations, and arms control in a region where every household is estimated to either own or have access to at least one weapon (Bonn International Center for Conversion, 2007).

Second, epistemic exclusion of those who are vulnerable has important ethical implications. In keeping with the fundamental commitments of CBCAR, consulting those who are in vulnerable positions has symbolic meaning by recognizing that their lived experiences are legitimate sources of knowledge. Echoing many feminist approaches to epistemology, inclusion of unheard voices signals an awareness of how dominant conceptions and practices of knowledge attribution have systemically disadvantaged the vulnerable people and a commitment to mitigate the impact of power hierarchy by balancing the epistemic authority of various stakeholders. As Susan Brison (2002) points out, women who have critical experiences are rarely part of the discourse about them. Those who are "most" oppressed or "differently" oppressed are often invisible to the researcher or the relatively powerful—they are spoken about, but not spoken with (Hoagland, 2009). Identifying and including them to the greatest extent feasible is thus a political and ethical dimension of research methodology (True & Ackerly, 2007). It acknowledges and affirms the value of the hitherto neglected and marginalized perspectives.

As part of our research, we had planned to speak with the police chief and other service providers regarding their experience working with people who endure gender-based violence. These individuals are familiar with the barriers facing those who are most vulnerable and can imagine or make inferences about the latter's experience. They also serve as advocates for the woman and others in similar situations by representing, arguing for, recommending, and acting in support or on behalf of them (Code, 2000). Such advocacy can be particularly helpful when those in vulnerable situations may not be able to speak for themselves. Nonetheless, these service providers hold a different vantage point and power privilege—the way they perceive the situation can be influenced by their own roles, agendas, or perceptions of those they serve, and their viewpoints may not fully represent the perspectives of local community residents (Green & Mercer, 2001; Wallerstein & Duran, 2003). Moreover, while advocates can be appropriately supportive and empowering in some situations, they may be underinformed, self-interested, and imperialistic in other cases (Code, 2000). Relying only on service providers' reports may thus reinforce the epistemic hierarchy by favoring their perspectives over the perspectives of those who have direct experience of vulnerability, or by assuming that these service providers can speak for their clients (Jones, 2002). It is also worth noting that some of these clients may have already been subjected to restrictions imposed by service providers or have concerns about how these limited services are delivered. Since people in vulnerable positions often have few venues to voice their concerns, rendering their needs and priorities unheard and neglected, it is particularly important for researchers to be mindful of how exclusion from participation based on concerns of vulnerability itself may further silence these individuals or dismiss them as knowers in self-advocacy (Hoagland, 2009). Even if these reasons in and of themselves are insufficient to justify recruiting the woman for the research, since autonomy-related factors also need to be considered, we need to bear in mind that our decision regarding who to include or exclude is partially determined by our attribution of epistemic authority. As some have pointed out, dominant groups tend to accord epistemic authority to themselves and those in similar positions but withhold it from others who are in marginalized positions. Such epistemic injustice may not only undermine the ability of the marginalized to participate in collaborative inquiry (Fricker 1998, 2003); it may also lead to biased and partial theories that tend to reinforce social inequality (Code, 2004).

Given the danger of reinforcing vulnerability by epistemic exclusion, researchers need to cultivate the virtue of what Miranda Fricker (2003) calls "reflexive critical openness." They need to strive for an awareness of how their privileges and experiences may condition their epistemology or their assessment of whose voices ought to be included in the inquiry, and ensure that any decision to exclude is not a prejudicial dismissal of the person's credibility, experience, and perspectives. Researchers have an ethical commitment to attend to the power of privileged epistemologies and seek to respectfully enter into constructive conversation with marginalized others to the largest extent possible. In situations where the capacity of the vulnerable to consent is doubtful, it may be helpful to seek advice from their advocates as feasible and appropriate. Researchers have the responsibility of deconstructing their own position of privilege and working towards transforming the power relations that support or reinforce that position (True & Ackerly, 2007). While it is important for researchers to carefully reflect on the woman's circumstances to evaluate the possibility of manipulation and coercion, refusing to listen to the woman's story before investigating her wishes and expectations regarding the research on the presumption of an inevitably compromised capacity for self-determination may ironically deny her agency and exacerbate our power hierarchy. A unilateral decision by the researchers at the outset to preclude the woman's involvement without consulting her regarding the most appropriate ways to address the power relations and promote her well-being may inadvertently dismiss her lived experience and deny the relevance of her concerns in the process of knowledge creation. As we shall see shortly, this approach also adopts the traditional view that recruitment and consent are singular events rather than ongoing processes.

Given that CBCAR is part of an "empowering and power-sharing process that attends to social inequalities" (Pharris, 2011), a categorical rejection of participation of individuals from impoverished backgrounds based on their presumed vulnerability without consideration of local perspectives may defeat the purpose of CBCAR. It may reinforce these individuals' disadvantaged position rather than promote the latter's autonomy. Since CBCAR promises to "[build] on strengths and resources within the community" (Pharris, 2011), it would be extraordinary to contend that desperate social conditions and the power hierarchy have destroyed vulnerable people's status as moral agents, rendering them *categorically* incapable of evaluating their own situation and exercising judgment accordingly. The assumption that researchers are active agents and participants are passive subjects waiting for others' advocacy to achieve autonomy may undermine the moral agency of the latter in research relationships (Code, 2000; Eckenwiler, Ells, Feinholz & Schonfeld, 2008). Given that those who are most oppressed are often silenced and thus invisible to the researcher, unilateral denial of participation of the marginalized is not only a form of epistemic injustice—it also contradicts the commitment of CBCAR to collaboratively define the research question and co-generate knowledge. Exclusion of participation based on presumptions of vulnerability is a methodological choice with deep ethical implications. In extending special protections, paternalistic measures that neglect to consult those to be excluded or override people's expressed wishes based on presumptions of vulnerability may inadvertently reinforce and yet conceal self-serving relationships of power and domination. Such measures might be questioned by the very groups for whom protection is sought (Macklin, 2003). After all, persons who are subject to oppression and highly restrictive environments may, nonetheless, still be able to express their autonomous agency and show resilience in some aspects of their lives (Mackenzie, McDowell, & Pittaway, 2007).

Our experience in Rwanda, for example, showed that many refugee women, despite their dire circumstances and systemic oppression, exercised their moral agency by speaking out about their experience and engaging in dialogues about how to improve the gender relationship in the refugee camp. Many of these women continue to experience gender-based violence in their daily lives, face multiple barriers in defending their human rights, and rely on the development community for support (Pavlish & Ho, 2009b). Nonetheless, those we met made their voices heard in our focus groups and key informant interviews—they spoke freely, candidly, spontaneously, and with passion. Certainly, we need to keep in mind that focus groups and interviews are social interactions that occur in highly controlled settings. Various parties have their specific goals—researchers wish to gather information on specific issues for academic and possibly social purposes, and participants wish to give testimony that could contribute to knowledge creation and possibly also advance their own interests. These interactions are performances that involve addressing audiences (Hoagland, 2009), and they occur within a socioeconomic–sociopolitical framework that can shape various parties' perception of their involvement and how they would participate in these interactive activities. Nonetheless, research participants we worked with had some control over the testimonial process. While the majority of the interview and focus group questions were structured and predetermined by the researchers with the input of community partners, they were open-ended, which allowed participants some degree of what and how much they would like to disclose. Participants also helped shape the discussion by prompting other questions and bringing up additional issues that they wanted to address. As these women repeatedly explained how their interests were often ignored by their respective spouses and others in the community (Pavlish & Ho, 2009b), their participation in the research might have been a rare opportunity for them to voice their concerns and contribute to potential policy and practice changes. It is interesting to note that male participants in Rwanda were less forthcoming with information than their female counterparts, who were full of ideas and appeared eager to share their experience and insight. While there may be multiple explanations or motives behind the different responses from the male and female participants, the women's forthrightness warns us of the danger of presuming that *all* members of a disadvantaged social group are incapable of advancing their interests. Exclusion of these women from participation in favor of only people who are not in vulnerable situations would not only skew the data; more importantly, it would deny the autonomy and epistemic legitimacy of these women who want their perspectives heard.

It is undeniable that researchers need to be mindful of the impact of economic desperation and insecurity on people's decision-making process, and to ensure that the autonomy language does not mask the power disparity between potential participants and researchers as well as other authority figures.

Such effort is particularly integral to CBCAR, given its purported commitment to "an empowering and power-sharing process that attends to social inequalities" (Pharris, 2011). Nonetheless, in places where most women occupy low socioeconomic positions and lack political power, the façade of the care discourse, which focuses on protection rather than empowerment, may inadvertently and ironically deny the "vulnerable" as moral equals. It constructs those in dire circumstances as inferior, in need of the paternalistic guidance and rule of more privileged positions to promote their welfare (Narayan, 1995). In this village in Southern Sudan, where many women experiencing violence would be afraid to seek help, the young mother exercised her agency and resistance by seeking a divorce from her abusive husband in a village that does not give women, let alone divorced women, high value. Presumptions of her inability to make informed and voluntary research decisions without engaging her in the process would be premature and condescending.

■ Taking Reciprocity Seriously

Ethical research, particularly in CBCAR, is argued to be about relationships founded on trust and reciprocity (Maiter, Simich, Jacobson, & Wise, 2008). Reciprocity, as a mode of social exchange, is defined as "exchange between social equals" (Kottak, 1986, p. 136). It is about promoting respectful research relationships and exchanges. Certainly, the reality of international research, including CBCAR, is often wrought with power disparity, demanding that researchers ensure that the reciprocity language does not conceal the barriers of oppression. It is because of such pervasive inequality that the feminist research ethic demands self-reflective attention to the power relationships that are a part of the research process and context. Nonetheless, restricting research participation, *particularly* for people labeled as vulnerable based on speculation about social manipulation, without considering the research context and local perspectives may ironically reinforce such defenselessness rather than promote trust or reciprocity.

In recognizing these ethical concerns of exclusion, a commitment to CBCAR's fundamental tenets of acknowledging "community as a unit of identity" and facilitating "collaborative, equitable partnership in all phases of research" reminds us that exclusion from participation may not be the most appropriate means to promote the autonomy of those who are vulnerable (Pharris, 2011). Those whose voices have often been neglected ought to be included and/or represented, not only because they may provide the missing pieces in knowledge co-creation, but also because they lend moral legitimacy to the research. By involving representatives of relevant stakeholders in developing the research program and committing to "bold conversation with partners and critics to uncover any coercive dynamics in the research process" (Pharris, 2011), CBCAR adopts a relational approach to research ethics. It seeks democratic and inclusive ways to address power relations to ensure that recruitment and other research processes and methods are respectful of community standards and expectations. Such collaborative deliberation can help researchers to work with marginalized groups to ensure that concerns of vulnerability and multiple barriers to participation are addressed (Boser, 2006).

The emphasis on attending to power relations and being inclusive in CBCAR can help to address the question of how to protect the autonomy and interests of members of impoverished social groups without being paternalistic in the research process. Instead of insisting on preset and potentially neocolonialist notions of protection and vulnerability, it would be more respectful for researchers to work with community stakeholders in sorting out the power dynamic and finding creative ways to solve ethical problems by attending to the community's priorities and its perception of risks, benefits, and voluntary participation. For example, in our research context, working with local representatives throughout the research process can help us identify appropriate key informants from various sectors of the society, attend to neglected perspectives, and manage unforeseen circumstances in a respectful and ethical manner. In encountering a surprising prospective participant, as with the young mother, a relational approach can help us to promote trust and ensure reciprocity. Instead of approaching recruitment and consent as one-time events, researchers in CBCAR can think of these elements as ongoing processes that involve reflective and collaborative deliberation throughout the research. For example, discussing with both UNPOL and the woman regarding concerns over involving her in a CBCAR, given the context and power dynamic surrounding her being in police custody, can help all sides to realize the value of the woman's perspectives and explore if there may be respectful ways for her to participate given the circumstances. The UNPOL officers were perhaps advocating for having the woman's concerns heard, and hoping that by virtue of the research, sustainable and responsive solutions would ensue to help people in similar situations. The woman might have also thought that this research could help her directly or others in the future. Honest discussions with the officers and the woman regarding whether this research topic is high on the woman's own agenda as well as the possibility of meeting with the woman another time or after she was no longer in police custody may help to explore and clarify each party's perception of the power dynamic, the purpose of the woman's involvement, and the practical and political implications of the research before determining the suitability of the woman's participation in her current circumstances. Instead of a one-time consent, a collaborative deliberation process can allow ongoing reflection of the research context. If all parties subsequently determined that inclusion of the woman's participation was appropriate, ongoing reflection and open dialogues throughout the interview process and thereafter would also allow the researchers and the young mother to reevaluate whether or how it might be appropriate to include her testimony in the data.

International field research, particularly projects carried out by academic and community collaborators with different socioeconomic, historical, and cultural backgrounds, can be ethically and politically complex. Even with informed consent, inherent power disparities and researcher privilege cannot be erased. Discussions of research ethics in North America often presume various Western notions of voluntary participation that, albeit well meaning, neglect the local contexts and realities. In preventing (the perception of) exploitation of people in dire conditions, responsible researchers can determine the most appropriate measures to promote participant autonomy by involving community members/partners in the research design, and ask whether and/or how the research may facilitate the agency of those who are most susceptible to undue pressure and harm. Instead of only focusing on an individual's consent process, researchers ought to consider the design, purpose, and impact of the research, such as how the research may benefit or address the priorities of the local community. Those from outside of the community should ask themselves if the purpose of the research is prompted by a genuine interest in the other person and situation as well as a commitment to work with local stakeholders (Häggman-Laitila, 1999; Eide & Kahn, 2008). They also need to consider if there is a promise of fair and reciprocal benefits (Mackenzie, McDowell, & Pittaway, 2007).

In many research projects, prospective participants who have individual opportunities to accept or reject particular invitations to enroll in the studies remain largely outside of the research enterprise, the function and operation of which are relatively nontransparent and unchallenged (Ho, 2008). They have minimal knowledge of or impact on how research priorities are set, how research protocols and data are assessed by various regulatory frameworks and funding agencies, and where and how data will be disseminated or used. In conventional, noncommunity based research, researchers generally predetermine the recruitment process according to guidelines from their home country and institution. They are also the ones who would seek consent from prospective participants, such that the responsibility and authority to determine vulnerability and ability to consent in any particular case generally fall solely on external researchers. While these requirements and processes help to promote researcher accountability, they also clearly distinguish researchers from participants and have the potential to reinforce the power hierarchy between them.

In its most appealing instances, community-based collaborative action research, which "facilitates collaborative, equitable partnership in all phases of research" and "fosters co-learning and capacity building among all partners" (Pharris, 2011), goes beyond the individual/micro model of special protection and considers how institutional/meso and societal/macro frameworks of research respond to community priorities and empower local residents. As Margaret Urban Walker (2007) explains, morality is an expressive–collaborative process. It is something people are actually doing together in their communities, societies, and ongoing relationships. Western approaches to autonomy, particularly in the context of international research, are open to criticism, refinement, and improvement by all stakeholders. Instead of imposing a unilateral and predetermined framework for recruitment and consent, CBCAR's commitment to respect for participants demands collaboration between researchers and local community members in designing and monitoring the research process. The collaborative team can determine how to best use the community resources to ensure participant safety, balance risks/benefits, and promote local priorities. It is only when research arises out of or responds to the priorities of those who bear the highest burden of research that potentially vulnerable participants are not only protected, but also respected.

■ Acknowledgment

I would like to thank our local partners and various community members we met in Rwanda and Southern Sudan for their valuable contribution to the community-based research project that informs much of this article. I also want to thank my research partner, Dr. Carol Pavlish, for her insight and support throughout this research process. Lastly, I am indebted to Suze Berkhout and Dr. Dave Unger for their constructive criticisms on earlier drafts.

■ Endnotes

1. For our purpose here, the terms "subjects" and "participants" are used interchangeably.
2. It is worth noting that while this ethnographic study in Southern Sudan was a collaborative project with the local ARC and was informed by input from some community

members, logistical factors prohibited *full* involvement with community members in the planning and data analysis phases. Nonetheless, the exemplar presents critical ethical considerations to guide CBCAR projects.

3. This document was established in collaboration with the World Health Organization.

4. While the Council for International Organizations of Medical Sciences mostly focuses on biomedical research, its guidance on fair distribution of risks and benefits among all stakeholders is also helpful for social science research.

■ References

Ackerly, B., & True, J. (2008). Reflexivity in practice: Power and ethics in feminist research on international relations. *International Studies Review, 10*, 693–707.

Bonn International Center for Conversion (BICC). (2007). *Communities safe from small arms in Southern Sudan: A handbook for civil society*. Germany: BICC. Retrieved from http://www.bicc.de/index.php/publications/other/communities-safe-from-small-arms-in-southern-sudan

Boser, S. (2006). Ethics and power in community–campus partnerships for research. *Action Research, 4*, 9–21.

Brison, S. (2002). *Aftermath: Violence and the remaking of a self*. Princeton, NJ: Princeton University Press.

Canadian Institutes of Health Research, Natural Sciences and Engineering Research Council of Canada, Social Sciences and Humanities Research Council of Canada. (1998). *Tri-council policy statement: Ethical conduct for research involving humans* (with 2000, 2002, and 2005 amendments). Retrieved from http://pre.ethics.gc.ca/eng/policy-politique/tcps-eptc/readtcps-lireeptc/

Code, L. (2000). The perversion of autonomy and the subjection of women: Discourses of social advocacy at century's end. In C. Mackenzie & N. Stoljar (Eds.), *Relational autonomy: Feminist perspectives on autonomy, agency, and the social self* (pp. 181–209). New York, NY: Oxford University Press.

Code, L. (2004). The power of ignorance. *Philosophical Papers, 33*, 291–308.

Council for International Organizations of Medical Sciences. (2002). *International ethical guidelines for biomedical research involving human subjects*. Geneva, Switzerland: CIOMS. Retrieved from http://www.cioms.ch/publications/layout_guide2002.pdf

Eckenwiler, L., Ells, C., Feinholz, D., & Schonfeld, T. (2008). Hopes for Helsinki: Reconsidering "vulnerability." *Journal of Medical Ethics, 34*, 765–766.

Eide, P., & Kahn, D. (2008). Ethical issues in the qualitative researcher–participant relationship. *Nursing Ethics, 15*, 199–207.

Fricker, M. (1999). Epistemic oppression and epistemic privilege, *Canadian Journal of Philosophy, Suppl. 25*, 191–210.

Fricker, M. (2003). Epistemic injustice and a role for virtue in the politics of knowing. *Metaphilosophy, 34*, 154–173.

Goodin, R. (1988). *Reasons for welfare.* Princeton, NJ: Princeton University Press.

Government of Southern Sudan. (2007). *Draft Interim Constitution of Southern Sudan.* Retrieved from http://www.gossmission.org/goss/index.php?option=com_content&task=view&id=268&Itemid=206

Green, L., & Mercer, S. (2001). Can public health researchers and agencies reconcile the push from funding bodies and the pull from communities? *American Journal of Public Health, 91*(12), 1926–1929.

Häggman-Laitila, A. (1999). The authenticity and ethics of phenomenological research: How to overcome the researcher's own views. *Nursing Ethics, 6*, 12–22.

Hawkins, J. & Emanuel, E. (2005). Clarifying confusions about coercion. *Hastings Center Report, 35*(5), 16–19.

Ho, A. (2008). Correcting social ills through mandatory research participation. *American Journal of Bioethics, 8*(10), 39–40.

Hoagland, S. (2009). Giving testimony and the coloniality of knowledge. Retrieved from http://www.cavehill.uwi.edu/fhe/histphil/philosophy/chips/2009/papers/hoagland2009.pdf

Jones, K. (2002). The politics of credibility. In L. Antony & C. Witt (Eds.) *A mind of one's own* (2nd ed., pp. 154–176). Boulder, CO: Westview Press.

Kottak, C. (1986). *Cultural anthropology* (4th ed.). New York, NY: Random House.

Mackenzie, C., McDowell, C., & Pittaway, E. (2007). Beyond "do no harm": The challenge of constructing ethical relationships in refugee research. *Journal of Refugee Studies, 20*(2), 299–310.

Macklin R. (2003). Bioethics, vulnerability, and protection. *Bioethics, 17*(5/6), 472–486.

Maiter, S., Simich, L., Jacobson, N., & Wise, J. (2008). Reciprocity: An ethic for community-based participatory action research. *Action Research, 6*(3), 305–325.

Miller, F., & Wertheimer, A. (2007). Facing up to paternalism in research ethics. *Hastings Center Report 37*(3), 24–34.

Minkler, M. (2004). Ethical challenges for the "outside" researcher in community-based participatory research. *Health Education & Behavior, 31*, 684–697.

Narayan, U. (1995). Colonialism and its others: Considerations on rights and care discourses. *Hypatia, 10*, 133–140.

Nuremberg Code, The (1947). Retrieved from http://ohsr.od.nih.gov/guidelines/nuremberg.html

Pavlish, C., & Ho, A. (2009a). Displaced persons' perceptions of human rights in Southern Sudan. *International Nursing Review, 56*, 416–425.

Pavlish, C., & Ho, A. (2009b). Pathway to social justice research on human rights and gender-based violence in a Rwandan refugee camp. *Advances in Nursing Science, 32*(2), 144–157.

Pharris, M. D. (2011). Community-based collaborative action research: Methodology unfolding. In C. P. Pavlish & M. D. Pharris, *Community-based collaborative action research: A nursing approach*. Sudbury, MA: Jones & Bartlett Learning.

True, J., & Ackerly, B. (2007, February). *Reflexivity in practice: Power and ethics in feminist research*. Paper presented at the annual meeting of the International Studies Association 48th Annual Convention, Chicago, IL, USA.

US Department of Health and Human Services, National Institutes of Health, Office for Human Research Protections. (2009). *Title 45 (Public Welfare), Code of Federal Regulations, Part 46 (Protection of Human Subjects)*. Retrieved from http://www.hhs.gov/ohrp/humansubjects/guidance/45cfr46.htm

United States National Commission for the Protection of Human Subjects of Biomedical and Behavioral Research. (1979). *The Belmont report: Ethical principles and guidelines for the protection of human subjects of research*. Retrieved from http://ohsr.od.nih.gov/guidelines/belmont.html#ethical

Walker, M. U. (2007). *Moral understandings: A feminist study in ethics*. New York, NY: Oxford University Press.

Wallerstein, N., & Duran, B. (2003). The conceptual, historical, and practice roots of community-based participatory research and related participatory traditions. In M. Minkler & N. Wallerstein (Eds.), *Community-based participatory research for health* (pp. 27–52). San Francisco, CA: Jossey-Bass.

Wertheimer, A. (1999). *Exploitation*. Princeton, NJ: Princeton University Press.

Wertheimer, A., & Miller, F. (2008). Payment for research participation: a coercive offer? *Journal of Medical Ethics, 34*, 389–392.

World Medical Association. (2008). *World Medical Association Declaration of Helsinki: Ethical principles for medical research involving human subjects*. Seoul, Korea: World Medical Association. Retrieved from http://www.wma.net/en/30publications/10policies/b3/index.html

CHAPTER

9

Preparing Grant Proposals for CBCAR Projects

*T*rees, of course, start small and grow tall. To stretch out from their small beginnings, trees absorb moisture and nutrients from the soil and participate in converting sunlight into energy through the process of photosynthesis. We often admire bold trees that root and thrive on mountainside rocks where moisture is scarce and weather can be harsh. We appreciate the struggles those trees push through to survive. We know that life is easier when nourishment is available—noting that the more nourishment the tree receives, the more productive it can be—it matures faster, stretches farther, lives healthier, and sustains its work longer. The same holds true for community-based collaborative action research (CBCAR) projects. These projects survive and sometimes even thrive without funding. However, the pathway is eased and the effect is often strengthened when funding is available to support the partnership's work.

Some funding agencies now recognize the importance of community–academic research partnerships and specifically request action-based research projects (Agency for Healthcare Research and Quality, 2009; Seifer & Calleson, 2004). For example, in 2009, the United States National Institutes of Health (NIH, 2009) convened a Summer Institute on Community-Based Participatory Research Targeting the Medically

Underserved. Objectives pertained to "addressing the conceptual, methodological, and practical issues inherent in planning and conducting research on health promotion, disease prevention, and health disparities that is conducted in partnership between communities and researchers" (para. 1). Realizing that strong partnerships with medically underserved communities generate more reliable research findings, organizers of the summer institute focused on preparing attendees to develop community-partnered research projects and fundable grant applications. The overall aim was to advance the NIH public health goal of improving health outcomes for populations experiencing disparities. After the summer institute, NIH posted the presentations on the course website, http://conferences.thehillgroup.com/si2009. This website offers many valuable suggestions for people who are interested

---

Box 9-1　Principles of Drafting Fundable CBCAR Proposals

- Partnership with community is historical, democratic, relational, genuine.
- Knowledge of community context is evidence-based.
- Research topic/questions emerge from the partnership and relate to grant objectives.
- Research design is rigorous yet flexible.
- Ideas are original and innovative.
- Protection for human subjects/participants is central and threaded throughout.
- Findings can be translated into action and measurable outcomes.
- Investigators are capable; environment is supportive.
- Benefits and challenges of CBCAR are addressed.
- Project and partnership are feasible.
- Budget is adequately justified; compensation is fairly distributed to all partners.
- Partnership and project are sustainable.

in pursuing federal funding for their community-partnered research projects and also provides links to specific NIH funding mechanisms.

This chapter provides general guidelines on writing grant proposals to support CBCAR projects. We first offer basic principles for writing CBCAR project proposals (see **Box 9-1**). Many of the suggested principles pertain to grant applications for all types of research; however, we particularize the principles for CBCAR projects. Within the explanation of each principle, we offer some suggestions. To illustrate the principles, we provide an NIH-funded CBCAR project proposal. Since funding opportunities vary extensively, the example should not be considered a model for other CBCAR grant proposals. The sample proposal simply illustrates key points in the proposed principles. We encourage readers to consider these principles, initiate community or organization-based partnerships, and together conceptualize their ideas for a CBCAR project aimed at enhancing human health and flourishing. The quest for grant support occurs alongside that creative and collaborative work.

■ Principles of Writing Grant Proposals to Support CBCAR Projects

Funding for CBCAR projects is available not just from federal agencies but also from philanthropic organizations and other institutions that support community-based initiatives. Agencies usually publish their guidelines in formal requests for applications (RFAs). These proposal requests might also be called funding opportunity announcements, program announcements, notices of funding availability, solicitations, or other names depending on the agency and type of program. In their RFAs, funding agencies describe specific grant objectives, features, and criteria.

Research partners should consider grant explanations carefully and be deliberate and explicit in describing how their proposed project fits the specific RFA and incorporates CBCAR principles. Also, each separate grant form should be closely studied; applicants need to consider how all completed grant forms fit together to describe their proposed project and its implementation. We also strongly encourage grant applicants to contact funding agency representatives with questions. In addition, consulting with those who have collaboratively applied for grants and administered their own action research projects is helpful. When writing grants, we urge readers to use the strengths of all collaborating partners and to think imaginatively. The following general principles are intended to help research partners prepare for the work of writing strong CBCAR grant applications.

Partnership with community is historical, democratic, relational, and genuine

Effective collaborative and working relationships develop over time. Funding agencies usually prefer partnerships that have a record of accomplishments such as successful program development, preliminary community assessments, or small-scale feasibility studies. Even one successfully partnered initiative is significant to many funders. Besides showing a shared and genuine interest in the research topic, setting, or population, these past accomplishments demonstrate that effective and productive group processes among partners already exist. Projects are generally viewed as more feasible and logistically easier to manage if prior relationships exist (Padgett & Henwood, 2009). Grant reviewers often view these past successes as important groundwork for launching the current proposal and a significant indicator for achieving future success.

If, however, a new partnership has formed and decides to pursue grant funding right away, we suggest that partners apply for a small grant. Another option for new partnerships is to collaboratively plan and implement a small-scale project before developing a grant application to fund a more substantial project. The newly-formed partnership might also consider creating a project proposal in which partnership formation is incorporated into project design. This design is illustrated in the NIH-funded example provided later in this chapter. Effective and collaborative relationships are central to CBCAR projects, and therefore, need to be part of the evidence that applicants provide in their applications.

Besides demonstrating a history of working together on previous projects, CBCAR partners need to demonstrate that their current working relationship is democratic. The proposal should detail how partners will collaborate to accomplish project objectives and outcomes. Memoranda of Understanding (MOUs) which were described in Chapter 4 (see Box 4-2), should be developed to illustrate shared decision making responsibility and accountability. Communication and decision-making transparency is important for promoting positive and productive working partnerships (Yonas et al., 2006). Additionally, research partners should consider creating a structure for resolving differences that arise in the collaborative process (Plumb, Price, & Kavanaugh-Lynch, 2004). MOUs should also clarify general funding streams and reflect partnered work, equitable distribution, and fair compensation—so both community and academic partners benefit from grant funds.

Additionally, appreciation for the context expertise of community partners, methods expertise of academic researchers, and content expertise of research participants should be evident in CBCAR proposals. Grant applicants should highlight their common bond of interest (frequently the research topic or population) and their plans for productive interactions that integrate all three types of expertise—content, context, and method. Communication and capacity building should clearly flow both ways—so all partners are listening and learning as much as they are talking and teaching (Seifer & Sisco, 2006). A work plan that demonstrates specific collaboration mechanisms and communication channels during all project phases should be clearly stated in the proposal.

Knowledge of community or organization context is evidence-based

Research partners should demonstrate that they are knowledgeable about community or organization context. Initiating a community advisory group is often a valuable mechanism for learning about and remaining grounded in the community context. This advisory group can also assist the CBCAR research team with project proposal by providing important and relevant contextual information. Evidence on the local context should not only highlight particular community assets but also identify significant need for the proposed project (Seifer, 2005). Data to clearly illustrate a community-derived priority, knowledge gap, existing disparity, or system inadequacy should be included. Local data should be provided (Seifer). National or state-wide data might help to establish project significance, recent trends, or related issues, but local data should be used to establish need. Careful attention to presentation of contextual data paints a vivid picture of community patterns that helps to justify the proposed project.

Another aspect of being knowledgeable about local context is clearly identifying a study population, sometimes called a *critical reference group* in action-oriented research (Genat, 2009; Wadsworth, 1997). The term refers to the group whose situation the CBCAR project is designed to improve. Critical reference groups could be African-born women and girls, men who perpetrate violence against women, obese children, or frail elderly. Some RFAs require that representatives of the critical reference group be part of the research team. Grant reviewers generally expect to see the critical reference group identified early in the grant application. Furthermore, reviewers anticipate reading existing demographic information about the group and important evidence that a local need exists. Information on community or organization context and critical reference group might be included in the "background" or "previous work/preliminary studies" section of a grant application.

To provide specific context and population information, research partners might need to collect some preliminary or pilot data prior to project development and grant application. Some partnerships conduct a baseline community health assessment or survey organization members' perspectives on the research topic. For example, to provide background information on risk factors and early indicators of ethical dilemmas in an organization, a research partnership conducted a critical incident study to learn whether nurses could describe factors that preceded ethical conflict. Researchers then used findings from this study to strengthen their grant application for a feasibility study on early nursing interventions for unfolding ethical dilemmas.

To further demonstrate knowledge of community context, research partners should identify key stakeholders. People who have an effect on or are affected by the research topic are considered stakeholders (Stringer, 2007). This is important for most CBCAR grant proposals and particularly important if an intervention is being tested within the proposed project. In this case, the research team should consult particular community or organization stakeholders who influence decision making (Israel et al., 2006). Because CBCAR projects occur in complex systems, awareness of key stakeholders is important to demonstrate.

Research topic/questions emerge from the partnership and relate to grant objectives

Project proposals should clearly show that the research topic pertains to issues of significance as identified within a particular group, community, or organizational context. Furthermore, CBCAR proposals should show that research questions were developed collaboratively by the partnership. In some CBCAR projects, significance emerges from within the project itself. In other words, critical issues emerge as research partners engage with organizational or community members. For example, in a CBCAR project with Somali women, community members identified significant health issues (Pavlish, Noor, & Brandt, 2010). These concerns became the foundation for a community forum where community members prioritized topics for project development. In other CBCAR projects, significant topics are determined by the partnership ahead of time and built into the project proposal. For example, community officials may be alarmed by a sudden rise in HIV infection and engage with researchers and community members to design a CBCAR project that formulates culturally appropriate prevention measures. The key issue is that CBCAR teams should clearly describe in their proposals the collaborative process of identifying the research topic and establish why it is significant for the community or organization.

To examine their project proposal for relevance to the RFA, CBCAR partners should consider the values embedded in their research question. For example, if the research question pertains to violence against women, embedded values include women's well-being, violence aversion, gender justice, and advocacy. The research team should also closely examine the grant objectives and their inherent values. Creating a persuasive argument that connects the research team's values to the funding agency's values is an important part of the project proposal. For CBCAR projects, persuasion is composed of pertinent evidence, pragmatic vision, and compelling optimism.

Research design is rigorous yet flexible

For all grant proposals, researchers must demonstrate internally consistent research designs and scientifically rigorous data collection and analysis. In addition, CBCAR teams should show that the design emerged from collaborative work. Bringing a preplanned design to a community partner and expecting to plop the project into a community setting will not work with CBCAR grant proposals. For some CBCAR proposals, design development might appear within the project proposal. These are sometimes referred to as formative research designs. For example, research partners might conduct focus groups to help plan a pilot program which could then be pilot-tested before large-scale testing or a randomized controlled intervention trial is planned. The CBCAR projects in Chapters 1 and 2 and the sample proposal that is included in this chapter are examples of formative design projects.

Another way to show design flexibility in CBCAR proposals is to use emergent designs, which usually refers to allowing early data collection and analysis to inform further data collection and analysis. As described in Chapters 4, 5, and 6, an emergent design allows for collaborative planning within the research process itself—not just during the design phase but also during implementation phases. The key for research partners using emergent or formative designs in their grant proposals is to be specific and transparent about their research procedures and strategies for rigor while being open and flexible to findings as the research process ensues (Padgett & Henwood, 2009). CBCAR teams should also explain how ethical guidelines for the protection of human subjects/participants will be rigorously observed in formative and emergent designs.

Emergent or formative designs usually pertain to CBCAR projects that are early in the collaboration phase of an academic–community partnership and where little information is known about the topic. As the research partnership becomes more established and more information about the research topic becomes known, then project designs might become more fixed, even to the point of including randomized controlled trials. Clearly describing a rigorous research method is an important component of CBCAR grant proposals.

Ideas are original and innovative

Most funding agencies seek projects that break new ground. Since CBCAR projects pursue change in current systems and structures by imagining and designing new futures, deliberate attempts to use group process for creative planning should be arranged. Being innovative can pertain to any aspect of the CBCAR project, such as forging a unique partnership, designing a novel program, creating a unique process, overcoming research challenges, or initiating an original data collection strategy. Research partners can also incorporate creative action planning and problem solving processes in their proposals. To be innovative, research partners need to be bold, forge new pathways, and produce grant proposals with uniqueness in mind.

Unfortunately, the human capacity for creativity and imagination is often untapped. Consequently, while designing CBCAR projects and grant proposals, research partners should plan opportunities to generate novel ideas (Viswanathan et al., 2004). For example, brainstorming stimulates people's imaginations, leads to swirling group dialogue, and often sets the foundation for creative co-thinking. Also, encouraging people to express divergent thoughts and ideas is important. However, divergence can sometimes make group members edgy and uncertain. Capturing people's differences and creating a unique tapestry of woven ideas can be one of the most challenging aspects of CBCAR. It can also be one of the most essential.

To work innovatively, research teams need to accept confusion, ambiguity, and disorder as normal aspects of inquiry (Heron & Reason, 2006). The importance of these "messy" inquiry steps should be discussed in early planning meetings. If group members are prepared for differences and potential tension, messy inquiry phases frequently progress to creative resolution (Heron & Reason, 2006). Innovation often emerges from these creative attempts to find new order in disorder. Synthesizing disparate ideas and constructing novel patterns is part of originality and innovation. Research partners should consider their own methods for unleashing human imagination during project design. If research teams are uncertain about the acceptability of their innovative ideas, they should consult with funding agency representatives.

Protection for human subjects/participants is central and threaded throughout

As stated frequently in this book, ethics is central to any research endeavor. Consideration of plans to protect participants and at the same time include a wide variety of participants is required in most grant applications. Research partners should be very familiar with all federal and institutional guidelines on the ethical conduct of research including issues surrounding conflict of interest. Because CBCAR projects often involve multiple partners in the research process, the research team should pay particular attention to potential conflicts of interest. The NIH Office of Extramural Research (2009) states that conflict of interest occurs when an institution or individual has "significant financial interest[s] that could directly and significantly affect the design, conduct, or reporting of NIH-funded research" (p. 2). Research partners should assess the CBCAR project for potential conflicts of interest and contact their ethics representative for further guidance. Current information is also available on an NIH website about conflict of interest (http://grants.nih.gov/grants/policy/coi/).

Because grant applications often require applicants to detail specific ethics procedures, the challenge for CBCAR partners is to assure funding agencies that ethical conduct of research is prominently observed in every step of the research—including steps that unfold from the process itself. The research team has to create a convincing argument that they are prepared to protect human subjects/participants and are vigilant about ethics during all iterative phases of the research process. Plans to prepare team and community members in the ethical conduct of research should be clearly stated. Ethics is vital to all research endeavors and plans to observe ethical guidelines must be visible in all grant applications.

Findings can be translated into action and measurable outcomes

Discovery is certainly the aim of many important research studies. However for CBCAR, discovery drives action planning, and action usually results in measurable effects. Most agencies that fund CBCAR projects examine proposals for evidence of project outcome, such as improved health, social change, practice improvement, learning promotion, policy shift, or system reform. Occasionally, programs developed and applied locally have the potential for becoming a national model. Findings from CBCAR studies are usually not generalized to broader contexts; however, processes and programs that are developed could pertain to other communities and organizations with similar contexts. So another project outcome could be the development of a national model to advance system improvement and health outcomes.

However, we should also acknowledge that many CBCAR projects follow a flexible and unfolding process, and for that reason, outcomes for some projects will be developed during the implementation phase (Waterman, Tillen, Dickson, & de Koning, 2001). This is particularly true for early-stage CBCAR projects. In these situations, if a research partnership predetermines specific outcomes in a grant application, these outcomes may, in turn, drive the project. Consequently, community voices and interests could be buried in the search to generate the specified outcomes promised to funders but which no longer represent the most pressing concerns of the community. For this reason, partners who plan early-stage CBCAR projects should acknowledge that general process outcomes, such as increased awareness or community engagement around the issue at hand, will be achieved. However, more specific outcomes will be determined as the CBCAR process ensues. These emergent outcomes allow communities to speak for themselves as they engage in dialogue, develop new insights, and plan follow-up actions and outcomes. The sample CBCAR grant proposal that appears at the end of this chapter identifies general outcomes for each phase of the formative project. Specific actions and desired outcomes were then designed in the follow-up community forums. Early-stage CBCAR project teams need to consider

---

Box 9-2   Project Outcomes in Specific Aims

A CBCAR partnership developed the Ubuntu-Human Rights Learning and Advocacy Program and its outcome measures in previous project steps. A follow-up specific aim with outcomes listed could be:

- Conduct a randomized intervention pilot study to assess the outcomes of 30 young adults (ages 19–25) who participated in the Ubuntu-Human Rights Learning and Advocacy Program at 6-month follow-up, as compared with a similar number of young adults who had just the formal human rights curriculum in school (usual care program) in terms of the following outcomes:
  - Improvement in knowledge about ubuntu and human rights principles
  - Empowerment in social interactions
  - Satisfaction with self in gender relationships
  - Increased awareness on gutter-based violence as a human rights violation

funding agencies that allow for community-developed outcomes within the project. Conferring with funding agency representatives is often helpful.

Once CBCAR projects have advanced through action planning and the research partnership has decided to develop and test the effectiveness of a specific community-based program, then predetermining specific outcomes is more appropriate. Outcomes in these situations can be written into grant proposals in a variety of ways. For example, outcomes might be listed within a specific aim (see **Box 9-2**). Outcomes could also appear in the proposal as hypotheses (see **Box 9-3**). The type of project design partially determines how outcomes are stated in grant proposals. In addition, RFA instructions may offer guidance on how to incorporate outcomes in project proposals.

Box 9-3   Project Outcomes in Hypotheses

This CBCAR project engaged RNs in developing a clinical practice program to strengthen nurses' voices in ethical dilemmas (Ethics Conflict Prevention Program). The following sample objectives for a preliminary controlled trial include outcomes in hypotheses:

1. To compare the effects of the Ethics Conflict Prevention Program (ECPP) and a control condition on nurses' use of ethics principles during clinical case discussions in weekly ethics rounds

   a. Hypothesis #1—Nurses participating in the ECPP will demonstrate increased use of ethics principles during clinical case discussions in weekly ethics rounds than those in a control condition.

2. To compare the effects of the ECPP and a control condition on number of ethics consultations

   a. Hypothesis #2—Nurses participating in the ECPP will initiate an increased number of ethics consultations than those in a control condition.

3. To compare the effects of the ECPP and a control condition on timeliness of ethics consultations

   a. Hypothesis #3—Nurses participating in the ECPP will initiate ethics consultation sooner than those in a control condition.

Establishing outcomes (and their measures if appropriate to the project) in CBCAR grant proposals enhances the accountability that many funding agencies require.

Whether designing general or specific outcomes, we encourage CBCAR teams to consider multidimensional outcome planning so changes are planned and measured not only for the critical reference group but also for other project stakeholders. For example, adopting a sociopolitical ecological perspective, Wadsworth (1997) encouraged researchers to include outcome measures not only for the people whose experience the project is designed to change (critical reference group) but also for those individuals and groups who need to be informed, convinced, and inspired to change systems and structures. Multilevel outcome planning is more likely to lead to effective social change (Emmons, 2000; Green & Kreuter, 2005; World Health Organization, 2008). If multiple stakeholders are considered and included when designing specific aims then their accompanying outcomes and measures, project and partnership sustainability is more likely (Israel et al., 2006).

Investigators are capable; environment is supportive

Content expertise is valuable in all research endeavors. In most participatory action projects, content expertise is provided by research participants as they engage with researchers to describe and find meaning in their experiences. So, in CBCAR grant proposals, research partners have to provide evidence that they are process experts and are capable of enacting many processes to implement the proposed research project. That means the research team should have expertise in processes such as the following:

- Creating productive dialogue
- Collaborating across differences
- Planning in dynamic, complex environments and amidst evolving events
- Being skilled in a variety of research methods and data collection and analysis strategies

- Facilitating emergent and formative processes
- Synthesizing differences to generate innovative ideas for action
- Evaluating group process and outcome achievement
- Thinking critically, reflectively, reflexively, and collaboratively

When research team members are skilled in these important processes, project sustainability is more likely to occur (Bradbury, 2006). So, to strengthen the grant application, research team members should highlight their past experiences in activities such as collaborating across disciplines, working with the study population or setting, facilitating participatory program development, and designing and implementing various research projects, particularly action-based research. If investigators are new to the CBCAR process, then the proposal should include mechanisms for consulting with necessary experts. Including letters of support from specific consultants strengthens project proposals.

CBCAR applications also need to demonstrate that the research partnership works in a supportive environment. The research team should consult with primary stakeholders before and during project design and grant applications. Letters of support from key stakeholders and gatekeepers are vital to most CBCAR grant applications. Investigators should also be able to show that research partners themselves work in supportive environments that will not pose barriers to project implementation (Israel et al., 2006).

Benefits and challenges of CBCAR are addressed throughout proposal

Collaborative, action-based planning is an important benefit of the CBCAR process. Research partners should convince funding agencies that collaboration is the best way to achieve RFA and project objectives. Collaborative partnerships not only assist with community needs assessments and recruitment and retention efforts, they also enhance research design, data collection, and analysis (Agency for Healthcare Research and Quality, 2009; Viswanathan et al., 2004). However, challenges to conducting CBCAR projects should also be acknowledged (Seifer & Sisco, 2006; Yonas et al., 2006). Research partners should consider potential barriers and convince funding agencies that they are prepared to implement alternative plans. For example, limited time and resources challenge many CBCAR processes (Israel et al., 2006). Therefore, research teams need to anticipate and be creative about potential solutions. Research partners' awareness of both benefits and challenges should be visible throughout the proposal.

Project and partnership are feasible

Feasibility is an important aspect of all funding applications. Partnership feasibility is especially important to emphasize in CBCAR funding proposals. One of the most significant ways to demonstrate partnership feasibility is by providing evidence of successful collaboration in the past. Strategies that advance partnership feasibility also strongly influence project feasibility. If partners are working effectively, logistical capability in implementing the project improves. Project feasibility is also enhanced by support from key stakeholders and organizations (Israel et al., 2006). Letters of support from a wide range of stakeholders and policy shapers strengthen grant applications.

Budget is adequately justified; compensation is fairly distributed to all partners

All researchers who seek financial support for their research must establish and justify a budget. However, in CBCAR budgets, there should be evidence that both academic and community settings are included in the budget and share resource management responsibilities (Seifer, 2005). Also, research participants should be fairly compensated for their contributions. Time release may be difficult to arrange for some CBCAR partnerships, especially in some community-based organizations with small staffs and limited resources. Applicants should consider hiring community members to fill some of the grant positions. Hiring and training community members tends to support project sustainability (Krieger, Allen, Roberts, Ross, & Takaro, 2005).

Partnership and project are sustainable

Grant reviewers are more likely to treat proposals favorably if project and partnership sustainability is addressed in the proposal (Seifer, 2005; Viswanathan et al., 2004). The architecture for sustainability should be created during the planning process. Bradbury (2006) suggested that the research planning team should attend to both the "rigor" of scientific inquiry and the "vigor" of work needed to promote sustainability (p. 242). Several ideas that advance sustainability should be incorporated into a CBCAR proposal (Israel et al., 2006). For example, providing for robust participation from multiple stakeholders promotes sustainability. Bradbury (2006) suggested that when research partners and stakeholders engage with one another, "Emergent change at the micro-level shifts the macro-dynamics of a system towards more sustainable practices" (p. 236). In other words, productive, dialogic interaction among a wide variety of stakeholders is likely to move change from microsystems, such as small group, neighborhood, or nursing care unit, outward to include larger systems, such as entire communities or organizations. Policy and practice changes in these larger systems and structures are more likely to be sustainable when there is strong partner engagement from the very beginning (Wallerstein, 2006).

Another mechanism for sustainability is developing shared vision and ownership (Rabiee, 2006; Seifer & Sisco, 2006). Asserting the importance of developing common goals, Bradbury (2006) suggested that initially research partners and participants are stimulated by self-interest to participate in an action-based project. Then, through dialogue, partners and participants progress toward shared vision and project ownership. As conversation about the project expands to other social networks, more people are invited into the conversation, and through interactive dialogue, visions for change expand and collaboration potentially widens. Bradbury emphasized the power of dialogue in promoting sustainability so engagement and dissemination become dynamic and move in many directions simultaneously.

CBCAR proposals should also incorporate opportunities for conversation and consideration of research lessons in public and professional forums. Ideally, community forums occur before wider dissemination; however, once again, we note the unique pathway for each CBCAR process. In some projects, preliminary results that shape action planning might be shared in meetings or conferences. This early dissemination of results could actually stimulate further ideas and support for change and action planning—which could make the project more sustainable (Bradbury, 2006). During CBCAR project development and grant writing, research partners should deliberately strategize—and advertise—the multiple ways they plan to sustain their partnership and project.

■ Some Challenges

As collaborative planning ensues and grant applications are written, a few cautions about funding mechanisms should be shared. First, managing timelines can be challenging. For example, communities might anticipate funding to address immediate needs. After action planning is complete and a feasibility grant is written, research partners are frequently ready to move forward. However, grant reviews take time. Delays are inevitable and can be difficult to predict. People who invested their time in project planning may lose interest by the time funding is secure (Plumb et al., 2004; Strong et al., 2009). There is a lag time that often is difficult for some CBCAR partners to keep fueled.

Second, when gaps are revealed or disparities uncovered, people's awareness and passions are heightened. People develop expectations that the research partnership will follow up with actions regardless of funding and timing. Sometimes people develop unrealistic or competing expectations, which can result in disappointment and frustration and hamper relationships (Strong et al., 2009).

Third, CBCAR funding often occurs in steps. If the research partnership implemented a funded pilot study in a community but loses funding to expand the program, community frustration can result (Strong et al., 2009). People invest valuable time and energy on projects that are not always funded, so research partners should state up front and often that funding is not guaranteed. Also, funding agencies might have limitations that narrow the scope or alter the direction of the intended project. This can also hamper partner and community relationships.

These cautions are best addressed through consistent, clear, multidirectional communication and dialogue (Strong et al., 2009). The advantages and limitations of funding have to be considered as part of the collaborative decision to apply for grant funds. Before people commit to work on grants, they should be informed that no guarantee exists. Communication mechanisms for handling frustration and tension should be developed as part of the partnership plan. Transparency about timelines, expectations, frustrations, and contingencies is vitally important. Keeping all communication channels between research partners open is essential.

■ Sample Proposal: Community Connections and Collaboration

During 2005–2008, the National Institute for Child Health and Human Development funded the following CBCAR project. The funding mechanism was particularly geared toward supporting research that was based in small college and university settings. The project followed a formative research design in which the specific intervention emerged from collaborative planning with community-based organizations and in focus group dialogue with African-born women. Several CBCAR principles are infused throughout the grant application. The intent is to provide readers some examples of how CBCAR principles are incorporated in project design. Even though this is a community-based project, similar principles pertain to organization-based projects.

Community Connections and Collaboration Project[1]

Project Introduction

The Community Connections and Collaboration Project intends to address health disparities, specifically the health disparities experienced by African immigrant women and girls. Health disparities refer to the "difference in health status between Populations of Color and American Indians and Whites" (Minnesota Department of Health, 2005, p. 3). Currently in Minnesota, populations of color and American Indians experience shorter life spans; higher rates of infant mortality; higher incidence of diabetes, heart disease, cancer and other chronic conditions; and poorer general health than the white population (Minnesota Department of Health, 2005). The Community Connections and Collaboration Project will examine the health experiences of African immigrant women and girls by establishing partnerships with community-based African immigrant and refugee organizations, identifying African women's and girls' perspectives on their health and health education priorities, and co-designing a community learning and translational research plan to address the community-identified priorities. The project goals are to:

- Form diverse and inclusive groups of collaboration and inquiry.
- Seek and examine multiple community-based perspectives.
- Weave those perspectives into community-based learning about the larger context of national health disparities and the NIH commitment to their elimination.
- Co-craft community-based strategic intervention plans that serve African immigrant girls, women, and their families.
- Co-create an agenda for community-based intervention research regarding outreach and health information dissemination.

The essential and ultimate goal of this academic–community partnership is community empowerment such that African women and girls and their families are empowered to express their health concerns and actively participate in finding and implementing solutions of crucial importance to their health and well-being.

As the largest Catholic college for women in the United States, the College of St. Catherine's[2] vision statement is *to be the world's preeminent Catholic college educating women to lead and influence.* The College is proud to have the most diverse student population of any private college in Minnesota. Of this year's undergraduate day students, 26% are the first generation of their families to attend college and 20% are students of color. The College's exceptional programs in nursing and allied health fields have been especially successful in creating a diverse workforce—27% of students are multicultural, 40% are the first generation in their families to attend college, and 38% are parents. The diverse student population and large representation of student parents indicate the strength and scope of the College's flexible programs, innovative education delivery systems, and supportive services for women with children.

The Department of Nursing is the largest academic department at the College of St. Catherine and offers certificate, associate, baccalaureate, and graduate degree programs on the Minneapolis and St. Paul campuses. Enrolling more than 650 nursing students and graduating more than 250 students annually from its nursing programs, the Department of Nursing is recognized as an innovator and leader in nursing and nursing education. Currently, 30% of the nursing students enrolled in the Associate Degree Program are students of color, the majority of whom are African-born immigrants. The College of St. Catherine is deeply concerned about the health of African immigrant women and girls and uniquely qualified to partner with them in the Community Connections and Collaboration Project.

Background and Significance

The Minneapolis–St. Paul area is rapidly becoming more ethnically diverse with African-American and African immigrants comprising the largest population of color (Minnesota Department of Health, 2005). The Minnesota State Demographic

Center (2004) reports that Minnesota has become a primary destination for refugees. For example, the largest number of Somali immigrants in the nation currently resides in the Twin Cities area (Minnesota Department of Health, 2003). In 2002, the highest number of immigrants came from Somalia (Minnesota State Demographic Center, 2004). Currently, this foreign-born population is experiencing rapid growth—both through natural increase and immigration. Refugees and immigrants account for approximately one-quarter of the student body in the Minneapolis schools (Minneapolis School District, 2004) and about one-third of the student body in St. Paul schools (St. Paul School District, 2004). The Somali population is estimated at 25,000 and the Ethiopian population is estimated at 7,500 (Minnesota State Demographic Center, 2004). Other African immigrants, composed of smaller numbers, also live in Minnesota. The State Demographic Center (2004) predicts that large numbers of African refugees will continue to arrive in subsequent years due to continued civil strife in many parts of Africa and immigration policies that support family reunification.

African immigrants have contributed their ambitions, talents, cultural values, and hard work toward helping Minnesota thrive. However, a recent report concluded that immigrants to Minnesota are among the least served by Minnesota's health and social service systems (Minnesota Department of Health and Minnesota Department of Human Services, Immigrant Health Task Force, 2005). The Task Force reported that:

■ Lack of insurance and difficult payment systems discourage immigrants from seeking needed health care resulting in poorer health for immigrants and increased expense to the healthcare system.

■ Immigrants who need screening and treatment for infectious diseases and chronic conditions, such as diabetes and depression often do not receive the required medical attention resulting in higher rates of chronic conditions for immigrants than nonimmigrant populations.

■ Healthcare professionals in Minnesota are primarily from cultures different from their immigrant patients and are often not aware of communication barriers resulting in lower rates of comprehension and adherence to medical treatments by immigrant groups.

■ Denied access to affordable health care or insurance, immigrants seek health care in emergency situations resulting in higher costs to the healthcare system and lower productivity in industries that employ immigrants.

The Minnesota Immigrant Health Task Force findings reinforce the reports of the Institute of Medicine (Smedley, Stith, & Nelson, 2003) that health disparities exist for many racial and ethnic groups. The well-being of the nation is critically dependent on solutions to the significant dilemma of health disparities.

Objectives for the Community Connections and Collaboration Project

The Community Connections and Collaboration Project seeks to:

1. Establish partnerships between the College of St. Catherine and community-based organizations. Specifically, we intend to:

   ■ Form effective inquiry partnerships between the College of St. Catherine (CSC), an international non-governmental refugee-assistance organization, three community-based African immigrant organizations, and African women and girls.

   ■ Apply the community-learning framework—Integrated Mindfulness for Participatory Action and Community Transformation—to guide the partnering process.

2. Identify and document the community's views of its health concerns and priorities. Specifically, we intend to:

   ■ Create an expanded, community-based dataset on health experiences, concerns, and priorities expressed by African immigrant women and girls through a series of focus group dialogue sessions.

   ■ Initiate key informant dialogue between *inquiry partners* and key stakeholders, such as community members, healthcare organizations, educational institutions, community groups, faith-based institutions, and service organizations to analyze the database and how the data pertains to community outreach and health information dissemination to African women and girls in the Minneapolis–St. Paul area.

■ Broaden community awareness of national and local health disparities and the NIH commitment to disparities elimination.

■ Extend community awareness about the health and information needs of African immigrant women and girls.

■ Gain deeper insights into the contextual factors pertaining to health concerns and health education needs for African immigrant women and girls.

3. Prepare an Intervention Research Plan for Phase II. Specifically, we intend to:

■ Establish a Community Connections and Collaborative Planning Committee. Members of the committee will include both inquiry and working partners, such as African immigrant women and girls and representatives from local schools, healthcare organizations, primary employers, faith-based institutions, service organizations, and other community groups. Committee members will:

a. Plan and conduct a series of community forums to share information on health disparities and African women's and girls' health concerns and to invite community participation and expanded perspectives.

b. Create a set of actions and research goals focused on community priorities pertaining to community outreach and health information dissemination to African women and girls in Minneapolis–St. Paul.

■ Apply for a Phase II NICHD Research Grant.

4. Advance the National Institute of Child Health and Human Development goal of conducting community-based research to increase the quality and years of healthy life and to eliminate health disparities.

The College of St. Catherine and community-based organization partners will accomplish these objectives through the implementation of a community-based, collaborative action and learning process called Integrated Mindfulness for Participatory Action and Community Transformation (IMPACT).

IMPACT: A Community Learning Model

The Integrated Mindfulness for Participatory Action and Community Transformations (IMPACT) Model will be used as a process framework for the Community Connections and Collaboration Project. IMPACT arises from the theoretical perspectives of transcultural nursing and adult learning as well as the practical experience of being with and learning from refugee and immigrant women. For example, IMPACT successfully guided the development of community learning initiatives for outreach and information dissemination on HIV prevention in refugee communities. The IMPACT model also effectively guided community-based research projects on women's health conducted with refugee women in a Rwandan refugee camp (Pavlish, 2005a; Pavlish, 2005b).

Three foundational principles are significant to the success of creating new knowledge and infusing learning into communities. First, since the IMPACT model is used across disciplines and cultures, a *mindful perspective* must be applied. Integrated mindfulness means "the readiness to shift one's frame of reference, the motivation to use new categories to understand cultural or ethnic differences, and the preparedness to experiment with creative avenues of decision making and problem solving" (Ting-Toomey, 1999, p. 46). Mindful transcultural and transdisciplinary communication involves constructing shared meanings that are mindful of both diversity and universality in identities, relationships, and goals. When community health professionals work across cultures and across disciplines, they must implement a mindfulness and a care perspective that represent a willingness and openness to co-construct meaning as opposed to imposing meaning.

Second, *community-based knowledge systems* are a vital aspect to consider when applying the model. Kamata (2000) described locally-based knowledge as "historically constituted [emic] knowledge instrumental in the long-term adaptation of human groups to the biophysical environment" (p. 55). Community-based knowledge represents the wisdom of local residents including socioeconomically marginalized groups. Criticizing Western approaches to research and development projects in low income countries, Sillitoe (1998) offered many examples of how expensive research and community projects imposed in a top-down fashion have collapsed. In contrast, participatory approaches to community-based learning acknowledge the significance of local knowledge and incorporate local wisdom into planning community learning to insure success (Chambers, 1997; de Koning & Martin, 1996; Hahn, 1999; Herda, 1999; Indra, 1999; Sillitoe, 1998; Smith, 2001; Snyder, 1995).

Much of community-based knowledge is embedded in practical wisdom and is often applied in solving practical problems (Sillitoe, 1998). However, this valuable aspect of locally-based knowledge is also one of the greatest challenges—the embeddedness of practical knowledge often makes the knowledge difficult for community health professionals to access. However, community health professionals must resist the temptation to stuff the gaps of inaccessible knowledge with their own. Continuous and patient attempts to learn community-based knowledge are necessary.

Third, *opportunities to co-create new knowledge* must be planned. The reflective process of co-creating and co-constructing meaning transcends personal and community-based knowledge systems and evolves into shared meaning systems. As stated by Litchfield (1999), "We are creating our worlds in the process of creating knowledge" (p. 70). Nonaka, Konno, and Toyama (2001) described a process that organizations use to continually create knowledge. Moving through four stages that vacillate between and expand upon tacit and explicit knowledge, people in organizations share mental models and in the process create new mental models. The authors claimed that an essential feature of continual knowledge creation is the deliberate creation of time and space for people to share, examine, and co-create new knowledge. Requiring an emergence from the self, collaborating across time and space results in shared experiences, collective reflections, and synchronous knowledge vision.

These three principles interact to guide implementation of the IMPACT Model. All knowledge systems are significant, productive, and creative and capable of expansion and change. By creating *inquiry* and *planning partnerships* with people who possess community-based knowledge, community health planners transcend simply understanding other knowledge systems and learn to co-produce and co-create new knowledge for community and organizational learning.

Community Connections and Collaboration Project: The Process

The IMPACT Model provides the procedural framework for implementing the Community Connections and Collaboration Project. As a guide for participatory inquiry and planning, IMPACT is composed of six stages around which activities can be planned. Being collaborative in nature and formative in design, specific steps within each stage will be planned by the participants. However, the overall objectives for each stage can be described. Stages 1–3 describe the *inquiry partnerships*, which are formed with people from inside the African immigrant community. The inquiry partnerships will establish the work of subsequent stages. Stages 4–6 outline how the planning and community learning phases might develop and proceed.

Stage 1—Inquiring: Inviting Participation
During the inquiry stage of the IMPACT Model, faculty representatives from the College of St. Catherine and community health educators, researchers, and advocates from an international non-governmental refugee assistance organization will meet to:

■ Exchange theoretical and philosophical perspectives on participatory methodologies to be implemented in the Community Connections and Collaboration Project.

■ Analyze the available literature on immigrant health disparities and African women's and girls' health concerns.

■ Inquire about which immigrant and refugee groups might be interested in participating in the Community Connections and Collaboration Project.

■ Invite African women's and girls' organizations to an information sharing meeting.

The outcomes of Stage 1 include: (1) insight into the current status of knowledge regarding African women's and girls' health concerns and, (2) a plan for developing community partnerships with various organizations interested in African women's and girls' health issues.

Stage 2—Meeting: Connecting with African Immigrant Organizations

A variety of African immigrant and refugee organizations will be invited to participate in meetings to:

■ Learn about each organization's mission and the work being done.

■ Converse about health disparities in African immigrant communities.

■ Begin to form a transdisciplinary and transcultural community of people interested in pursuing questions about African women's and girls' health concerns and health disparities.

■ Dialogue about the partnership possibilities in initiating further inquiry into African women's and girls' health concerns and health disparities.

■ Determine what additional data is required and the best methods with which to collect data.

McKay, Scotchmer, Figueroa-Melendez, and Huq (2000) researched barriers and opportunities for increasing leadership in immigrant and refugee communities and concluded that programs are more successful and have their greatest impact when the "programs are developed and run by immigrant or refugee-led organizations or overseen by a project steering committee that reflects the participant population" (p. 22). Including African immigrant-led organizations in the *inquiry partnership* is vitally important to the success of the Community Connections and Collaboration Project.

The outcomes of Stage 2 include: (1) effective *inquiry partnerships* between organizations interested in examining African women's and girls' health concerns, (2) formulation of critical questions to investigate further, (3) plan for reaching into and connecting with African women and girls, and (4) a set of networks to incorporate into subsequent stages.

Stage 3—Partnering: Connecting with African Immigrant Women and Girls

Based on methods developed during Stage 2, some informal gatherings with African women and girls will be implemented during the partnering stage. The African immigrant organizations that indicate interest in continuing with the Community Connections and Collaboration Project will co-plan with CSC and the nonprofit refugee assistance organization a series of community gatherings whereby organizers and African women and girls will:

■ Create a shared awareness and attention to immigrant health disparities and the need for community outreach to learn more about African women's and girls' perspectives of their health.

■ Develop a shared commitment to inquire into and address immigrant health disparities—especially those experienced by African women and girls.

■ Review the available literature and work already completed pertaining to African women's and girls' health.

■ Develop and implement strategies (focus groups, community meetings, surveys) to collect more data about the nature and extent of health concerns within the community of African women and girls.

■ Determine the best methods to expand the dialogue.

In the process of connecting across cultures and disciplines and reaching into communities to dialogue and learn about the health concerns of African immigrant women and girls, existing knowledge is expanded and reexamined. New knowledge is co-constructed, and that knowledge will impact subsequent stages of the Community Connections and Collaboration Project. Seeking *inquiry partnerships* and active participation by African-led organizations and African women and girls before expanding the dialogue to include institutions and organizations within the broader community is a significant departure from traditional hierarchal structures often imposed by academic institutions. However, the IMPACT process model requires grassroots participation at the initial and all subsequent stages of the process. The strong community link is vital to the success of the Community Connections and Collaboration Project.

The **Stage 3 outcomes** will be: (1) an effective capacity to work across disciplines and cultures in addressing the expressed health concerns of African women and girls, (2) a database to share with an expanded community regarding women's and girls' perspectives of their health concerns, (3) an organized structure for subsequent planning, and (4) expanded networks from which to implement Stage 4.

Stage 4—Acting Imaginatively: Expanding the Dialogue

Drawing on work initiated by the *inquiry partnerships* in the first three stages, subsequent stages of the IMPACT Model expand into working with community institutions and organizations. During Stage 4, organizers from CSC, nongovernmental refugee assistance organization, African immigrant organizations, and African women and girls (i.e., *inquiry partners*) will invite more people into the ongoing dialogue about African women's and girls' health concerns. Representatives from local schools, healthcare institutions, service organizations, and primary employers of African women will be invited to a series of participatory workshops. Information about the Community Connections and Collaboration Project will be presented at the workshops and activities designed to enhance participation of workshop attendees will be planned. The primary objective of the participatory workshops is to provide opportunities for dialogue between African women and girls and members of community institutions, such as local schools and healthcare providers. Specifically, the workshop participants will:

■ Learn about the African immigrant community in the Minneapolis–St. Paul area.

■ Learn about national and local health disparities and the NIH commitment to their elimination.

■ Learn about the Community Connections and Collaboration Project.

- Explore existing community resources and institutional services for African women and girls.

- Analyze the contextual factors that impact African women's and girls' health, including both strengths and challenges in existing services, delivery systems, working and learning conditions, community resources, and formal and informal political and social structures.

- Develop goals for addressing information and service gaps.

- Organize into a Community Connections and Collaborative Planning Committee.

The Stage 4 outcomes will be: (1) a more complete picture of health issues for African women and girls, (2) transdisciplinary and transcultural dialogue and shared analysis, (3) expanded networks, and (4) a committee structure for planning a series of community forums.

Stage 5—Crafting: Transforming Problems into Priorities

The Community Connections and Collaboration Planning Committee will collaborate to reach even more deeply into the community and plan a series of community forums. Composed of African immigrant women and girls, educators, researchers, community health professionals and advocates, members of organizations working with immigrant groups, and community members, the Planning Committee will organize for a series of community forums to disseminate information found during the previous stages of the Community Connections and Collaboration Project. Specific topics will be determined by members of the Planning Committee and shaped by the participatory work conducted in Stages 1–4.

The Stage 5 outcome will be the community forums implemented in Stage 6.

Stage 6—Transfusing: Creating Community Learning

The Community Connections and Collaborative Planning Committee will:

- Conduct a series of community forums to disseminate information on national and local health disparities and the NIH commitment to their elimination and share information pertaining to the Community Connections and Collaboration Project.

■ Invite community input into developing community intervention projects for advancing the health of African immigrant women and girls.

■ Create an intervention research agenda that sets priorities for community intervention projects.

The open community forums will be held in various Minneapolis and St. Paul neighborhoods and will focus on disseminating information and gathering community responses and perspectives. Subsequent to the community forums and based on participant responses to the community forums, the Planning Committee will then prepare a grant application for Phase II of the Academic–Community Partnership Conference Series.

The Stage 6 outcomes include: (1) research questions that address a community-developed research agenda on health questions and concerns raised during the Community Connections and Collaboration Project, (2) community-developed, strategic intervention plans for outreach and health information dissemination to African women and girls, and (3) application for Phase II of the Academic–Community Partnership Grant opportunity offered by NICHD.

Project Summary

The Community Connections and Collaboration Project focuses effort on creating effective *inquiry partnerships* to think intently, care collectively, and communicate effectively about African women's and girls' health priorities and concerns. We intend to participate actively with community members to achieve better-informed and more action-oriented citizenry in communities, healthcare organizations, educational institutions, faith-based organizations, and community service professionals. In addition, we intend to promote leadership capability in African immigrant community members and organizations as well as ourselves, and co-construct community-based research goals focused on community outreach and health information dissemination to African women and girls.

Project Conclusion

The Community Connections and Collaboration Project implements IMPACT as a process for community health professionals who, in partnership with interested community members, inquire about community health concerns (such as health disparities), develop a shared commitment to address the concern, actively participate in the work of planning and organizing for community and organizational learning, and reflectively and reflexively infuse new ideas into communities, organizations, and institutions. The participatory nature of the model is not the usual way of community learning in many cultures and requires thinking "not as usual" (Yershova, DeJaeghere, & Mestenhauser, 2000, p. 39). The skills of critical, reflective, reflexive, and comparative thinking enhance transcultural and transdisciplinary collaboration and "go well beyond the individual level; they influence institutional decisions, policy making, international relations, and so on" (Yershova et al., 2000, p. 65). These thinking skills are the basis for the type of participatory and collaborative learning described in the Community Connections and Collaboration Project.

Connecting meaningfully and partnering effectively with diverse communities are central factors in improving the health of communities and require individual as well as community learning. When community health professionals envision themselves and the immigrant women and girls with whom they work as inquiry partners in the health promotion of individuals, families, populations, and entire communities, the whole nature of their mission transforms—from providing to learning, from giving to sharing, from producing to innovating, and from reaching to connecting. The Community Connections and Collaboration Project seeks to learn, inform, and transform with that vision in mind.[3]

■ Summary

Padgett and Henwood (2009) suggested that, overall, project proposals should be "convincing, feasible, and worthwhile" (p. 870). In other words, grant applicants have to provide a strong argument that their project will specifically and sustainably improve people's situations, and that the project partnership is well qualified and positioned to accomplish their specific aims. Additionally, a CBCAR grant application must adhere to all methodological assumptions behind the CBCAR process. **Table 9-1** offers a matrix that encourages CBCAR research teams to

Table 9-1 Self-Evaluation of CBCAR Proposals: Intersecting Criteria with CBCAR Tenets

	Relevance and significance	Innovation originality	Scientific rigor	Feasibility	Sustainability
Community-based	Community priority, need with evidence provided Community assessment complete	Other community models leave gap which is filled with this research	Expertise exists within community to assure rigorous research design	Letters of support demonstrate a web of community support	Sustaining community Support is evident Stakeholders represent many community sectors
Collaborative	Benefits and challenges to partnership/project included Equal participation in planning/ implementing Project benefits all partners	Unique partnership Expanding margins	Partners are skilled in essential CBCAR processes Partners are educating one another on context and methods	Partners possess the resources to carry out proposed project Partners have been successful in past collaborations	Strength of partnership and partners evidence long-term commitment

Action	Outcomes are important to community members and community well being Action plan has wide impact	Unique plan/outcome Unique outcome measurement	Action plan relates to research findings Action plan impact evaluation is rigorous	Capacity exists to generate funds for emerging action steps	Action plan aims at multilevel change and includes structural changes (policy and practices)
Research	Research topic is worthwhile Project promotes human flourishing	Unique design Potential for becoming model for other CBCAR projects	Project design adheres to CBCAR assumptions	Methodological and logistical capacity is evident	Research design engages community in all steps

Consider focus and clarity in each aspect of proposed project

Consider coherence—all grant sections fit together to form whole

Consider ethics in parts/whole

These sample criteria are general; exact criteria would emerge from particular funding agency consider how well their project proposal adheres to common evaluation criteria for grants and intersects with CBCAR's methodological assumptions. As stated previously, CBCAR pathways are unique in every project; however, the methodological assumptions are common to all projects and should be evident throughout the project proposal and grant application.

Endnotes

1. The authors wish to thank Beth Koenig, JD, Director, Office of Research and Sponsored Programs, St. Catherine University for her sage advice on grant preparation.
2. The College of St. Catherine officially became St. Catherine University in 2009.
3. Partial findings from this research can be found in Pavlish, Noor, & Brandt (2010). Follow-up projects on health literacy and violence prevention are being planned.

References

Agency for Healthcare Research and Quality. (2009). *AHRQ activities using community-based participatory research to address health care disparities.* Retrieved from http://www.ahrq.gov/research/cbprbrief.pdf

Bradbury, H. (2006). Learning with *The National Step*: Action research to promote conversations for sustainable development. In P. Reason & H. Bradbury (Eds.), *Handbook of action research* (pp. 236–242). Thousand Oaks, CA: Sage.

Chambers, R. (1997). *Whose reality counts?: Putting the first last.* London, UK: ITDG Publishing.

de Koning, K., & Martin, M. (Eds.) (1996). *Participatory research in health.* Atlantic Highlands, NJ: Zed.

Emmons, K. (2000). Health behaviors in social contexts. In L. Berkman & I. Kawachi (Eds.), *Social epidemiology* (pp. 242–266). New York, NY: Oxford.

Genat, B. (2009). Building emergent situated knowledges in participatory action research. *Action Research, 7,* 101–115.

Green, L., & Kreuter, M. (2005). *Health program planning: An educational and ecological approach.* Boston, MA: McGraw-Hill.

Hahn, R. (1999). Anthropology and the enhancement of public health practice. In R. Hahn (Ed.), *Anthropology in public health: Bridging differences in culture and society.* New York, NY: Oxford University Press.

Herda, E. (1999). *Research conversations and narrative: A critical hermeneutic orientation in participatory inquiry.* Westport, CT: Praeger.

Heron, J., & Reason, P. (2006). The practice of co-operative inquiry: Research "with" rather than "on" people. In P. Reason & J. Heron (Eds.), *Handbook of action research* (pp. 144–154). Thousand Oaks, CA: Sage.

Indra, D. (1999). Not a "room of one's own:" Engendering forced migration. In D. Indra (Ed.), *Engendering forced migration: Theory and practice* (pp. 1–22). New York, NY: Berghahn Books.

Israel, B., Krieger, J., Vlahov, D., Ciske, S., Foley, M., Fortin, P. . . . Tang, G. (2006). Challenges and facilitating factors in sustaining community-based participatory research partnerships: Lessons learned from the Detroit, New York City, and Seattle Urban Research Centers. *Journal of Urban Health, 83,* 1022–1040.

Kamata, Y. (2000). Indigenous knowledge, cultural empowerment and alternatives. *Contributions to Nepalese Studies, 27,* 51–70.

Krieger, J., Allen, C., Roberts, J. Ross, L., & Takaro, T. (2005). What's with the wheezing? Methods used by the Seattle-King County Health Homes Project to assess exposure to indoor asthma triggers. In B. Israel, E. Eng, A. Schultz, & E. Parker (Eds.), *Methods in community-based participatory research for health* (pp. 230–250). San Francisco, CA: Wiley.

Litchfield, M. (1999). Practice wisdom. *Advances in Nursing Science, 22,* 62–72.

McKay, E., Scotchmer, K., & Huq, S. (2000). Research on barriers and opportunities for increasing leadership in immigrant and refugee communities. Retrieved from http://www.hyamsfoundation.org/documents/Mosaica%20Reprot%20April%202000.pdf

Minneapolis School District. (2004). An overview of Minneapolis public schools. Retrieved from http://www.mpls.k12.mn.us

Minnesota Department of Health. (2003). *Refugee health information.* Retrieved from http://www.health.state.mn.us

Minnesota Department of Health. (2005). *Eliminating racial and ethnic health disparities initiative.* Retrieved from http://www.health.state.mn.us/ommh/publications/legislativerpt2005.pdf

Minnesota Department of Health and Minnesota Department of Human Services (2005). *Immigrant health: A call to action.* Retrieved from http://www.health.state.mn.us/divs/idepc/refugee/topics/immhealthrpt.pdf

Minnesota State Demographic Center (2004). *Estimates of selected immigrant populations in Minnesota: 2004.* Retrieved from http://www.demography.state.mn.us/PopNotes/EvaluatingEstimates.pdf

National Institutes of Health. (2009). Community-based participatory research targeting the medically underserved. Retrieved from http://conferences.thehillgroup.com/si2009

National Institutes of Health, Office of Extramural Research. (2009). *Financial conflict of interest.* Retrieved from http://grants.nih.gov/grants/policy/coi/tutorial/fcoi.pdf

Nonaka, I., Konno, N., & Toyama, R. (2001). Emergence of "ba": A conceptual framework for the continuous self-transcending process of knowledge creation. In I. Nonaka & T. Nishiguchi (Eds.), *Knowledge emergence: Social, technical and evolutionary dimensions of knowledge creation.* (pp. 13–29). New York, NY: Oxford University Press.

Padgett, D., & Henwood, B. (2009). Obtaining large-scale funding for empowerment-oriented qualitative research: A report from personal experience. *Qualitative Health Research, 19,* 868–874.

Pavlish, C. (2005a). Action responses of Congolese refugee women. *Journal of Nursing Scholarship, 37,* 10–17.

Pavlish, C. (2005b). Refugee women's health: Collaborative inquiry with refugee women in Rwanda. *Health Care for Women International, 26,* 880–896.

Pavlish, C., Noor, S., & Brandt, J. (2010). Somali immigrant women and the American health care system: Discordant beliefs, divergent expectations, and silent worries. *Social Science & Medicine, 71,* 353–361.

Plumb, M., Price, W., & Kavanaugh-Lynch, M. (2004). Funding community-based participatory research: Lessons learned. *Journal of Interprofessional Care, 18,* 428–439.

Rabiee, F. (2006). Sustainability in local public health nutrition programmes: Beyond nutrition education, towards community collaboration. *Proceedings of the Nutrition Society, 65,* 418–428.

Seifer, S. (2005). *Tips and strategies for developing strong community-based participatory research proposals.* Retrieved from Community–Campus Partnerships for Health website: http://depts.washington.edu/ccph/commbas.html

Seifer, S., & Calleson, D. (2004). Health professional faculty perspectives on community-based research: Implications for policy and practice. *Journal of Interprofessional Care, 18,* 416–427.

Seifer, S., & Sisco, S. (2006). Mining the challenges of CBPR for improvements in urban health. *Journal of Urban Health, 83,* 981–984.

Sillitoe, P. (1998). The development of indigenous knowledge: A new applied anthropology. *Current Anthropology, 39,* 223–253.

Smedley, B. D., Stith, A. Y., & Nelson, A. R. (Eds.). (2003). *Unequal treatment: Confronting racial and ethnic disparities in health care.* Washington, DC: The National Academies Press.

Smith, L. T. (2001). *Decolonizing methodologies: Research and indigenous peoples.* New York, NY: Zed.

Snyder, M. (1995). *Transforming development: Women, poverty, and politics.* London, UK: IT Publications.

St. Paul School District. (2004). *Demographics of the school district.* Retrieved from http://ell.spps.org/Demographics.html

Stringer, E. (2007). *Action research.* Thousand Oaks, CA: Sage.

Strong, L., Israel, B., Schulz, A., Reyes, A., Rowe, Z., Weir, S., & Poe, C. (2009). Piloting interventions within a community-based participatory research framework: Lessons learned from the Health Environments Partnership. *Progress in Community Health Partnerships, 3,* 327–334.

Ting-Toomey, S. (1999). *Communicating across cultures.* New York, NY: Guilford.

Viswanathan, M., Ammerman, A., Eng, E., Gartlehner, G., Lohr, K., Griffith, D. . . . Whitener, I. (2004). *Community-based participatory research: Assessing the evidence.* Retrieved from Agency for Healthcare Research and Quality website: http://www.ahrq.gov/downloads/pub/evidence/pdf/cbpr/cbpr.pdf

Wadsworth, Y. (1997). *Everyday evaluation on the run.* Crows Nest, Australia: Allen & Unwin.

Wallerstein, N. (2006). Commentary: Challenges for the field in overcoming disparities through a CBPR approach. *Ethnicity & Disease, 16,* 146–148.

Waterman, H., Tillen, D., Dickson, R., & de Koning, K. (2001). *Action research: A systematic review and guidance for assessment.* Retrieved from http://www.hta.ac.uk/execsumm/summ523.shtml

World Health Organization. (2008). *Closing the gap in a generation: Health equity through action on the social determinants of health.* Retrieved from http://www.who.int/social_determinants/en

Yershova, L., DeJaeghere, J., & Mestenhauser, J. (2000). Thinking not as usual: Adding the intercultural perspective. *Journal of Studies in International Education, 4,* 39–78.

Yonas, M., Jones, N., Eng, E., Vines, A., Aronson, R., Griffith, D. . . . DuBose, M. (2006). The art and science of integrating "Undoing Racism" with CBPR: Challenges of pursuing NIH funding to investigate cancer care and racial equity. *Journal of Urban Health, 83,* 1004–1012.

Chapter 10

A Whispered Dream: CBCAR in More Hands

*T*his book is the fruit of a partnership that took root 6 years ago when we began teaching a *Global Search for Justice: Women's Health* course together in southern Mexico. As part of the course, we ventured with students to live and learn with Mexican women and their families. This past January one of us was with a group of 10 students in San Cristobal de las Casas in the Mexican state of Chiapas. We were sitting in a large garden on the grounds of the museum of Mayan medicine, exhausted yet inspired, at the end of a day of intense learning about different healing modalities. Each garden tree and shrub was labeled in Tzotzil, Tzeltal, and Spanish for its healing properties. As we sat in a circle on the ground with the museum's curator, surrounded by healing plants, one of us stated in awe, "Just think about the hundreds of years of trial and error the labels on these trees and plants represent." Miguel, the curator, smiled and paused for a moment before saying, "Yes, there was some trial and error, but mostly the knowledge came through observation, intuition, and being in relationship with the plants. For this, you need more than Western, linear and positivist thinking. You need to open yourself to broader ways of knowing." He then continued by asking if any of us had dogs. One woman said she did, and he asked what her dog does when sick. She responded that the dog goes outside and eats grass. He said, "Just as dogs have the knowledge of which plants are healing and what to do, so do we. We simply need to slow down and use all of our senses to be in relationship so that we can take in the learning that is presented to us." He urged us to observe carefully and act out of our interconnectedness with all living things so we can learn what they have to teach us.

In this book we have offered a new way of being in relationship with what is around us—a unique process of research that allows for insights to arise out of the interactions and situations in which we are critically engaged. We have stressed the importance of being fully present and open, without judgment or predetermined notions so that new insights can be revealed, recognized, and acted upon. We have presented community-based collaborative action research (CBCAR) as a rigorous, scientific process for producing innovative, essential, and context-relevant knowledge. We have provided a forest of examples from which readers can choose just the right location to sow the seeds of their own CBCAR project.

In this chapter, we review why this collaborative work is important and offer ideas for further development of CBCAR. We have faith that readers will push this process even further and create stories yet untold of methods to promote human health and flourishing, improve systems, and create just structures and policies. Finally, we add impetus to these endeavors and close the book by launching readers on their own journeys.

■ The Important Work of CBCAR

The CBCAR process provides a novel, robust vehicle to move through uncharted and troublesome situations, specifically in the area of addressing health disparities, coping with complex health conditions, and reorganizing inefficient, ineffective, or failing systems. Currently in health care, the majority of empirically-supported health interventions focus on individual and team level variables. The results have created important, evidence-based best practices that suggest how patients, nurses, and other healthcare providers can improve outcomes. Many of these suggestions involve pharmaceuticals, healthcare products, and other advancements that improve health. Additionally, research studies have created standardized clinical pathways that maximize benefits and minimize risks for healthcare organizations, insurers, and some populations.

However, persistent problems remain. In many areas, nurses are increasingly torn between their commitments to patients and the constraints and demands of the complex systems they work in. Moreover, health outcomes have not improved for all groups. Significant knowledge gaps on how to address intersecting, contextual factors that contribute to disease and suffering continue. The World Health Organization noted profound and persistent health disparities within countries and around the world (Commission on the Social Determinants of Health, 2008). Although we know more about health disparities, our knowledge about how to address these disparities lags (Horowitz, Robinson, & Seifer, 2009). Additionally, when the Institutes of Medicine (IOM) panel on health disparities met to analyze the hundreds of studies done on the subject, they concluded that when all else was controlled for—i.e., income, insurance, access, and exposure—it was unequal treatment in the healthcare encounter that is the focus of concern. For this reason they named their report, *Unequal Treatment: Confronting Racial and Ethnic Disparities in Health* (Smedley, Stith, & Nelson, 2003). Other IOM studies revealed inadequate healthcare delivery—prompting a call for research agendas that increase healthcare quality for all (Adams & Corrigan, 2003; Chao, Anderson, & Hernandez, 2009; Committee on Quality of Health Care in America, 2001).

CBCAR produces knowledge that addresses many of these issues. By engaging patients, healthcare providers, marginalized people, policy makers, and other key stakeholders, CBCAR examines areas of concern from a wider ecological perspective—to see the pattern of the whole so that efforts can be strategically targeted at root causes. CBCAR studies, such as the ones that are described in Chapters 1 and 2 and the numerous examples that are referenced in this book, uncover needed actions within local contexts to address such issues, with action steps reaching wider and deeper to address ecological structures impacting health.

■ Nudging CBCAR Forward

The CBCAR framework provides a structure for nurses to partner with interested and involved others from multiple sectors to address the root causes and branching impacts of health inequities, social injustices, and system inadequacies. With this in mind and somewhat urgently, we challenge more nurses to collaborate with colleagues in nursing and other fields to move the community-partnered, action-based research process forward. Although we provide some suggestions on how we might move forward, this is by no means an exhaustive list. Many initiatives are needed; we invite multiple voices into dialogue about advancing the science and impact of CBCAR. We trust that conscientious nurse researchers will shape and extend the application of CBCAR in profound ways.

Practitioners Improving Care: Learning Communities

Action science, which refers to communities studying their own situations and practices, holds promise for healthcare professionals and organizations. Other professional fields such as organization development, management science, and education have used action research to improve quality, but few examples in health care exist (Friedman, 2006). This application involves gathering diverse groups to initiate collaborative inquiry and become knowledge-creating systems (Bray, Lee, Smith, & Yorks, 2000). Reed and Lawrence (2008) challenged the nursing profession to harness practice-based knowledge by using deliberate, theory-based, meaning-making strategies. Walsh, Moss, Lawless, McKelvie, and Duncan (2008) suggested that nurses collaborate to study persistent and "puzzling practice" issues; through study and collective reflections, innovative actions result (p. 95). Moreover, practice-based research networks that form to study common health and healthcare experiences can be strengthened by incorporating community-partnered research (Macauley & Nutting, 2006). Networks that incorporate community voices can maximize process knowledge across settings while honoring the contextual differences that shape organizational change at the local level. The CBCAR framework could guide many of these knowledge-producing efforts.

Similarly, Senge and Scharmer (2006) described "learning communities" in which diverse partnerships form to create space for collective reflections on scientific and pragmatic knowledge (p. 197). Specifically, in learning communities, healthcare providers gather with stakeholders and beneficiaries to create a community of inquiry that explores the experiential and scientific knowledge systems that operate in everyday clinical practices. In this vein, Barrett (2006) reported on her experience with collaborative inquiry that included a gathering of midwives with expectant and new mothers to examine birthing experiences and current midwifery practices. Together these mothers and midwives identified assets and concerns, discovered substantive patterns, and developed a critically-oriented action plan that changed midwifery practices and policies. Using CBCAR to frame these inquiry groups leads to unique partnerships within and among complex healthcare organizations. The novel blending of ideas that occurs in these partnerships can transform practice by initiating innovative solutions to address complex problems such as recurrent disparities and system inadequacies. Nurses possess unique abilities to drive these social and organizational change efforts.

Communities Constructing and Testing Theory

Future CBCAR projects might also explore opportunities for communities to theorize. Partnered dialogue that considers CBCAR findings usually includes shared reflection on relationships and patterns. For example, in a human rights research study, community health workers analyzed how various findings interconnected to influence susceptibility to or protection from human rights violations. **Figure 10-1** emerged from these community discussions and provided a community-based theoretical framework that could be further refined and tested in steps using analytic techniques such as structural equation

Figure 10-1 Community Theorizing on Human Rights

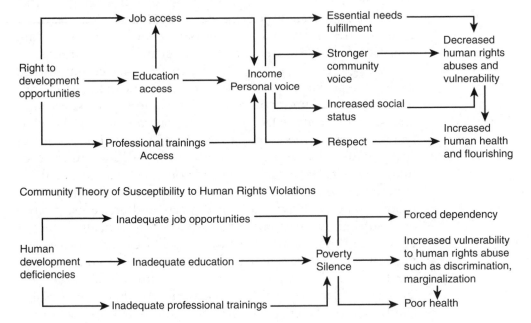

modeling. Theorizing everyday ways of being offers communities a voice in constructing deeper understandings about life experiences and naming intermediary and intersecting variables. Community-developed theory could also provide intriguing insights into health determinants—especially how they intersect to create synergistic and recalcitrant forces that impact health.

Developing reliable and valid measures is critical to the strength of theoretical models. Few measures—especially for underserved populations and groups experiencing disparities—have been developed and refined. CBCAR projects could contribute valuable information for the development of measurement tools. Community theorizing and testing is on the CBCAR horizon, and nurses can be among those innovative researchers and clinicians who make progress in encouraging community voices to develop their own theories of experiences.

Communities Developing, Testing, and Disseminating Interventions

According to Hebert, Brandt, Armstead, Adams, and Steck (2009), using CBCAR strategies to develop interventions ensures relevance to high-risk populations. The Institute of Medicine's Committee on Comparative Effectiveness Research (2009) called for increasing participation of consumers, patients, and caregivers in the development of intervention research. In Chapter 7, we described a community-developed, human rights intervention that will be tested in a clinical trial (see Box 7-2). Some researchers distinguish explanatory clinical trials, which test intervention effectiveness in ideal situations, from pragmatic clinical trials, which test intervention benefits in actual settings (Fransen et al., 2007; Godwin et al., 2003; Maclure, 2009; MacPherson, 2004). Using CBCAR strategies in intervention studies produces robust designs—especially for disadvantaged populations (Burns & Grove, 2005). However, clinical trials in CBCAR projects should be cautiously designed to:

- Account for health determinants and individual preferences.
- Incorporate local ideas and community capacity-building.
- Avoid ethical dilemmas associated with delivering substandard treatment to some participants (Rapkin & Trickett, 2005).

These authors called for more comprehensive and dynamic intervention designs and suggested new avenues for incorporating community voices in intervention research. We would add that it is especially essential to assure that the critical reference group has a strong voice in shaping and guiding these studies.

Translation of research findings into community initiatives is also informed and strengthened by CBCAR strategies (Becker, Stice, Shaw, & Woda, 2009; Hebert et al., 2009; Horowitz et al., 2009; Lindamer et al., 2009; US Department of Health and Human Services, 2007). For example, communities provide valuable insights on effective methods for information dissemination and can help reduce disparities in health promotion and education efforts. Community participation in research also helps to ensure study validity—both internal and external (Hebert et al., 2009). Moreover, collaborative partnerships between researchers, health service organizations, and healthcare providers optimize pragmatic clinical trials and dissemination research (Sussman, Valente, Rohrbach, Skara, & Pentz, 2006). The future is bright for community–academic partnerships to test elements of implementation feasibility and treatment effectiveness for community-developed interventions and programs (Burns & Grove, 2005; Lindamer et al., 2009; Pequegnat, 2005). Nurses who use CBCAR to develop and test novel interventions can contribute significantly to research agendas that promote health, health equity, and health system effectiveness.

Standards for Evaluating CBCAR Quality

Process flexibility and method diversity are important features that allow CBCAR partners to engage communities in developing and investigating research questions of local importance. The challenge is to find meaningful standards for evaluating CBCAR quality while still respecting its relational, participatory, pragmatic, and emergent characteristics. The International Collaboration on Participatory Research for Health is a new initiative whose goals include providing an international forum for considering research quality and standards (Wright, Gardner, Roche, von Unger, & Ainlay, 2010; Wright, Roche, von Unger, Block, & Gardner, 2010). As a versatile process, CBCAR may employ single or mixed method designs that can complicate the selection of appropriate criteria for assuring scientific rigor. Moreover, CBCAR projects require additional criteria that evaluate the unique features of CBCAR such as partnership and pragmatic action. Bradbury and Reason (2006) implored action researchers to seek common standards for "getting valuable work done well" (p. 343) without restricting the uniqueness in each action research process. This challenge provokes several questions. How do we characterize quality in developing a praxis of relational participation? How do we assess inclusivity and plurality of knowing in CBCAR projects?

What are quality measures of reflexive pragmatism? How do we assess project and partnership worthiness? How do we assure quality endpoints for projects that are part of an emergent process that aims for sustainability? How do we measure sustainability and determine its appropriateness over time? Assuring research quality is an important and evolving area of CBCAR that requires new questions and expanded thinking.

Developing the Science and Art of CBCAR

Nurses are in an ideal position to learn and implement CBCAR projects—whether trying to improve health practices, policies, and systems or attempting to address health inequities, injustices, and social structures. Nurses already embrace health as part of larger life experiences, engage in relational practice, collaborate in providing quality care, apply evidence-based knowledge and pragmatic wisdom, and aim for sustainable health outcomes and quality improvements. As part of healthcare teams, nurses have developed strong voices for evidence-based change. Scientific research and reflective practice have strengthened those voices. With this book, we add CBCAR to the mix of sciences that strengthen nurses' voices.

Our challenge now is to further develop the art and science of CBCAR and conduct research on the process itself. Many questions arise as we do so. What are the attributes of effective CBCAR researchers? What partnership techniques provide impetus to CBCAR processes? How do we measure teams' effectiveness in identifying and minimizing power differentials? What type of infrastructure supports CBCAR? What recruitment and data collection efforts are effective in engaging with multiple and diverse populations? How do we assure adequate participation of people from the critical reference group without overburdening or exploiting them? How do we simultaneously promote autonomy and minimize vulnerability of CBCAR participants? What techniques engage stakeholders in CBCAR projects? How do we measure effectiveness and efficiency of CBCAR strategies/process? How do CBCAR findings compare to research findings using traditional research methods? What are effective action planning and evaluation methods for small and large CBCAR projects? What are effective knowledge diffusion techniques for CBCAR projects? How do CBCAR results impact policies, practices, and systems to create meaningful, structural change for health? What characterizes effective and sustainable partnerships—both large and small? What barriers exist at different phases of CBCAR projects? Who listens to CBCAR results and changes as a result? In what manner do CBCAR projects alter health disparities and improve quality of health care? These are only a few of the questions that CBCAR scientists should address as they develop and further improve the method.

■ Let's get started....

We started most chapters in simple awe of mother earth's graceful gifts to us—the trees that arise from invisible rootings to surround, nourish, and shelter us while also decorating our world. In CBCAR, trees can become an analytic tool that initiate a CBCAR journey as people cluster in hallways and gather around tables to consider unfair disparities, inefficient systems, or structural gaps that leave human health and flourishing a distant goal. So, imagine an issue that concerns you. Think of the issue as a tree trunk; consider what is known about root causes and deliberate on branching impacts for individuals, systems, and communities. Reflect on ways in which root causes perpetuate and sustain branching impacts. Think about how branching impacts often nourish and sustain root causes—similar to tree branches that eventually drop their leaves, fertilize the soil, and perpetuate roots. Let's examine an example.

Suppose you are concerned about the marginalized experience of dying in an acute care setting (Pavlish & Ceronsky, 2007). Consider this issue as the tree trunk. You notice that your dying patients receive less attention from physicians and fewer visits from other healthcare providers. Nurse staffing patterns reflect little regard for the intricate care that dying patients and their families often require. Sociocultural norms discourage open discussions about death so even family members are uncomfortable talking with their loved ones (root causes). As you think further, you consider branching impacts and notice that your dying patients are lonely even if surrounded, families suffer, grief and pain set in, healthcare providers distance care, and quality of life diminishes. As these impacts continue, they tend to contribute to root causes—contributing to dying patients receiving even less attention and healthcare providers enacting even more avoidance.

CBCAR projects start as people consider issues of concern, examine and address contributing causes, and alter their impacts. Reflect back to Figure I-1 where a tree is surrounded by the CBCAR steps. Initiating partnered inquiry into issues that are significant to people in their everyday lives, analyzing the meaning of the patterns discovered, and enacting effective solutions provide new ways of seeing and being. Our tree is transformed; the trunk becomes solutions, roots become resources, and branching impacts are the vital and diffusive energy that sustains and nourishes equitable and quality care. Human health can flourish with such attention—even, and perhaps especially, in the days and hours before death. Life is to be lived fully and attentively; nurses are uniquely able to stay with people through complicated and uncomfortable situations to discover the way to health for that person, that family, that community. Most often this involves intense relationships and includes rearranging the environment (contextual rearrangements). CBCAR is simply taking the nursing process to a wider contextual level so that problems can be solved at their roots, clearing the ground for a flourishing environment in which health becomes a reality for all and healthcare delivery becomes less like being impeded on a congested freeway and more like walking along a clear, unfolding pathway.

We conclude this book with a worksheet that invites your ideas (see **Figure 10-2**). We welcome all voices into the CBCAR framework and appreciate all hearts and hands in advancing the process. We wish for you: illuminating vision to enlighten your insights and an abundance of good and critical friends for your journey.

Figure 10-2 Starting the CBCAR Process: Root Causes and Branching Impacts

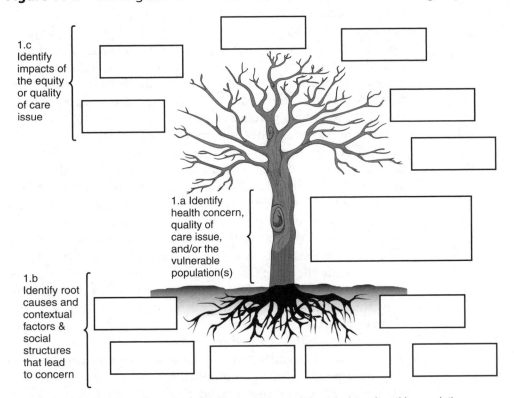

1.c
Identify
impacts of
the equity
or quality
of care
issue

1.a Identify
health concern,
quality of
care issue,
and/or the
vulnerable
population(s)

1.b
Identify root
causes and
contextual
factors &
social
structures
that lead
to concern

1. a) Imagine a health concern, quality of care issue or a particular vulnerable population as the tree trunk; b) Using the tree metaphor, describe the root causes and contextual factors/social structures that lead to the concern; c) Then imagine the branches as the impacts of the health/equity concern or, quality of care issue and identify specific impacts—especially the health and well being impacts.
2. Consult with potential collaborators and review what is known about the issue.
3. Consider critical reference group, stakeholders, and organization who might be interested in pursuing a partnership to explore and address concern.
4. Formalize partnerships and use suggestions in Chapters 3, 4, 5, 6, & 7 to proceed.

References

Adams, K., & Corrigan, J. M. (Eds). (2003). *Priority areas for national action: Transforming health care quality.* Washington, DC: National Academy of Sciences.

Barrett, P. A. (2006). The early mothering project: What happened when the words "action research" came to life for a group of midwives. In P. Reason & H. Bradbury (Eds.), *Handbook of action research* (pp. 228–235). Thousand Oaks, CA: Sage.

Becker, C., Stice, E. Shaw, H., & Woda, S. (2009). Use of empirically supported interventions for psychopathology: Can the participatory approach move us beyond the research-to-practice gap? *Behaviour Research and Therapy, 47,* 265–274.

Bradbury, H., & Reason, P. (2006). Conclusion: Broadening the bandwidth of validity: Issues and choice-points for improving the quality of action research. In P. Reason & H. Bradbury (Eds.), *Handbook of action research* (pp. 343–351). Thousand Oaks, CA: Sage.

Bray, J., Lee, J., Smith, L., & Yorks, L. (2000). *Collaborative inquiry in practice.* Thousand Oaks, CA: Sage.

Burns, N., & Grove, S. K. (2005). *The practice of nursing research: Conduct, critique, and utilization.* St. Louis, MO: Elsevier.

Chao, S., Anderson, K., & Hernandez, L. (2009). *Toward health equity and patient-centeredness: Integrating health literacy, disparities reduction, and quality improvement.* Washington, DC: National Academy of Sciences.

Commission on Social Determinants of Health. (2008). *Closing the gap in a generation: Health equity on the social determinants of health.* Retrieved from http://whqlibdoc.who.int/publications/2008/9789241563703_eng.pdf

Committee on Comparative Effectiveness Research Prioritization, Institute of Medicine. (2009). *Initial national priorities for comparative effectiveness research.* Washington, DC: National Academy of Science.

Committee on Quality of Health Care in America, Insitute of Medicine. (2001). *Crossing the quality chasm: A new health system for the 21st Century.* Washington, DC: National Academy of Science.

Franson, G., von Marrewijt, C., Mujakovic, S., Muris, J., Laheij, R., Numans, M. . . . Knottnerus, J. (2007). Pragmatic trials in primary care. Methodological challenges and solutions demonstrated by the DIAMOND-study. *BMC Medical Research Methodology, 7,* 16–26. doi:10.1186/1471-2288-7-16

Friedman, V. (2006). Action science: Creating communities of inquiry in communities of practice. In P. Reason & H. Bradbury (Eds.), *Handbook of action research* (pp. 131–143). Thousand Oaks, CA: Sage.

Godwin, M., Ruhland, L., Casson, I., MacDonald, S., Delva, D., Birtwhistle, R. . . . Sequin, R. (2003). Pragmatic controlled clinical trials in primary care: The struggle between external and internal validity. *BMC Medical Research Methodology, 3,* 28–34.

Hebert, J., Brandt, H., Armstead, C., Adams, S., & Steck, S. (2009). Interdisciplinary, translational, and community-based participatory research: Finding a common language to improve cancer research. *Cancer Epidemiological Biomarkers and Prevention, 18,* 1213–1217.

Horowitz, C., Robinson, M., & Seifer, S. (2009). Community-based participatory research from the margin to the mainstream: Are researchers prepared? *Circulation, 119,* 2633–2642.

Lindamer, L., Lebowitz, B., Hough, R., Garcia, P., Aguirre, A., Halpain, M. . . . Jeste, D. (2009). Establishing an implementation network: Lessons learned from community-based participatory research. *Implementation Science, 4,* 17–23.

Macauley, A., & Nutting, P. (2006). Moving the frontiers forward: Incorporating community-based participatory research into practice-based research networks. *Annals of Family Medicine, 4,* 4–7.

Maclure, M. (2009). Explaining pragmatic trials to pragmatic policymakers. *Canadian Medical Association Journal, 180,* 1001–1003.

MacPherson, H. (2004). Pragmatic clinical trials. *Complementary Therapies in Medicine, 12,* 136–140.

Pavlish, C., & Ceronsky, L. (2007). Oncology nurses' perceptions about palliative care. *Oncology Nursing Forum, 34,* 793–800.

Pequegnat, W. (2005). Toward the next generation of AIDS interventions with community impact. In E. Trickett & W. Pequegnat (Eds.), *Community interventions and AIDS* (pp. 278–285). New York, NY: Oxford.

Rapkin, B., & Trickett, E. (2005). Comprehensive dynamic trial designs for behavioral prevention research with communities: Overcoming inadequacies of the randomized controlled trial design. In E. Trickett & W. Pequegnat (Eds.), *Community interventions and AIDS* (pp. 249–277). New York, NY: Oxford.

Reed, P. G., & Lawrence, L. (2008). A paradigm for the production of practice-based knowledge. *Journal of Nursing Management, 16,* 422–432.

Senge, P., & Scharmer, C. (2006). Community action research: Learning as a community of practitioners, consultants and researchers. In P. Reason & H. Bradbury (Eds.), *Handbook of action research* (pp. 195–206). Thousand Oaks, CA: Sage.

Smedley, B., Stith, A., & Nelson, A. (Eds.). (2003). *Unequal treatment: Confronting racial and ethnic disparities in health care.* Washington, DC: National Academy of Science.

Sussman, S., Valente, T., Rohrbach, L., Skara, S., & Pentz, M. (2006). Translation in the health professions. *Evaluation and the Health Professions, 29,* 7–32.

US Department of Health and Human Services, National Institutes of Health, National Cancer Institute. (2007). *Transforming translation: Harnessing discovery for patient and public benefit.* (NIH Publication No. 07-6239). Retrieved from http://www.cancer.gov/aboutnci/trwg/finalreport.pdf

Walsh, K., Moss, C., Lawless, J., McKelvie, R., & Duncan, L. (2008). Puzzling practice: A strategy for working with clinical practice issues. *International Journal of Nursing Practice, 14,* 94–100.

Wright, M., Gardner, B., Roche, B., von Unger, H., & Ainlay, C. (2010). Building an international collaboration on participatory health research. *Progress in Community Health Partnerships, 4,* 31–36.

Wright, M., Roche, B., von Unger, H., Block, M., & Gardner, B. (2010). A call for an international collaboration on participatory research for health. *Health Promotion International, 25,* 115–122.

Index

Note: page numbers followed by f or t denote figures or tables respectively.